THE MEDICAL TOURISM

Your Complete Reference to Top-Qua
Cosmetic, Medical Care & Surgery Overseas

Library of Congress Cataloging-in-Publication Data

Gahlinger, Paul M.
  The medical tourism travel guide : your complete reference to top-quality, low-cost dental, cosmetic, medical care & surgery overseas / Paul Gahlinger.
    p. cm.
  ISBN 978-1-934716-00-7
  1. Medical tourism--Handbooks, manuals, etc. I. Title.
  RA793.5.G34 2008
  362.1--dc22

                          2007052009

ISBN-13 978-1-934716-00-7
SRP600

SUNRISE River Press

39966 Grand Avenue
North Branch, MN 55056 USA
(651) 277-1400 or (800) 895-4585

Medical Tourism — traveling abroad for medical care — is quickly becoming part of how Americans choose to get medical treatment. For most people, however, it is an unfamiliar process and difficult to find reliable information on how to go about it. Paul Gahlinger has now filled that void with the first authoritative, comprehensive, and trustworthy book about medical tourism. It will be invaluable to patients and health-care providers alike.

Medical tourism is becoming an increasingly vital healthcare alternative for all Americans. Still, in order to realize the savings offered by this formerly unimaginable solution, much more information needs to be available — and presented in a straight-forward manner by someone who really knows the industry. Dr. Gahlinger brings his extensive experience as a physician, anthropologist, hospital director, and professor of public health to the challenge. The result — this book — is an excellent overview of the key issues related to medical tourism: quality, process, destinations, medical fa-cilities, financing, and — not least — cautions for the consumer. In doing so, he con-vincingly dispels the common misperception that the only reliable medical care is that which is found in the United States or Europe.

America's business leaders, union directors, hospital administrators, and health in-surance executives are starting to discuss this new phenomenon and how to integrate medical tourism into the complex web of healthcare. As this industry builds, Dr. Gahlinger's authoritative book will provide the foundation.

Sparrow Mahoney
CEO, MdTrex Corporation
Publisher, MedicalTourism.com

Paul Gahlinger has spent more than 30 years in medicine, in virtually every area. He began as a paramedic in northern Canada, then studied medical anthropology (Ph.D.) and epidemiology (Master of Public Health), after which he taught as a professor at San Jose State University, California. He left to pursue a lifelong dream to be a country doctor. After completing his M.D. degree at the University of California, Davis, he did residencies at the University of Hawaii and University of Utah. He has been a hospital director, Chief Medical Officer for a military base in the Pacific Ocean, and worked or traveled in over 120 countries — as well as a stint as a physician in Antarctica. He is currently adjunct professor at the School of Medicine, University of Utah, and consultant in bioastronautics for NASA. He can be reached at pgahlinger@gmail.com.

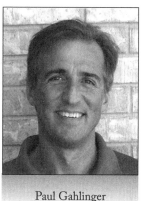

Paul Gahlinger

ACKNOWLEDGMENTS

My explorations of medical tourism would not have been possible without the hundreds of people who shared their expertise and experiences with me. I am deeply grateful to the hospital administrators, physicians, international patient directors, travel agents, hotel owners, government immigration and customs officials, and countless patients who took considerable time — often hours — to educate me on the intricacies and concerns of the medical tourism industry in their countries. I have traveled, and sometimes worked, in all but a few of the 46 nations described in this book and have been very fortunate to meet government officials, hospital directors, and the executives of the travel industry. During these travels, I also took every opportunity to talk to people who are often closest to medical tourists: taxi drivers, waitresses and waiters, hotel concierges and staff, and nurses and other caregivers.

When I began to interview the medical tourists themselves, I broached the subject gingerly, concerned that they might be reticent to talk about such a personal and private experience. On the contrary! Almost everyone I met described their surgeries or other therapies in detail. Some were eager to share their initial worries and their surprised delight when they found the level of care and professionalism so much higher than they expected.

Perhaps because I am a physician, or perhaps because I simply enjoy talking with patients, many medical tourists came to me to talk about their travel — some of whom were overseas for the first time — and encourage my work on the book, offering their photos and even their names for publication.

I also got an earful of their exasperations with the U.S. medical system. I often, as a token American doctor, reluctantly served as a lightning rod for tourists venting tirades about the frustrations of medical care at home.

Aside from personal impressions, I gained an insight into the economics of medical tourism from executives who were kind enough to provide access to proprietary data of their facilities. In particular, I would like to thank Dr. Ravindra Karanjekar, Manager, and Pradeep Thukral, Head of International Marketing, of Wockhardt Associate Hospital of Harvard Medical International; Barbara Seet, Manager of International Medical Services at Singapore General Hospital; Dr. Saw Aung, Serene Tan and Phan Nhung, Managers of International Marketing of the Raffles Medical Group; Ravi Chandran, Corporate Communications Executive of Singapore National Eye Centre; Joshua Goh, Vice President of International Operations at Parkway Group Healthcare; Alice Pang, Programme Development Manager, and Angeline Tan, Manager of Marketing Communications, of SingHealth; Peter Davison and Kenneth Carlson, International Services Managers at Phuket International Hospital; Dr. Sompach Nipakanont, Medical Director of the International Medical Center, Bangkok Hospital; Dr. Ivo van der Vegt, Director of MedicalThailand.com; Dr. Thein Htut, Marketing Director of TheraVitae; Dr. Niran Thaweekul, Director of the Wongsada Skin & Cosmetic Clinic; Tac-Whei Ong, Head of Marketing at BNH Hospital; M. Zakariah Ahmed, Manager of Corporate Marketing International of Fortis Healthcare; Dr. Anand Parihar, Treasurer of the Association of Medical Consultants, Mumbai, India; Nitin Sibal, Vice President of Warburg Pincus, India; Dr. Mandakini Parihar, Director of Mandakini IVF Centre in Mumbai, India; Vishal Bali, Vice President of Wockhardt Hospitals; Dr. Parag Rindani, Microbiologist of Wockhardt Hospitals; Ronald May, Senior Executive of Wockhardt Hospital & Heart Insitute, Bangalore, India; Paulami Karnwal, Marketing Manager, and Anil Maini, President of Corporate Development, at Indraprastha Apollo Hospitals.

I am very thankful for the advice and encouragement of Dr. Robert Clark, President and Chairman of Theravitae; to Janese at the Bodyline Retreat in Phuket, Thailand, who graciously and patiently explained the needs of medical tourists; and to her extraordinary manager, Ms. Fareda "Da" Susimanon, who gave me an insight into medical tourism from a Thai perspective.

The Internet research in this book was greatly facilitated by the brilliant Ms. Sparrow Mahoney, of medicaltourism.com, whose zeal for the subject is unmatched.

Finally, I deeply appreciate the patience of the staff of Sunrise River Press with such a complex book, especially my editor Ms. Karin Hill.

I greatly prefer books with lots of illustrations — and I believe other readers do, too. However, good illustrations can be expensive; otherwise it is very time-consuming and difficult to secure permission for their reproduction. Although about one-third of the photos in this book are my own, it was necessary to obtain permission from others, or find photos that are not copyrighted or available under common-use agreements. I owe an enormous debt to Wikipedia, from which much information and many photos are taken. Wikipedia provides a tremendous service by allowing publication of certain illustrations under the GNU Free Documentation License (GFDL). Flikr, an online photo repository, posts images by photographers who sometimes allow reproduction of their photos under the Creative Commons License. Wayne Chan Kian Jin, of the Parkway Hospitals International Group, Singapore, kindly gave permission to use photos of many hospitals in Singapore, Malaysia, and Brunei. The BFC clinic provided two photos of its medical center in Barbados. The classic car and other photos of Cuba were provided by Ken Beaune. Permission was granted to use a number of images from major medical tourism referral websites treatmentabroad.net and privatehealth.co.uk. Photos of Hungary are from the Hungarian Health Organization. The American University of Beirut also kindly gave permission for numerous photos; unfortunately, Lebanon's incipient medical tourism industry, headed by the American University, was devastated by the terrible war of 2006 and therefore not included in this book. Photos of bariatric surgery were provided by the Miguelangelo Plastic Surgery Clinic, in Cabo San Lucas, Mexico, and by the International Surgery Center (surgery4obesity.com). Mike O'Keefe was extraordinarily courageous to post his experiences of plastic surgery online (www.okeefe.ukf.net) and very supportive of my efforts. It is rare for an individual to post photos of such a personal experience for no compensation, just the simple desire to help others considering overseas plastic surgery. Photos of Tunisia and Turkey were provided, respectively, by the El Menzah Clinic and Jinemed. Finally, random cultural and medical photos were provided by Lilivati Hospital, the Krishna Heart Institute, Linda Briggs, and Professional Capital. The appeal of this book is largely due to their kind contributions.

COUNTRY AND PROCEDURE

	Argentina	Barbados	Belgium	Brazil	Brunei	Bulgaria	China	Costa Rica	Croatia	Cuba	Cyprus	Czech Republic	Dominica	Dominican Rep.	Dubai	Egypt	Finland	Germany	Greece	Hong Kong	Hungary
abdominoplasty	•		•	•		•		•		★		•		•		•		•	•		•
abortion							★			•								•		•	
acupuncture							★													★	
algaetherapy									★												
alternative medicine						•	★			•		★				•				★	★
antiaging programs						•				★			•	•					•		
aromatherapy						•	•			•											
assisted reproduction		★																	•		
ayurvedic medicine																					
balneotherapy						★		•				•									
blepharoplasty			•	•		•		•	•	•		•		•		•		•	•		★
bone-marrow transplant																•					
Botox treatment	•		•	•		★		★		•		•		★		★		•	•		★
breast augmentation	•	★	•			•	★	•	•	•		•		•		•		•	•		•
buttock implants	•	★	•			•	•	•	•	•		•		•		•		•	•		•
cancer treatment	★	★	•	•		★				•							★	•		★	
cardiac bypass	★	★		•						•					•			•			
cataract removal	•				★					•		•						•			•
collagen injection	•		•	•		•		•	•	•		•		•		•		•	•		★
cosmetic surgery	•		•	★		★		★	•	★		★		★		★		•	★		•
cryotherapy										•		★									
dental care	•					★		★	•	★		★						•			•
dialysis											★							•			
ear pinning	•		•	•		•		•	•	•		•		•		•		•	•		•
electrotherapy									★												
epilepsy surgery																	★	•			
eye surgery	•				•			•		•		•						•			•
eyebag removal	•		•	•		•		•	•	•		•		•		•		•	•		•
facelift	•		•	★		•		•	•	•		•		•		•		•	•		•
fangotherapy									★												
fertility assistance		★																	•		
gastric bypass surgery	★																	•			
glaucoma	•					★		•		•								•			•
hair transplant											★					•		•			
healing mud										•											
heart surgery	•			•		•		•							★			★			
hemorrhoidectomy	•					•												•			

- • This medical tourism service or procedure is readily available in this destination.
- ★ This is a top destination for this service or procedure, known for facilities offering exceptionally high-quality care.

CROSS-REFERENCE CHART

India	Iran	Israel	Italy	Jordan	Latvia	Malaysia	Malta	Mexico	New Zealand	Panama	Philippines	Poland	Saudi Arabia	Singapore	S. Africa	S. Korea	Spain	Syria	Taiwan	Thailand	Tunisia	Turkey	Venezuela	Vietnam
•			•					•		•	•	•		•	•	•	•			•	•	•	•	
•														•						•				
														•		★			★	•				•
																					•			
★	★	★						★				★		•			•			★	•			★
	•							•				•								•	•			
												★								•				
★		★						•						•	★		•			•		★		
•														•						•				
	★											★								•				
•			•			•	•	•		•	•	•	•	•	•	•	•			•	•	•	•	•
★		•		•										★	•					•				
•			•					★		•	•	•	•	•	•		•			•	•	•		
•			•					•		•	•	•	•	•	•		•			•	•	•		
•			•					•		•	•	•		•	•		•			•	•	•		
•		•				★	•	•						•						•		•		
★		•	•			★				•				•	•					•		★		
•		•						•	•	•				•	•		•			•		•		•
•			•					•		•	•	•		•	•		•			•	•		•	
•		★						★		★	★	★	★	★	★	★	★			★	★	•	★	•
												•												
•				★			★	•	★	★		•		•	•			★	★	•	★	★	★	•
•		•	★				★				•			•	•					•		•		
•		•						•	•		•	•	•	•	•		•			•	•	•	•	•
•														•						•				
★			★			•		•	★	★	★			•	•		•	★	★	•		•		•
•		•					•	•		•	•	•	•	•	•		•			•	•	•	•	
•		•						•		•	•	•	•	•	•		•			•	•	•	•	
•	•					•				•				•	•		★			•				
•	•					•				•				•	★					★	•			
•	•			•		•		•		•	•			•	•		•		•	•	•			•
•			★					•						•						•				
																					★			
•		•		★		•				•				★	★					★		•		
•		•				•	•			•				•	•				•	•	•			

(procedures continued on page III)

	Argentina	Barbados	Belgium	Brazil	Brunei	Bulgaria	China	Costa Rica	Croatia	Cuba	Cyprus	Czech Republic	Dominica	Dominican Rep.	Dubai	Egypt	Finland	Germany	Greece	Hong Kong	Hungary
herbal treatments						•		•					★		•					★	
hip replacement	•		•		★				•						•			★			
hip resurfacing			•												★			•			
hymenoplasty																					
hypobaric therapy									•												
Ilizarov procedure																					
in-vitro fertilization		★																	•		
kidney transplant							•											•			
knee replacement	•		•	•					•						•			•			
labia reduction	•		•	•		•		•	•			•		•		•		•	•		•
laetrile therapy																					
lap-band surgery																		•			
LASIK vision correction								•								•		•			
liposculpture	•		•	•		•		•	•			•		•		•		•	•		•
liposuction	•		•	•		•		•	•			•		•		•		•	•		•
magnetotherapy							•														
male cosmetic surgery	•		•	•		•		•	•			•		•		•		•	•		•
massage						•		•		•	•							•			
mineral springs						•		•		•	•							•			
minimally invasive spinal surgery			•		•											•		•			
mommy makeover	•		•	•		•		•	•			•		•		•		•	•		•
organ transplant							•											•			
panchakarma																					
plastic surgery	•	★	★			•		•	•			•		•		•		•	•		•
reconstructive surgery	★	★	★			•		•	•			•		•		•		•	•		★
reflexology																			•		
rhinoplasty	•		•	★		•		•	•	•		•		•		•		•	•		•
spa						•		•			•	•	•	•							•
stem cell therapy																		•			
thalassotherapy						•		•		•									•		
thermotherapy								•													
titanium implants	•					•		•	•	•		•						•			•
traditional Chinese medicine							★													•	
veneers	•					•		★	•	•		•						•			•

• This medical tourism service or procedure is readily available in this destination.

★ This is a top destination for this service or procedure, known for facilities offering exceptionally high-quality care.

India	Iran	Israel	Italy	Jordan	Latvia	Malaysia	Malta	Mexico	New Zealand	Panama	Philippines	Poland	Saudi Arabia	Singapore	S. Africa	S. Korea	Spain	Syria	Taiwan	Thailand	Tunisia	Turkey	Venezuela	Vietnam
•								•						•						•	•			
★		•				★				★				★	•	★				★		★		
•		•				•				•				•	•	•				•		•		
•														•						•				
														•										
•																				•				
•		•				•				•				•	•		•			•		•		
•		•		•								•		•						•				
•		•				•				•				•	•	•				•		•		
•			•						•		•	•	•	•	•	•	•			•	•	•	•	
									•															
•						•				•				•						•				
•				•					•					•	•		•			•				
•		•							•		•	•		•	•	•	•			•	•	•	•	
•		•							•		•	•		•	•	•	•			•	•	•	•	
•									•		•	•		•	•	•	•			•	•	•	•	
•												•								•				★
	•											•									•			
•		•		•		•				•				•	•	•				•		•		
•		•						•		•	•	•		•	•	•	•			•	•	•	•	
•		•		•							•			•	•					•				
•														•						•				
•		•							•		•	•	•	•	•	•	•			•		•	•	•
•		•							•		•	•		•	•	•	•			•		•	•	
•	•													•						•				
•		•					•	•		•	•	•	•	•	•	•	•			•		•	•	•
•		•						•			•			•		•		•		•	•			
•		•												•		•				•				
		•									•										•			
											•										•			
•					•			•		•				•	•					•		•		
														•		•			•	•				★
•					•			•		•		•	•	•	•		•			•		•	•	•

Imagine a spotlessly clean hospital staffed by the world's best doctors — who give you their home and cell phone numbers to call any time. The air is fragrant with frangipani and bougainvillea that bloom by your bed, while a swarm of smiling nurses and attendants care for all your needs — not just providing medications, but also back rubs and foot massages, bringing you a Starbucks coffee or a DVD movie you requested, or simply showing you how to use the 250-channel 40-inch plasma TV in your hospital suite — which can be large enough accommodate your family should they choose to accompany you.

Because they can afford it, presidents, royalty, and Hollywood stars are accustomed to getting this level of care in a prestigious facility that caters to their requests for luxury and privacy. You may not know that you can get it, too. And, incredibly, you can get it for about one-fifth of the cost of a hospital stay in the United States.

It is called medical tourism. Simply put: people traveling for healthcare. The concept is not new, but it is just starting to become a major global industry. A primary reason for this is the failure of the American medical system, which has dropped the ball on providing good care for a large part of the population. Another reason is the fast-growing and futuristic development of medical care overseas. The first of these reasons is well known, and the second is what this book is about.

Everyone agrees that the U.S. medical system is failing. The problem is not a lack of quality or technology — we are quite good at that. The problem is that few people can afford our medical care. Healthcare costs are now the number one cause of personal bankruptcy, and they are getting more expensive every year.

Medical care is not like other business. In a free market, consumers make demands and suppliers pop up to fill them. Doctors, like other suppliers, were once able to respond to people's needs. But this is no longer true for healthcare in the United States. Now, other agencies control your care. Television shows love to portray compassionate doctors, caring nurses, and patients who are given the most advanced medical treatment. The reality is different. Your doctor is likely an employee of a managed care organization, which means your treatment may actually be determined by a clerk at a computer in some remote office. Doctors are so disgusted by the loss of their authority, the paperwork, and the constant threats of malpractice liability, that more than half say they would not again choose medicine as a career. As for nurses — good luck actually finding one.

Managed care — which I prefer to call "mangled care" — functions by taking your money first and then giving back as little healthcare as possible, since any "care" they give comes right out of their profit. The whole system is a mess — one of the few issues on which Democrats and Republicans heartily agree.

But there is good news on the horizon. Airline travel and the Internet have turned the world into a global village. Most people in the U.S. can travel to almost any country for less than two weeks' wages, and it doesn't take long. From New York to Europe is just five hours, and you can travel from Los Angeles to Asia in about 12 to 18 hours. Central America and the Caribbean are even closer, and you can travel there without suffering jet lag. Medical tourism has brought opportunities to Americans for healthcare overseas at a far lower cost — and often of better quality — than in the United States.

Around the world, countless hospital and clinical services are developing to provide the very best medical care to foreigners. Most of their doctors have trained at top-notch American medical schools. In overseas hospitals there is far less paperwork, no argument over services, and just a single flat price. You can recover from your treatment in a resort, if you like, or follow it with a sightseeing vacation. And the total cost will still be a fraction of what you would pay at home.

Unbelievable? Yes — until you experience it. As one woman said, after medical visits in the United States and overseas: "There is just no comparison."

Three years ago, I was in Singapore for meetings at several hospitals. The buzz was all about medical tourism. I was surprised to discover that their hospitals — which are equal to the very best in the U.S. — were rapidly expanding to attract "international patients." I began to study the new industry. I was invited to tour the major hospitals in Thailand and India, where I spoke to their presidents, chief executive officers, chief finance officers, medical tourism directors, and countless patients. I traveled to dozens of other countries to look at smaller medical-tourism clinics that focused on cosmetic surgery, dentistry, assisted reproduction, alternative healthcare, and even stem-cell therapy not yet available in the United States.

Meanwhile, former travel agents, Internet entrepreneurs, and scam artists have not been asleep. As medical tourism becomes more popular, hundreds of advertisements and Internet sites are springing up to try to cash in on it. These sites usually try to steer you to a hospital or clinic that will pay them the most kickbacks (pardon me, "referral fees"), regardless of quality. There are many horror stories of medical treatment in foreign countries, and frankly, when you use the Internet to research overseas healthcare, you will not necessarily find the top clinics. You will find the top marketers, promoters, advertisers, and hustlers.

The purpose of this book is to cut through the ads, the scams, and the nonsense. My goal is to make American healthcare better by making you aware of your growing number of options. For that, I have tried to answer every question I've heard on medical tourism and provide the most thorough information to help you choose what is right for you.

In the long run, the inefficient and high-profit U.S. healthcare system will benefit from overseas competition. Ford and GM needed a kick in the butt from Toyota to improve their products. Medical care needs the same — competition is good. I am convinced that eventually U.S. healthcare will again become the best in the world.

But that will not happen anytime soon.

Meanwhile, this book will guide you to far more healthcare possibilities than you ever dreamed of.

PART I

What Your Doctor Doesn't Know About Medical Tourism

Very few doctors know much, if anything, about medical tourism.
Those who do may see it as a threat to their livelihood.

One doctor, quoted in the *New York Times*, said:
*"You're asking me to discuss the outsourcing of my business overseas.
I think it's understandable that I would not want to do that."*

Another wrote:
"The increasing appeal of 'medical tourism' is a dangerous prospect."

To such doctors, I can only suggest:
If you care about your patients, read this book.

Why Should I Go Overseas For Health Care?

Last year, two million tourists visited India for a special purpose. They didn't go to see the ancient temples, shop at the colorful markets, or to ride elephants through the jungle. They went to have surgery and other medical care.

India is not the only country with this attraction. Tourists with the same goal went to dozens of other lands — 230,000 to Thailand, 200,000 to Singapore, 160,000 to Malaysia, and thousands more to another 40 nations, from Argentina to Vietnam.

Why?

Savvy Americans know that they can go overseas to get surgery, medical and dental treatment, and many other types of healthcare for a fraction of the cost in the United States — and be treated like a Hollywood star. They are picked up at the airport by limousine and taken to a posh hotel suite, where they are greeted with a soothing massage, freshly cut flowers, and are given complimentary native handicrafts. The next day, they are brought to a medical center — often brand new and rivaling the best facilities in the United States. In fact, the surgeons were probably trained at top-ranked universities in the U.S. and use the latest techniques. Unlike surgeons in the U.S., however, these doctors give the visitors courteous, attentive, and personal care unimaginable at home —

> *They'll come for hip replacement or knee replacement or cataracts and, yup, while they're here they'll take a vacation. They get their cosmetic surgery or their dental work and, boom, they're off to the beach."*
>
> ~ Ruben Toral, director of international programs at Bumrungrad Hospital, Bangkok, Thailand.

typically giving them the doctor's private home and cell phone numbers to call if needed. Patients get first-class, 24-hour concierge service throughout their stay, spending their recovery time relaxing at a five-star hotel, or on the beach, or taking in the sights and pleasures open to every other tourist. When they get home, they look relaxed and refreshed. Few of their acquaintances or co-workers would suspect that they had just had breast implants, stomach reduction, a hip replacement, or a complete medical makeover.

Meanwhile, their neighbors at home in the U.S. might have had the same treatments, in the usual manner. They checked into a regional hospital, dealt with endless hassles and paperwork from their health insurance (if they were lucky enough to have insurance), and still paid heavily out of pocket for various copays, deductibles, and uncovered services. If they did not have insurance, they paid a small fortune for the procedure. Then they were treated by harried doctors, exhausted interns, and stressed-out nurses. They had a one-in-five risk of getting seriously sick because of their hospital stay, with medication errors alone killing an estimated 100,000 patients every year. Then they were sent home to recover without nursing care or support, sometimes pushing an IV-pole with a bag and catheter still dripping into their arm. And if they woke up at night in pain or with a fever and needed to talk to their doctor? Good luck trying to reach someone.

Now, which would you prefer?

Traveling for Medical Care Makes Sense, Financially and Otherwise

Medical tourism involves travel to other countries to obtain medical, dental, and surgical care. Because tourism suggests recreational or frivolous activities, it is sometimes called "medical value travel," and the travelers are referred to as "international patients." Regardless of the label, it has become a major world industry, growing at 30 percent annually. Already, medical tourism accounts for a phenomenal *seven percent* of the entire world health industry outside of the United States. The greatest motivation is cost saving. In developing countries, medical procedures can be performed for as little as one-tenth the cost of that in the United States. For example, a hip replacement that would cost $53,000 in the U.S. is about $5,000 to $8,000 in India.

The trade-off used to be that treatment was provided in lower-class facilities. That has changed. Specialty hospitals in India, Thailand, and elsewhere are now newly built with medical tourists in mind, and they are state-of-the-art facilities, as modern and technologically equipped as the best in the world. They are mostly staffed by doctors and surgeons trained in the U.S. or Europe, and they provide quality care equal to that in American hospitals. In many cases, they offer even *better* care. For example, consider hip replacements. In the United States, this surgery is usually done by a standard method. Because of government regulations, the newer, much improved technique of hip resurfacing is not yet generally available. However, the improved technique is available and can be performed quickly and inexpensively at a number of specialized orthopedic surgery centers in India. In this case, India is ahead of the U.S. by a few years, and even the wealthiest Americans sometimes prefer to travel there for treatment.

Medical tourism hospitals tend to regard healthcare in the full meaning of the word — they provide not just medical treatment, but full-body care that can include daily massage and skin care, excellent food, and patient rooms that have all the comforts of a quality hotel — many even have Starbucks with room service, free high-speed Internet, global satellite television and other amenities. I have visited hospital rooms in Thailand that are equipped with 40-inch plasma-screen televisions featuring 250 channels and a wide selection of DVD movies. These hospitals go all-out to attract patients, joining with tour operators to develop all-inclusive packages that provide travel, sightseeing, shopping, and admission tickets to popular attractions.

This kind of medical care — high quality, luxurious, personal, and private — used to be available only to the rich and the powerful. Now it can be had by anyone who can afford a Disney World vacation. This is quite a change from previous years, when it was the United States that attracted international patients for the highest-quality care.

How did this come about?

Basically, the same trend that took place in the automobile industry in the 1970s is taking place now in the American healthcare industry — the main players think they control the market and become overconfident. They become less responsive to consumers. During the gasoline crunch of 1973, people clamored for smaller cars, but Detroit continued to crank out fuel-guzzling monsters. American automakers almost went under — but then they finally adapted to consumers' preferences and produced a much better-quality line of cars. Recently, the same thing is happening again. The big American automobile manufacturers initially dismissed demands for electric cars and continued to manufacturer highly profitable SUVs. Now, GM and Ford dealers have vast parking lots of unsold SUVs while the electric hybrid Toyota Prius has an almost year-long waiting list. Every business student learns that competition improves quality and ultimately benefits everyone.

> ## Don't People Come *To* the U.S. for Healthcare?
>
> When I was a surgical intern in Hawaii, my hospital had a distinguished patient — deposed Philippine President Ferdinand Marcos. His wife Imelda often brought us baskets of deli foods and desserts (definitely a way to an intern's heart). We loved her, even though we knew the two were accused of stealing hundreds of millions from the poor country. Naturally, President Marcos was given top-quality treatment.
>
> Now, ironically, it is Americans who go to the Philippines to get the most luxurious care.

I believe that medical tourism, by offering lower-cost and higher-quality care, will eventually have a positive effect on the United States healthcare industry.

People still do come to the U.S. for specialty healthcare — medical tourism is not a one-way street.

Jordan is now developing its profitable medical tourism industry (see *Jordan, page 229*), but when Jordan's King Hussein needed treatment, he went to the renowned Mayo Clinic in Rochester, Minnesota. Dubai, one of the United Arab Emirates (UAE), is also promoting its medical tourism industry with ultra-sophisticated billion-dollar facilities, overseen by Harvard University, that promise to be among the best in the world (see *Dubai, page 180*). Nonetheless, Dubai's President, Sheikh Zayed bin Sultan Al Nahyan, preferred to be treated in the United States, choosing to have his kidney transplant at the top-rated Cleveland Clinic in 2000. When such world leaders choose to come here for quality care, the U.S. reaps a great economic benefit: the Sheikh arrived with an entourage of hundreds and stayed for four months. All of them needed to be fed, transported, and housed during that time — and I doubt that they stayed at the Motel 6.

However, this book is not concerned with such high rollers, but is directed at regular people who have found that overseas medical care can be as good as that in the U.S., much less expensive, and far more welcoming. The trend of medical tourism is only just beginning, so most Americans have not yet heard of this new phenomenon. There have been a few TV special reports covering it, and major newspapers such as the *New York Times* and the *Wall Street Journal* have run articles on medical tourism economics — they can't very well ignore a multi-billion dollar industry. But the fact is, there has been little publicity outside of New York or Los Angeles, and there is no reliable literature on traveling for healthcare. You are holding the first complete guide to medical tourism.

Medical Tourism Is 21st Century Healthcare

Within five years, the question will no longer be "Why?", but "Why not?" American healthcare is slow, inconvenient, and frustrating beyond belief as patients struggle with everything from insurance approval to the shortage of quality nursing care. This will soon change — and this book will show you how.

Within the next five years, medical tourism will be as well known as liposuction and dental veneers. In other words, just about everyone except the Amish brethren and Montana hermits will know about it — and may be making plans to do it. Among this publicity, there will no doubt be a tremendous amount of nonsense. There will be frightening stories of rip-offs by unscrupulous agents, and of people carved up and poisoned by incompetent doctors in shabby foreign hospitals. In this book, you will find the accurate information you need, based on the authenticated experiences of real people and verified facts.

Consider the computer industry. Just 20 years ago, personal computers were entirely made in the United States. Now, every component is outsourced: the microchips, the displays, the keyboards, the assembly, the packaging, the software to run the whole works, and even the call centers to answer questions. In Bangalore, India, you can see enormous industrial plants with names like IBM, Intel, Microsoft, and other major computer firms. That's why we no longer pay $5,000 for a computer with only as much power as those tiny chips now inserted in greeting cards. We continue to design them, but we let the manufacturing be done where labor is cheaper. It makes sense for everything from athletic shoes to cell phones. Outsourcing has brought tremendous efficiency to American industry, which continues to be the world leader in the development of new and innovative technology.

The same will become true of medical care.

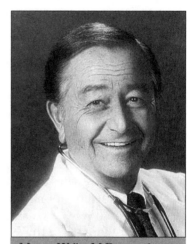

The American medical system is a $1.7 *trillion* industry, but it is overburdened with restrictive ties to the insurance industry and tangled procedural codes. Medical tourism will help everyone by giving patients options they would not otherwise have. At this time, however, doctors are locked into a system that does not allow such practices. Healthcare has changed for the worse since the days of the family doctor who practiced independently and could advise whatever was best for his or her patients.

Medical tourism is traveling for the purpose of medical care, so usually that involves combining healthcare with a vacation. Sometimes the medical component is foremost, such as having heart surgery in a foreign hospital, followed by sightseeing excursions. Other times the vacation is the priority, such as a stay at a tropical beach resort paid for by taking advantage of hugely discounted local dental care. The primary motivation determines which country you choose. For a hip replacement, you cannot do better

Marcus Welby, M.D., *was the most popular television show of the early 1970s. It featured a wise, compassionate, always-available doctor who worked independently. The show was a hit because, even then, such doctors were becoming a relic of the past.*

than a top-notch hospital in India, Thailand, or Singapore. If a vacation is the major goal, the list of destinations is much greater. More than 50 countries are now promoting packages that combine healthcare with recreation and other activities. You can get excellent cosmetic dental treatment in Costa Rica, and the most skillful hair transplants in Cyprus. South Africa, on the other hand, specializes in medical safaris — you can go on a week-long big-game safari with a stop for cosmetic eye-bag removal surgery or dental restoration.

In this book, you will find out how to get inexpensive yet high-quality surgery, dental care, weight-loss treatments, assisted reproduction, and many other therapies. Some of these — such as stem-cell therapy — are not even available yet in the United States. All the major newspapers, *Time* and other magazines, and TV shows such as *60 Minutes* have reported on medical tourism. But none of these can answer the most important question: Is this something for *you*?

Traveling for Healthcare is Not a New Phenomenon

Medical tourism is as old as humanity itself. People have always traveled to visit special healing places or skilled healers. In prehistoric times, mineral hot springs were known to be curative for many conditions, especially arthritis, muscular injuries, and skin diseases. Archeological evidence shows that some spa resorts were popular tens of thousands of years ago. Even animals will travel long distances to get to places with healing plants or salt licks.

The earliest written records of medical tourism are from ancient Greece, about 5,000 years ago, describing people with eye diseases who journeyed to Tell Brak, Syria, to temples where miracle cures were available. In the following centuries, many other temples to healing gods sprang up around the Mediterranean, often located at propitious sites such as mineral springs, waterfalls, and mountaintops. It is now recognized that these sites do, indeed, have healthful properties, and many feature modern resorts. Ancient Romans traveled as far as the distant lands of Britain to take waters at a place now known as the city of Bath.

The most famous of the ancient sites was Epidauria, a small territory in Greece. It was believed to be the home of the god of health, Asclepius.

From the Mediterranean, healing resorts spread throughout Europe. The same was happening in Asia, but the European phenomenon was more pronounced and much more documented, largely because of a single trend: the aristocratic practice of tourism. After the Renaissance — the "rebirth" of science and culture in the 15th century — it became very fashionable for wealthy young British men to travel to the classical lands of Italy and Greece. Their grand circuit was called a *tour*, after the Greek instrument to draw a circle, and the aristocratic travelers called themselves tourists. Along the way, they discovered mineral springs and countless other healthy places to restore and rejuvenate — or just hang out for a while. Baden Baden, Wiesbaden, Carlsbad, and countless other towns with *bad* ("bath") in their name, sprang up to service these well-appointed tourists.

Napoleon triggered the next big development in medical tourism when he rode into Egypt, and his soldiers eagerly sampled the new sights and therapies. The end of the Napoleonic Wars in 1815 brought a flood of Europeans to the shores of Africa and the Near East for convalescence. Later that century, the railways opened up the continent even more. Places that had formerly just been visited developed into long-stay areas. Healing resorts became sanatoria for tuberculosis and other conditions, where

The Legend Of Asclepius

According to Greek legend, Asclepius was a renowned surgeon and healer, able even to revive the dead. His name, meaning "to cut up" has given us the modern word scalpel. Statues of Asclepius show him holding a staff, to signify authority, wrapped by a single snake.

Snakes were both feared and revered in ancient Greece. While vipers were poisonous, the rat snake was appreciated for exterminating the vermin that brought plague and other diseases. Snakes periodically shed their skin, a symbol of death and rebirth. In the temples of Asclepius, non-poisonous snakes were allowed to slither among the dormitories where the sick and injured slept.

The god Zeus was angered when Asclepius revived the dead — an ability that should be reserved only for gods and violated the natural order. He killed Asclepius with a thunderbolt. But then, realizing how important Asclepius had been to humanity, he turned him into the constellation Ophiuchus ("the serpent bearer").

By 300 BC, the cult of Asclepius had grown very popular and thousands of people traveled to the healing temples built in his honor. There, patients would sleep and then tell their dreams to trained physicians, aesclepieion, who prescribed medicines or exercises according to their interpretations. Socrates's last words, as reported in Plato's Phaedo, are a reminder to sacrifice a cock to Asclepius.

The father of modern medicine, Hippocrates, was one of these aesclepieion. The original Hippocratic oath begins with the invocation, "I swear, . . . by Asclepius," to uphold the selfless principles of medical practice.

Meanwhile, the Staff of Asclepius, with a single serpent, has now become a symbol of medicine around the globe. However, it is very often confused with the Caduceus of Mercury, the Roman god of commerce, with its two intertwined winged serpents. How ironic that the mix-up of these two symbols should so reflect the change in medicine from healing to commerce!

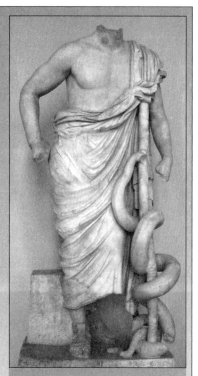

Asclepius was a mythical demigod of ancient Greece, the son of a human mother and the god Apollo. Assisted by snakes, he was considered the greatest healer and forerunner of modern physicians. This statue shows him holding his characteristic staff with a single serpent.

Often confused with Asclepius, the Caduceus is the symbol of the Mercury, the god of commerce. How ironic that so many modern medical facilities prefer this symbol!

people might stay for months or years. In fact, medical tourism became the driving force for the economic development of Europe.

The modern era of medical tourism can be said to have started with the collapse of the economy in Thailand in 1997. The country had long been a favored destination for tourists from around the world, so it already had a huge number of hotels and hospitality services. The economic crisis hit medical care particularly hard, since hospitals depended on government funding. Hospitals needed money to stay open, so they started catering to foreigners, who could pay in hard cash. The peculiar Thai combination of sun, sea, and anything-goes culture led to an explosion of cosmetic surgery services. Nearby Malaysia and Singapore followed suit, while India focused particularly on its medical expertise and cheap labor to provide major surgery at huge discounts. These four countries now dominate medical tourism — and they plan to keep it that way. Each of them is pouring billions of dollars into constructing massive new hospital complexes that are as technologically advanced and luxurious as any in the world.

The trend is accelerating around the world, with ever more high-tech healthcare facilities and specially designed convalescent accommodations. Dubai has plans to join the ranks of the top medical-tourist countries, and other countries from Argentina to Vietnam hope to do the same. One of the more remarkable of these new facilities is the planned development of Munich International Airport as a healthcare hub. You will be able to land in Munich, be taken directly from the airplane to the hospital, have surgery and other advanced treatment and never leave the airport or even go through customs! The airport hospital already has a magnetic resonance imaging (MRI) facility on the premises. This futuristic development is a sign of the globalization of healthcare.

Affordable Care, Vacation Included

In the summer of 2004, Howard Staab got some bad news. The 53-year-old carpenter from Durham, North Carolina, was an athletic bicycle rider and had always been in good health. He was a private contractor — as his own boss, he did not have health insurance from an employer, and the enormous premium of private insurance for an individual in his age group did not seem worth it. When the rugged, pony-tailed man was told he had a potentially fatal heart condition, he was surprised. But the real shock came when he was told that without health insurance, he had to pay the $200,000 bill himself — with a $50,000 up-front deposit, please.

His story, picked up by the *Washington Post*, reveals a problem faced by many Americans — and Howard's clever solution. First, the *Post* reporter confirmed the cost. Hospital spokeswoman Katie Galbraith explained that Mr. Staab would not quality for charity care, and without his cash payment the hospital would be stuck with the bill.

As a self-employed contractor, Howard was used to hunting for the most economical deals. He did some research and decided to fly to New Delhi, India, and undergo treatment at the renowned Escorts Heart Institute & Research Centre (see *India, page 200*). Accompanied by his partner, Maggi Grace, the two stayed in a luxurious private suite in the hospital. After the surgery, they went sightseeing, which included a trip to the Taj Mahal. The total cost — their combined airfare and hotel, his complete medical care, medications and rehabilitation therapy, and even the side trips — came to about $10,000.

"The Indian doctors, they did such a fine job here, and took care of us so well," said Staab. As for the experience of having major surgery in India: "Nobody even questions the capability of an Indian doctor, because there isn't a big hospital in the United States where there isn't an Indian doctor working."

Cost saving is clearly the most prominent attraction of modern medical tourism. With American medical costs spiraling out of control, each year more people have to do without life-saving surgery, or else go bankrupt trying to pay for it. At this time, the number one cause of U.S. home foreclosures and personal bankruptcy is medical expenses. The hue and cry by politicians and the news media about this embarrassing state of affairs doesn't help much if you are the one facing the crisis, and no matter how alarming the news headlines become, this is not going to change anytime soon. So the best solution is increasingly being seen as going overseas for care.

Let's consider some comparative costs:

- A bone-marrow transplant that costs $250,000 in the United States is just $25,000 in India.
- Heart-bypass surgery in the U.S. costs $60,000 to $80,000; it is around $10,000 in Asia. Open-heart surgery can cost as little as $3,000 in India.
- Stomach-reduction surgery in the United States costs $20,000 and as high as $70,000, with expensive follow-up treatment if needed. Overseas it can be done for well under $5,000, with free follow-up treatment.
- For knee-replacement surgery in the U.S., you are often looking at about $50,000, whereas the same procedure in a high-tech hospital in the Philippines performed by Western-trained surgeons might cost you $6,000.
- Laparoscopic adrenalectomy (an operation to remove an adrenal gland) typically costs $30,000 in the U.S., but just $2,600 — less than one tenth the cost — in Thailand.
- A full facelift that would cost $20,000 in the U.S. runs about $1,250 in South Africa.
- In the United States, a comprehensive check-up, sometimes called an "executive physical," runs about $500 and up to $2,000 or more. In Malaysia, the same thorough examination, using the same diagnostic instrumentation, can run as little as $84.

- Dental, eye, and cosmetic surgery in the United States typically cost about three to 10 times as much as in dozens of other countries that now advertise these services to foreigners.

Even if you have health insurance, your share of the cost for medical treatment is often more than the total cost would be overseas. Your insurance may not cover physical therapy, which can be an additional substantial cost. Depending on your insurance, there may also be copays, administrative fees, outpatient costs, and uncovered medications. And despite all those out-of-pocket costs, you might still be liable for 20 percent of the insurance-covered portion. The overall result is that Americans pay an estimated 32 percent of their healthcare costs out of pocket. That means even medical tourists *with* insurance will usually come out ahead.

How can overseas hospitals offer services at so much lower prices?

There are many reasons, beginning with the most oppressive part of practicing medicine today in the United States: the paperwork. I can't tell you how many doctors I know who constantly complain about this. Some are so frustrated that they are at the point of quitting the profession. Indeed, surveys show that less than half of all doctors would recommend a medical career to their children. And it is even worse for nurses, who spend much more time at the computer desk than they do in patients' rooms. It is so bad that few young people now want to enter the nursing profession — the average age of U.S. nurses is 49, and fresh nursing school graduates typically burn out within five years. Their biggest complaint is paperwork. Almost 80 percent of our healthcare bill goes to paperwork of various sorts. Hundreds of thousands of clerks are employed in health professions just to shuffle paper around. It is a staggering inefficiency, an enormous waste of time and effort, and a source of frustration to everyone.

> ## First-World Treatment at Third-World Prices
>
> Bradley Thayer, a 60-year-old retired apple farmer from Okanogan, Washington, tripped in his orchard and badly tore the ligaments in his knee. Without health insurance, he faced a six-month wait and a $35,000 bill for the surgery. So he flew to Mumbai (formerly Bombay) in India, got his knee fixed, had a wonderful time traveling, and the total cost of the trip was less than a third of the surgeon's fee alone had he had the procedure done in the United States.

When Meghan Stone received a magnetic resonance imaging (MRI) test a few years ago, she thought her insurance company would pick up the bill. Instead, the Chicago resident was charged 40% of the cost, or roughly $3,000. In Thailand, the same MRI scans can be had for a couple of hundred dollars.

The fundamental problem is that U.S. medical care does not follow a normal economic pattern of supply and demand. In economic systems, there are generally two players: provider and consumer, or seller and payer. Instead, the American medical system has three players — the patient, the doctor, and the health insurance payer — and each of the three is pitted against the other two. This absurd situation reminds me of when I traveled in the former Soviet Union. If you wanted to buy groceries, you stood in line, found what you wanted (if you were lucky), got approval from the state to pay for it, and then picked up your supplies. Since the state paid for it, you tried to get the best food possible, regardless of price. Since you were not the one paying the grocery store, the service was abysmal. And since the government was the one paying the store, they balanced the budget by leaving supermarket shelves bare. Each of three economic players — citizen, food market, and government — were pitted against each other to try to get ahead. The result was a disaster. This is exactly what is happening in the U.S. healthcare system.

As a medical tourist, you eliminate the paperwork. You pay a fee that goes directly to the providers. That's it — simple and efficient. The hospital and doctors do a good job not because of the threat of litigation but because you provide their income — if you are satisfied, they prosper; if you are unhappy, they are out of business.

There are further reasons why overseas care is less expensive than in the U.S. These hospitals, clinics, and doctors do not suffer from the other plagues of American healthcare: the outrageous greed and corruption of the CEOs of major health insurance plans, and skyrocketing malpractice insurance premiums to protect against frivolous claims. Richard Scrushy, the CEO of HealthSouth, the largest U.S. healthcare services provider, was convicted in 2006 of bilking his investors out of $2.7 billion, much of which went into his pocket. Where did that money ultimately come from? The patients. This sort of gross fraud rarely occurs in Asian and other countries, where personal integrity is considered more important than life itself. As for frivolous lawsuits, what do you think the reaction would be in India to a restaurant customer claiming the coffee was too hot? Probably an apology — if not a stomachache from fits of laughter at the silliness of our legal system. In the United States, that absurd lawsuit cost McDonald's over $2 million — paid for, eventually, by its customers.

When you pay for healthcare in the U.S., you are paying not only for your care but also a portion of the care for others who have not paid their bill or were treated by charity. After all, the hospital has to balance the books somehow, and if it is legally required to treat the poor, it will do so by over-charging the paying patients. In 2005, uninsured patients racked up $43 billion in unpaid medical bills. This amount was simply parceled out and added to the invoices of those who paid. The average family paid an extra $922 in health insurance premiums to subsidize healthcare for other people without insurance. Perhaps it is fair to consider that the well-off should help pay for those who are destitute, but a little-known fact is that the majority of the uninsured are middle-class individuals with incomes over $50,000 per year. Nonetheless, they can't always pay their medical bills because even a middle-class person cannot afford $300,000 for a liver transplant. These people would have been far better off to consider medical tourism — had they known about their options.

In other words: when you pay for a procedure overseas, you pay the true cost of your care. When you pay in the U.S., you also pay for other people's care. The same is true for your insurance premium. You also, of course, pay for all the marketing and advertising and corporate jet airplanes for the hospital administrators (like Scrushy), and, naturally, a substantial profit for the private investors. Overseas, there is little marketing or advertising, the administrators are usually doctors, and they fly coach.

Cost Comparison of U.S. and Overseas Care

On average, costs overseas run about 25% to 50% less than in the United States. There are many variables affecting this — the country, the relative value of the U.S. dollar, the amount of competition, the development of new technology, etc. — but you can find really exceptional deals on some types of medical care, while others are not that much cheaper overseas. One problem in comparing costs is that the stated price of U.S. medical procedures is often just the doctor's or surgeon's fee — and does not include anesthesiology, physical therapy, medications, or even room and board at the hospital. The result is that quoted U.S. fees are typically just one half of the final total cost.

A few countries offer really good bargains. For example, a comprehensive check-up, sometimes called an "executive physical" in the U.S., runs about $500 and up to $2,000 or more. In Malaysia, the same thorough examination, using the same diagnostic instrumentation, can cost as little as $84. Laparoscopic adrenalectomy (an operation to remove an adrenal gland) typically costs $30,000 in the U.S., but just $2,600 — less than one tenth the cost — in Thailand. A full facelift that would cost $20,000 in the U.S. runs about $1,250 in South Africa. Stomach-reduction surgery in the U.S. ranges from $20,000 to as high as $70,000, and may need expensive follow-up treatment. Overseas it can be done for well under $5,000, with free follow-up treatment. For knee-replacement surgery in the U.S., you are often looking at about $50,000, whereas the same procedure in a high-tech hospital in the Philippines performed by Western-trained surgeons might cost you $6,000. Heart bypass surgery in the U.S. costs $60,000 to $80,000; it is around $10,000 in Thailand and as little as $3,000 in India. In-vitro fertilization (IVF) is seldom covered by U.S. insurance and costs about $10,000 for each cycle, when all fees are added. In Barbados, on the other hand, all fees — including transportation, hotel, and luxury spa treatments — are bundled into a single low price. Perhaps the greatest saving, however, is acupuncture treatments, which cost about $75 per session in the U.S. and as little as $1 in China — from a far better practitioner!

Typical Procedure Costs	United States	Overseas
Abdominal surgery		
Colonoscopy and polyp removal	$1,200	$750
ERCP and gallstone extraction	$2,000	$1,000
Gall bladder removal	$4,000	$555
Hemorrhoidectomy	$3,800	$1,000
Hernia repair	$2,800	$1,000
Clinical laboratory		
Bone metabolism (osteoporosis)	$190	$94
Kidney function	$150	$66
Liver function	$140	$63
Cosmetic surgery		
Blepharoplasty (eyelid)	$4,400	$2,300
Breast reconstruction	$7,000	$3,000
Cervicoplasty (neck lift)	$4,800	$2,150
Chemical peel	$1,000	$600
Dermabrasion	$3,100	$1,500
Facelift	$11,000	$6,800
Fat injections	$900	$400
Rhinoplasty (nose reshaping)	$4,900	$3,100
Dental care		
Smile designing	$8,000	$1,000
Metal-free bridge	$5,500	$500
Dental implants	$3,500	$800
Porcelain bridge	$1,800	$300
Porcelain crown	$600	$80
Impacted tooth removal	$500	$100
Root canal	$600	$100
Tooth whitening	$350	$110
Tooth-colored composite fillings	$200	$25
Periodontal plastic surgery	$1,125	$500
Periodontal regenerative procedure	$1,350	$600
Free gingival graft	$1,150	$450
Eye surgery		
Cataract removal	$2,000	$1,250
Glaucoma surgery	$5,500	$2,000
Heart disease		
Echocardiogram	$750	$300
Stress echocardiogram	$900	$500

Echocardiogram with dobutamine	$1,000	$450
Holter monitor	$500	$200
Exercise stress test	$450	$200
Heart function and coronary risk	$110	$61
Lung disease		
Bronchoscopy	$800	$350
Percutaneous lung biopsy	$2,500	$1,000
Thoracentesis	$250	$150
Orthopaedic surgery		
Arthroscopy	$10,000	$5,000
Carpal tunnel release	$7,000	$3,000
Herniated disc repair	$20,000	$6,500
Hip or knee replacement	$25,000	$4,500
Transplant		
Bone marrow transplant	$250,000	$30,000
Liver transplant	$300,000	$40,000
Women's health		
Breast lump removal	$3,200	$700
Choosing the sex of your baby	$3,250	$960
Hysterectomy	$3,000	$511
In-vitro fertilization (IVF) cycle	$10,000	$1,800
Intrauterine insemination	$1,500	$850

We expect patients to be responsible when shopping for affordable care. But how can they be? Most hospitals cannot, or will not, quote a reliable price. Sure, they love to tell you about how good they are, with tables of figures on successful recovery and frequency of infections and other data that you would have to be an epidemiologist to critically evaluate. But they simply will not tell you the exact price. And don't expect the doctors to discuss these issues at all — they do not know, and often do not *want* to know, the answers.

But let's say you are persistent and manage to get the prices from the hospital's comptrollers. These numbers will turn out to be a fiction. According to a *USA Today* article, "Even when prices are quoted, the data given might be nearly useless if they reflect 'charges,' which few people pay, rather than actual negotiated rates." In other words, you — the naïve customer — may pay the fictitiously exaggerated amount, but the insurance companies all negotiate lower prices. The hospital's answer is that you, too, should negotiate. That's absurd! How are you supposed to negotiate when you are in an emergency room? Even if you have lots of time and energy, are you

" *A*sk 3 hospitals how much a knee operation will cost…and you're likely to get a headache."

~ *USA Today* headline, May 9, 2006

knowledgeable enough to juggle numbers with an MBA healthcare finance specialist? Not surprisingly, few patients try to negotiate price. As *USA Today* notes: "Riding in the back of an ambulance is no time to do price comparisons." That is not the time or place to haggle or dispute unnecessary items — the shock comes later, often as much as a year later, when the invoices arrive.

Hospitals discourage talk about the cost of care, and they make their bills difficult to interpret because they really do not want you to know the total cost. If you did, you might not use their services.

This is what Dr. David Brailer, interviewed by the *New York Times* in 2005, has to say about the "explanation of benefits" (EOB), a standard health insurance itemization of your bill:

"I'm the president's senior adviser on health information technology, and when I get an EOB for my four-year-old's care, I can't figure out what happened, or what I'm supposed to do."

Although Dr. Brailer is National Coordinator for Health Information Technology, with an office in the Department of Health and Human Services, he admits: "I can't figure out what care it was related to or who did what." If the top dog in the government kennel cannot make head or tail of these numbers, what are the rest of us supposed to do?

One reason hospitals don't quote prices is because there *are* no real prices! The official prices are fictional, and everyone in health administration knows this. To illustrate this, let's say, for example, a hospital needs to get $10,000 for a gall bladder surgery in order to cover all costs and break even. It will list the procedure at $15,000, the insurance company will pay $12,000, and uncollected bills average $2,000, which is written off as free care. Therefore, the hospital ends up with $10,000 and everything works out, right? Sure, except that if you happen to be paying cash, you will still pay the official $15,000. So the result is that you are paying 50 percent more in order to cover the insurance discount, the charity cases, and the deadbeats.

An article in the November 2007, *Wall Street Journal* described just how much hospitals inflated prices. Leg-compression stockings, commonly used to prevent blood clots, were billed at $791, even though they could be bought on the Internet for $12. When the *Journal* reporter asked why the charges were so high, the hospital's Chief Medical Officer, Dr. Allan Pont, called the prices "Disneyland numbers," and explained: "I do not deny that our charges look insane. But all hospitals operate the same way. It is the reality of the industry." The reality in the United States, anyway.

This practice does not take place overseas. There, fees are typically fixed. At the Apollo Medical Group in India, an outpatient consultation is generally less than $10. A complete cardiac examination, including a full range of tests, costs about $100. The average hospital bed costs $50 a night. And this is at a top-ranked facility. It is even cheaper in other cities.

The direct billing and simple efficiency of foreign hospitals result in lower prices. Other factors include reduced labor costs — which are still much higher than the local average — and lower costs for building and maintenance. The doctors also earn much smaller salaries. I spoke with many surgeons throughout Asia who told me they gave up a $300,000 annual salary in the United States to return to their home country where they earn a $30,000 salary but can live among family and friends in a less stressful work and social environment. Dr. Naresh Trehan, executive director of Escorts Heart Institute and Research Centre, earned nearly $2 million a year from his Manhattan practice before returning to India. He told me the money was not worth a heart attack, which is what his lifestyle was pushing him toward.

For a long time, the United States benefited from an international "brain drain" by luring the best professionals from around the world. Now it is increasingly common for the very best foreign surgeons trained in the U.S to return to their home country.

No Waits, No Hassle, and No Attitude

In the 1950s, the majority of doctors practiced medicine in a small office and made house calls. They knew their patients personally, accepted cash or other payment, and were respected members of society. That was a long time ago. Now, the typical doctor is a salaried employee of a huge health management firm, and specialists are often corporations in themselves. They do not have much authority, and they are so regimented that they cannot give you ideal personal care even if they wanted to, which they seldom do because they do not get paid for the extra work. Financial clerks, not the doctor, determine who gets care, what they get, and when they get it. The insurance companies have to put the lid on care to hold down their costs.

In Canada, with its wonderful and highly praised socialized heathcare system, the situation is even worse. Waits for surgery can go on for years. When my mother, who lived in Ontario, developed cataracts in her eyes, she was put on a three-year waiting list for the surgery. (My siblings and I ended up paying a private ophthalmologist for her cataract removal, but if I had known about medical tourism then, I would have sent her on a vacation to Costa Rica for a fraction of the cost.) The situation is so bad that the official government approval letter includes an apology if the patient has died during the wait!

Waits are also lengthy in the United States, where we have our own version of the Canadian socialized health plan, called Medicare. For example, Boston has more doctors per capita than almost any other American city, but the waiting time for a specialist averages about four months. Why so long? It is because the Medicare administration wants to hold off as long as possible, figuring that many of these patients will move away, get treated privately, or die. It is not just an American problem; socialized health insurance plans face the same problem everywhere. Either they hold the line on costs (by delaying treatment, for example) or they go bankrupt. In 2000, the European Court of Justice defined healthcare as a service, and thus required health insurance to pay for medical tourists' care if they were subject to "undue delay" at home. In Great Britain, the National Health Service even encourages its patients to go to India for care, since it is much cheaper for everyone in the long run.

 If you wait six months for a heart bypass you may not need it anymore."

~ Prathap Reddy, cardiologist and founder of Apollo Hospitals, India

At this time, the average waiting time to be seen in a typical U.S. emergency department is 6.2 hours. If you are a senior, it is 10.6 hours, and if your annual income is under $20,000 and you qualify for Medicaid, it is 13.3 hours. Once you are seen, you begin your journey through the maze of healthcare that involves talking with a dozen employees, none of whom knows exactly what the others are doing. I am not exaggerating: although I am a faculty physician at a sophisticated university medical hospital, my own lab test was lost, requiring two unnecessary repeat blood samples, and no one could explain why.

Now let's compare this to service overseas. There is no wait whatsoever. Typically, you are met at the airport and taken directly to the hospital. You may not even see a waiting room. If you opt for luxury service, you will be picked up in a limousine and may be taken first for a relaxing bath and whole-body massage before going to the hospital. Once there, you often have private nurses, dedicated to you, around the clock. This is unheard of in the United States, where you are lucky just to get a nurse's attention. Overseas nurses are trained in a level of personal care long ago lost in the U.S., when nurses became more highly trained professionals and left the basic care duties to lowly paid medical assistants who have just months of training and little real concept of healthcare.

In India, and many other countries, your doctors will give you their home and cell phone numbers and encourage you to call if you have any concerns. Countless times,

I met patients discharged from overseas hospitals who were just incredulous at the service they received. One elderly man swore he would never again set foot in a U.S. hospital after what he experienced in Thailand.

Access to Treatments That Aren't Available in the United States

Besides the lower cost, another major attraction for medical tourists is the availability of procedures, medicines, and treatments not available in the United States These range from newer surgeries that are not yet approved in the U.S., to exotic treatments such as ayurvedic medicine, acupuncture, and other alternative healthcare. While some of these can now be found in the U.S., the quality is better in the country where the therapy originated.

One example is hip resurfacing. American surgeons still favor the traditional method of hip replacement, mainly because that is what they were trained to do, and the prosthetic hip manufacturers are a powerful lobby and want to keep their business. The newer treatment does not involve replacing the hip — which is loaded with consequent problems and a lengthy recovery — but just replacing the worn-down surface of the existing hip with an extremely durable chrome alloy cap. The result is a superior procedure with a much shorter recovery. Resurfacing is not suitable for everyone, but if you have the opportunity, I would unhesitatingly recommend it over a full hip replacement. However, you will probably have to travel overseas to get it.

Numerous other surgeries that are difficult or impossible to arrange in the U.S. are available overseas. Stem-cell therapy is a new type of medicine in which the U.S. lags three to four years behind Thailand and Singapore. Another surgery, not performed in the U.S., involves a peculiar leg-lengthening process to give short people (usually

---

After years of working as a mountain guide, Tom Raudaschl developed osteoarthritis in his hip. He was told by an orthopaedic surgeon that he needed a hip replacement, and then discovered that the operation would probably cost about $21,000. Raudaschl decided to fly to Apollo Hospital in Chennai (see *India, page 200*) to undergo hip resurfacing. The total cost was about $5,000.

Not everyone was happy that he went overseas for his care. "As soon as you tell people that you're going to India, they frown," Raudaschl said, but he could not have been more pleased with the service. "They picked me up at the airport, did all the hotel bookings, and the food was great, too." His private room was equipped with Internet service, a microwave, and a refrigerator. Best of all was that he recovered quickly and was back skiing a month later.

---

men) an extra few inches of height. Throughout this book, you will find odd procedures and therapies that are only available outside the U.S. The benefit of medical tourism is that you, rather than the medical system, can determine your choice of therapy.

Countless medications are also available only in other countries. Many have not yet been, or will never be, approved by the FDA. Others simply fall outside the American pharmaceutical marketing system. For example, according to a *Time* report, Eli Lilly was the last U.S. manufacturer of animal insulin. This type of insulin, extracted from the pancreatic tissue of cows and pigs, was just no longer profitable for Lilly, so it stopped selling the drug on March 31, 2006. Lilly now produces only synthetic human insulin produced by recombinant-DNA technology. The problem is that up to 10 percent of diabetics cannot tolerate synthetic insulin. They develop resistance to it, or they suffer reactions that can be severe, even fatal. Since they need animal insulin, their only option is to get it abroad — another class of medical tourists who have little choice but to travel for adequate healthcare.

Family Medical Tourism Packages: Something For Everyone

Healthcare has become demystified in the last few decades. Historically, medical care had more in common with religion than it did with other types of vital services, such as getting food, clothing, or shelter. Medical procedures were shrouded in secrecy. Your family might have just the vaguest notion of what was going on, and even you might not be told the truth by your doctor. Now, healthcare is more like other types of services. We expect to be told everything, we demand to be in control, and we talk about surgery as if we were having the car repaired or the house painted.

Cosmetic surgery is at the forefront of this new approach. Like legal services or auto repair, there are phonebook ads and TV infomercials for cosmetic procedures. It might seem crass to people who think healthcare should be more private and intimate, but it is definitely the way of the future. Medical tourism facilities, especially, see little difference between marketing a hotel or a hospital. Some overseas medical centers, especially those in Thailand, are bundling packages for friends, couples, and entire families. It is definitely less miserable to have surgery when a close friend or relative is going through the same procedure and knows how you feel. You can see this at Bumrungrad Medical Center in Bangkok, where clutches of shy, veiled women from Saudi Arabia arrive to have their cosmetic surgery or other care. There is comfort in numbers.

Couples can have "his and hers" medical care — perhaps one has a hip replacement and the other has liposuction. Why not? The savings of having the work done overseas are doubled. Moreover, it is an experience to be shared — an adventure to go through together and laugh about later. It is the new sort of romantic vacation — the man recovering from a hair transplant and the woman recovering from a face-lift, both of them swathed in bandages, sipping cocktails, and watching the sun set on the ocean.

The ultimate package is for entire families. When a child needs a major medical procedure, it can be frightening and alienating. But what if the entire family is having some sort of medical care? Few things are more terrifying to a child than heart surgery. Yet this can be turned into an almost normal vacation when the whole family shares a hospital suite and all are undergoing some form of treatment. You might think that it is unlikely that every member of the family would need hospital care. But one of the remarkable benefits of Asian hospitals is that they often include dental and cosmetic clinics, alternative medicine, and even beauty makeovers, all in the same lavish hospital complex. While a child has surgery, the parents can use the opportunity to have teeth restored, or LASIK vision correction, or any number of procedures that would be impossible to have done at the same facility in the United States. Asian hospital rooms and suites are expansive to accommodate families. Some have several bedrooms, a living room, private balcony, and multiple bathrooms.

Treating the whole family at once takes a lot less time than attending individual medical appointments. Let's say your tousle-haired boy is blessed with those Prince Charles ears that look like miniature microwave antennas. Ear pinning is a very common, minor cosmetic surgery in the United States But it is amazing how much time can be consumed to get it done — shuttling the kid to various doctor appointments, etc. On a medical vacation, it takes no extra time whatsoever since you are already there, and no transportation is necessary. And it is quite likely that this sort of minor surgery will be done for free if you are already there for some other procedure.

If you don't need to be in the hospital, there are many other options. Rather than being cooped up in a hotel, the family can stay at a whole new type of lodging: the medical tourism recovery resort. The pioneer of these is Bodyline Resort in Phuket (see *Thailand, page 286*). This ingenious resort is run by twin sisters from Australia, and it caters to people who have surgery at any of the nearby medical tourism hospitals. All of the fully equipped cottages are specially designed for someone who has come from the hospital, and each of the staff is trained to care for these tourists. It is a unique experience to have a communal dinner in the large open-air atrium, with some people in wheelchairs and others swathed in facial bandages. No one feels stared at, or like they are attracting the uncomfortable attention of others who wonder what happened. Residents at Bodyline often become friends and keep in touch long after they have returned to their home countries.

What About Quality of Care?

The first question everyone has about medical tourism, once they learn about the heavily discounted cost, is about the quality of these procedures. Are the hospitals safe? Are the doctors competent? What are the recourses if something goes wrong? All of these questions are more thoroughly answered further along in this book. But consider this: fully one third of the doctors in the United States were trained overseas, especially in Mexico or the Caribbean, where medical schools are vastly inferior to those in the U.S. Conversely, almost all of the doctors at major medical tourism hospitals were trained in the U.S. This seeming contradiction points out a curious fact: when you have surgery at home you are receiving average medical care, but when you have surgery overseas you are getting the very best. In India or Thailand, your surgeon will be among the most highly regarded in the country. In the U.S., however, your surgeon will be someone who has managed to pass his or her residency — if he or she has even gotten that far. It is actually more likely that you will have a surgical resident in training, especially if your procedure is done at a university-affiliated medical center. Ironically, if you want the best of American healthcare, you might have to go to India to get it!

We had an old saying in medical school: "C = MD." In other words, if the student can scrimp a passing C grade, no more is necessary to get the degree. A pass is all that matters, since patients rarely do a thorough study of their surgeon's experience and competence. In fact, patients usually have no choice in the matter since the surgeon is assigned by availability or by the insurance plan.

When you have surgery in the U.S., therefore, you might get a great surgeon or you might get a surgeon who barely passed by getting Cs throughout medical school and squeaked through a residency. This is not true overseas, because only the best and brightest end up working at the most sophisticated hospitals — the medical tourism centers. Indeed, some of these centers are affiliates of renowned institutions such as the Mayo Clinic and the Cleveland Clinic, or even run directly by Harvard, Johns Hopkins, and other major universities.

Which would you prefer: a highly experienced U.S.-trained doctor overseas, or a tired resident at your regional hospital who might have gone to an unaccredited medical school in the Caribbean? American doctors increasingly tend to be overworked as they are caught in the competitive economics of managed-care conglomerates. Quality suffers as a result.

A landmark study by the Rand Corporation, published in 2003, found that adults in the U.S. received, on average, just 54.9 percent of the recommended care for their

Who Has the Better Doctors?

At U.S. hospitals, one in three doctors was trained overseas because his or her college grades were too low to get into an American medical school. At medical tourism hospitals in India, Thailand, and elsewhere, the doctors were likely trained at top U.S. universities like Harvard and Stanford.

conditions. The shortfall was due to restrictions on their care in order to save costs. Of course, you would not be told about these restrictions and would have no way of knowing without being a medical specialist yourself. The ruthless cost cutting has often led to horrific stories, such as this one from Dr. Donald Berwick, a pediatrician. When his wife was hospitalized with a rare spinal-cord problem, he wrote, "No day passed — not one — without a medication error. Tests were repeated, data misread, information lost. And this was at a top hospital. The errors were not rare; they were the norm."

In contrast, medical tourism doctors cater to their patients and are dedicated to their care no matter how much time it takes. The results show up in medical quality evaluations. In 2002, the World Health Organization's first worldwide analysis of health systems ranked Singapore, a top medical tourism destination, as the best — ahead of Japan (which ranked 10th) and the United States (which ranked 37th).

 I tell the story of my experience to everyone . . . the efficiency and the speed. What happened to me was just the absolute opposite to anything that could happen in the United States."

~ Medical tourist from Carmel, California.

Medical tourism hospitals in the Philippines and other countries actually have to meet a higher standard than in the United States because their entire survival is on the line. If you have a bad experience in the U.S., nothing will come of it. If you are unhappy with your care in the Philippines, however, you might tell 20 people about it, and cause that hospital to lose 20 customers. Since the Philippine hospitals and clinics depend on medical tourists for their income, they will do their absolute best to make sure that you have a wonderful experience.

There is no comparative incentive in the U.S. When insurance pays, it does not matter if the patient is disappointed. In fact, from the insurance provider's point of view, it might even be *better* for you to be uncomfortable, so you won't be so quite so eager to go through an expensive hospitalization again. Certainly, the staff won't be too concerned; they get paid regardless of whether the patients are happy.

Medical tourism hospitals are paid directly by you, which means they listen intently to what you want and try their best to serve you. That includes having the most advanced technology. I was astonished in India to see a Toshiba 64-slice CT angiography machine — the same used by Johns Hopkins Medical Center and far better than that available at hospitals near my home. At major medical tourism hospitals, all equipment is top-of-the-line and FDA-approved.

All this quality doesn't mean something can't go wrong. With any surgery, it is inevitable that there will be an adverse outcome in the course of thousands of procedures. Approximately one percent of all people undergoing gastric bypass surgery die on the operating table. That's going to happen in any country. It is not because the procedure is dangerous, but because many of these patients are very sick and already at risk of dying. The presence or lack of malpractice lawyers will not change that. The only way to ensure that you are getting the highest quality is to examine the hospital according to recognized standards of excellence, further explained in the next chapter.

Talking to Your Doctor About Medical Tourism

Q: What is my doctor going to say when I mention that I am considering going overseas for surgery?

A: American doctors know even less about medical tourism than the American public, which is to say, almost nothing. Naturally, they will be skeptical. They understand the system here; they know the checks and balances and quality control. In the best of circumstances, your doctor can refer you to a trusted colleague or a specialist if needed. But they do not have this knowledge about doctors and hospitals in other countries. Your doctor will most likely try to talk you out of it — not because medical tourism poses a higher risk, but simply because it is unfamiliar and seems uncertain.

Q: I did mention it to my doctor, and she was horrified. She warned me strongly against going off on my own. Should I trust her on that?

A: Traditionally, patients have placed complete trust in their doctors, essentially handing over all decision-making regarding their health. This is no longer advised. While it is good to have a certain degree of trust, you also need to retain responsibility for your decisions. It is especially important to consider all the issues that influence a decision. Your doctor is licensed by the state, credentialed by one or more hospitals and employers, has membership in medical societies, and pays fees to a malpractice insurance carrier. Each one of these institutions is not happy about medical tourism because, frankly, they are losing money and power. If your doctor encourages you to go overseas, she can be reprimanded by the state for "inappropriate medical advice," and she can also lose her malpractice insurance. She may get into trouble with the local hospitals, since they are directly losing your business, and she may even be fired by her employer for sending you to the competition. How long do you think a Ford salesman will last if he tells his customer to buy a Toyota, even if the choice is in the customer's best interest? Unfortunately, your doctor is no longer a free agent, but part of a system. Primary care doctors, in particular, are needed to funnel patients into lucrative specialty practices and hospital stays. These institutions look very unfavorably on doctors who send their patients elsewhere.

Q: *My doctor says American healthcare is the best in the world. Isn't he right?*

A: In general, yes. But this is changing right now. Very few physicians are aware of the tremendously sophisticated new facilities popping up everywhere from Argentina to South Africa, all of them competing to offer the very best, most advanced treatment in the world. Even I, who have spent the majority of the last two years studying medical tourism, was astonished to discover these new hospital complexes. I have never seen anything like it, and when I tell my medical colleagues about it, they are equally amazed. We are entering a new world of healthcare. This will be generally recognized in five years, but for now, your doctor probably has very little idea of the care available overseas. For example, at Escorts Heart Institute and Research Centre (see *India, page 200*) the death rate for coronary bypass patients is 0.8 percent. In contrast, the death rate for the same procedure at New York-Presbyterian Hospital, where former president Bill Clinton recently underwent bypass surgery, is 2.35 percent, according to a 2002 study by the New York State Health Department. The lower death rate at Escorts is partially due to its status as one of only a handful of treatment facilities worldwide that specialize in robotic surgery. This type of surgery is the way of the future: it is less invasive than conventional surgery because it relies on tiny, remote-controlled instruments that are inserted through a small incision and manipulated with computerized precision. In this regard, Escorts has taken the lead in international quality.

Q: *Won't medical tourism hurt U.S. hospitals?*

A: Medical tourism hospitals owe their fortunes almost directly to the failure of the medical system in the tourist's home country. The American medical system is failing in its duty to provide rapid, high-quality care at a reasonable cost. It is a tragedy. But sometimes, you need competition to foster change. The U.S. medical system has been stagnant for a long time, locked to obsolete systems by for-profit hospital management that takes the patients for granted, and often racks up outrageous profits. Competition from overseas will force change here for the better.

Q: *Won't medical tourism harm the U.S. economy by outsourcing services?*

A: Outsourcing can actually strengthen American companies and the overall economy. Take computers, for example. Soon after the home computer was invented, virtually all computer makers shipped their manufacturing operations overseas, keeping only the design and final assembly in the U.S. The result was that computers became so cheap that they soon were household items. Meanwhile, the overseas factories in turn spawned a demand for further American ingenuity. The overall result was a tremendous gain for the U.S. economy — the high-tech boom of the 1990s — that could never have been achieved if manufacturing had stayed within the U.S. Computers would have remained too expensive for personal use, and the entire industry would have been limited to a technological niche.

Outsourcing creates wealth. It is occurring in almost every service industry. Medical care is no different. The more that can be outsourced, the cheaper it will become, and the more Americans will prosper. This is further explained in Chapter 4.

Q: I have heard that the sophisticated hospitals in India that cater to medical tourists drain much-needed doctors and services from the poorer population. Is that true?

A: There is no evidence of this, despite much investigation and research. In fact, the infusion of money from medical tourists has created a tremendous development of new hospitals. All of these are committed, to varying extents, to improving the health of the local population as well. For example, the renowned Hyderabad Eye Institute (see *India, page 200*) devotes one half of all its revenue to providing free eye care for lower-income Indians who come long distances for specialized treatment that would not otherwise be available. Virtually the entire medical system of Thailand is underwritten by its medical tourism services. Medical tourism throughout Asia is providing major gains in quantity and quality of healthcare to the local population.

Q: Should I really consider combining surgery with a vacation? My doctor said I should stay out of the sun and avoid activities.

A: Planning a medical tourism trip involves a lot of issues (see Chapter 3). In general, surgical incisions should not be exposed to strong, direct sunlight in order to prevent unattractive darkening of the skin. This is especially true of cosmetic surgery, where the incisions tend to be in sun-exposed locations and appearance, naturally, is a priority. However, given proper precautions, there is no reason *not* to have a vacation after surgery, and there are many good reasons to do so. A relaxed, happy person heals better. Enticing food and a pleasant environment go a long way toward maximizing the body's ability to recover from surgery. With proper planning, the combination of medical care and a vacation is, in fact, ideal.

Chapter 2

How Do I Decide Where To Go?

What You'll Find When "Googling" Medical Tourism

Type "medical tourism" in an Internet search engine, and you will find a staggering amount of junk. This is the problem with the Internet — the amount of information you can access is virtually endless, but good, usable information can be surprisingly difficult to find. Countless websites provide healthcare advice. The problem is that most of it is nonsense. A major study showed that the vast majority of medical information was of poor quality or flat-out wrong. In fact, most people who used the Internet for healthcare advice actually made their condition worse!

In general, you should be suspicious of any Internet information about medical tourism. Wikipedia (www.wikepedia.com) has one of the few objective descriptions. One problem is that the medical travel industry is so new that reliable sources have not yet had time to thoroughly separate sense from nonsense. Meanwhile, there are a lot of people trying to sell you something, and giving you accurate information is not their top priority. Almost all the sites that pop up are commercial operations. You really have to dig deep to find anything useful. For all its shortcomings, however, the Internet is still the quickest and by far the broadest, most easily accessible and up-to-date source of information on any subject, and it's becoming more so every day.

This is what you will find when searching "medical tourism:"
- Newspaper, magazine, and TV articles and features about medical tourism, with catchy headlines such as "Sun, surf, and surgery."
- Headlines on medical tourism-related conferences and events around the world, especially new government proclamations about how they will be promoting their countries for international patients.
- Hundreds of medical tourism referral sites. All of these promise to handle everything for you. These sites swamp any search for good information. Instead, they

focus on catching your attention and selling you a product. Online medical tourism referral sites have become the new travel agencies. In fact, many people from the travel industry who lost their jobs to the Internet (with the advent of quicker and cheaper online booking) have now gone into the medical tourism business. Should you use one of these agencies? You'll find your answer below, because you first need to decide exactly what it is you want.

Determine Your Priority: Cost, Availability, Pleasure, or Privacy?

Before you take any action whatsoever regarding a trip for healthcare, it is very important to get your priorities in order. Most people skip this step and go right into exploring what is available. This is a big mistake! If you do not clearly define what you want to accomplish, the referral agency will do it for you. It is not a good idea to have a salesperson determine your healthcare — in fact, that's a big part of the problem with managed care in the U.S., where some administrative clerk decides whether to approve your doctor's recommended care. If you don't have a clear sense of what you want, you will probably become distracted by all the amazing offers and possibilities, and you may end up booking a trip that is very different from what you first wanted.

You have to have a single priority. For most medical tourists, it is cost saving. You already have some idea of what the procedure will cost at home. You may not know the exact dollar figure (which can be maddeningly difficult to find out), but you know one thing: it will be expensive — perhaps prohibitively so. For example, let's say you are overweight and have been considering the new stomach-banding procedure. This is a remarkably efficient method of dramatic weight loss that does not involve cutting into the stomach. Unfortunately, it is generally not offered in the U.S., where surgeons prefer the more traditional stomach-reduction surgeries. Also unfortunately, it is extremely expensive, costing $25,000 and up (you may see surgeons advertising the procedure for less, but that is just their fee — you need to double the cost to add the hospital fee, and then add the anesthesiology, GI consult, dietetics, medications, and post-operative care). If your priority is weight loss, it makes sense to explore stomach banding overseas and compare total costs, and not get distracted by all the other features. It reminds me of the first time I bought a new car. I was thinking about a sporty sedan, while the salesman tried his damnedest to sell me a pick-up truck (on which the dealer made a higher profit). If I hadn't been clear on what I wanted, I would have driven home a utility vehicle. Be as specific as you can in your priorities, but stay open-minded and don't limit yourself to familiar procedures. You will find many innovative procedures that you have not heard of, and many that are not available in the U.S.

Although some countries tend to be cheaper than others — for example, India is notably less expensive than Singapore — the discounts are not the same across the board. A country might have excellent deals on one procedure, but not particularly good deals for another procedure. The LASIK corrective vision surgery, for example, may actually be cheaper in the United States than it is in Asia. It is best to shop for the specific procedure or care that you want.

Availability is another priority in medical tourism. You are traveling because whatever you want (for example, the banding procedure) is simply not available in the U.S. A different priority might be to find a nice place for a vacation with the added benefit of healthcare, or to be able to receive treatment far from the attention of acquaintances, neighbors, and coworkers.

You can have secondary priorities. Write out all your desires in order of importance before you begin your search. Don't limit yourself here just because you think something is out of reach. Put down everything on your wish list. It doesn't matter if the desires are contradictory. For example, you can put down stomach surgery, scuba diving, tropical beach, and snow skiing. These make no sense if you look at everything on the list together. Obviously, you cannot go diving after having surgery, and there are very few places in the world where warm beaches are located near ski resorts. But put it all down anyway, and then re-order them according to what you want the most. Add every feature you can think of. Want to practice your high school Spanish? Savor the best Thai food? Visit the land of your ancestry in Hungary? Go on a safari? These are all features that can add immeasurably to your medical vacation.

Here is an example of a priority list:
- Inexpensive, high-quality stomach banding
- English-speaking country
- Sightseeing, especially big wildlife
- Warm climate, but not too hot

Given this list, you can start your search. There are many excellent hospitals around the world that offer stomach banding. This is a very common procedure. According to the American Medical Association, less than one percent of all Americans who would benefit from stomach reduction go on to have it, almost always because of the cost and availability (rarely will insurance pay for it). Your list will include countries in Europe, South America, Africa, and Asia. All will be less expensive than having

---

It is amazing how many different services are offered. Even funerals can now be outsourced overseas, saving thousands of dollars. Polish crematoriums lure foreign clients with cut-price deals — just BYOB (bring your own body).

---

the surgery in the U.S., but not equally so. For example, Argentina will be much cheaper than Chile, and both will be cheaper than countries in Europe. India and Thailand will be the cheapest. But you won't be able to determine the total cost until later, when you get to the details.

The next item on your list is a desire for an English-speaking country. Many people prefer this. It is unsettling enough to have surgery in a foreign hospital, without waking in the night and being unable to talk to the nurse. The truth is that almost all medical tourism facilities around the world have staff who speak at least passable English. However, you may desire an English-speaking country not only for the treatment but also for travel, shopping, meeting locals, etc. In some countries where English is not the national language, it is nonetheless spoken almost universally,

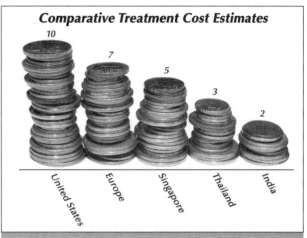

Comparative Treatment Cost Estimates

Even when standardized for quality and other features, treatment costs vary dramatically among different countries.

such as India and the Philippines. Having English-speaking as a feature will narrow your list to South Africa, India, New Zealand, and Philippines. All of these also offer wildlife sightseeing opportunities, but the best are in South Africa and India. If you don't like hot climates — and I mean really insufferably hot — I would not recommend India except for the northern part of the country during the winter. The remaining choice is South Africa, which can be hot inland, but most of the country has a pleasant climate like coastal California. South Africa costs a bit more than Asia, both for travel and for medical care, so your ultimate choice will be based on your personal preference and the importance of cost in your decisions.

Here is another priority list:
- Inexpensive, high-quality hair transplant
- Privacy! No other tourists gawking at you
- Inexpensive, high-quality dental work for partner
- Quiet, pleasant spa-type location

High-quality hair transplants in the U.S. can run up to $8,000 or more. Why pay that much when you can have it done for a fraction of the cost in a beautifully relaxing environment? Because quality hair transplants depend mostly on skill, the specialty clinic does not require a huge investment for infrastructure and equipment. Therefore, many poorer countries have entered this level of medical tourism. The same is true of dentistry. Although a high-tech dental office requires substantial investment, it is still much less costly than a hospital. Your list will first focus on countries that provide quality hair-transplant services — and there are a lot of choices here! Most of them are in popular tourist destinations, however. You can focus on the more discreet locations, but this characteristic is more specific to the individual facility rather than the country. Some resorts excel in privacy, and you may cross paths with celebrities who have the same interest. All those movie stars and politicians with a full head of hair — they must have been very lucky to be born with such favorable genes, right? Sure. And their hair color is natural, too.

For overall privacy, Dubai is an excellent choice. Situated on the Persian Gulf, the new Dubai Healthcare City will cater to those who want the highest-quality treatment away from the regular tourism circuit. You definitely won't see the Disney Land crowd here. A different type of privacy is offered by the Bodyline Resort in Phuket, Thailand, where you can recuperate along with fellow medical tourists at a private beach, pool, and restaurant.

Once you have your list of priorities, it is easy to focus on a few destinations that provide the ideal combination. If you desire multiple procedures, you'll find that certain types of care are often found together, such as hair transplant and dental work, along with minor cosmetic surgery. This is one of the peculiarities of the medical tourism industry. In the U.S., typically, dental and cosmetic healthcare services tend to be located individually and without much proximity, if any, to a major medical facility. Medical tourism, however, thrives off the synergy of having multiple services. In Thailand, for example, you may find a major hospital with dental care, hair transplant, cosmetic surgery, massage and spa, beauty parlor, and many services nearby or even in the same building! This, of course, makes it much easier to get a variety of treatments for yourself and your companions.

Other preferences might include standards for quality, such as having Joint Commission International (JCI) accreditation. If travel is a concern and you don't want to spend endless hours on the airplane, Central American and Caribbean countries offering medical tourism can be closer to your home than New York or Los Angeles.

Should You Use a Referral Agent?

At this time, you have just two ways to go about getting medical care overseas: you can arrange it yourself with the facility, or you can use a referral agent. This will change in the future, when medical tourism becomes more integrated with American healthcare (see Chapter 4). For now, you need to decide yourself how to go about it. The easiest way to do so is by using a referral service.

The majority of referral agents are people who were medical tourists and decided to get into the business themselves. Many of them had barely returned from their experience before setting up a website and offering referral services. It is one of the easiest businesses to get into. What other home business requires just a few hours and a hundred dollars to open — with immediate profit and no risk? It reminds me a bit of the real estate boom, when seemingly everyone who had bought a house was considering getting a license as a real estate agent and flipping properties — except that medical tourism is far easier to get into.

How easy is it? Let's say you had a hip replacement in Bangalore that cost just $5,000. You know that hospitals in India will pay as much as 10 percent as a referral fee to get new patients. So you decide to put up a website and make the "arrangements" — which is nothing more than steering your customers to the Bangalore hospital. If you manage to refer just 10 people to the hospital, you have earned back the cost of your own surgery!

Because referral sites are so easy to set up, they are popping up everywhere. Most are coy about giving out useful information, and they do not disclose which hospitals they are working for or how they make money. They don't want you to contact the hospital directly, which you could do very easily by going to the hospital's website (given in this book).

Commissions? Fees? Kickbacks? All of these come into play. Many referral agents do not have a physical address, just an email address, or perhaps only a mail drop. This is the sign of an Internet entrepreneur whose business exists only in "cyberspace." Don't expect them to be around if you have a problem. One website goes so far to advise: "In case your intervention cannot take place for any reason; you cannot pretend to any refund. Due to our sharp regulations regarding request handling this case is of very weak probability." In other words, you pay your money and hope for the best.

How Easy is it to Become a Medical Tourism Agent?

In a coffee shop in Phuket, Thailand, I met a young man from Holland. He had little education and few skills, preferring a life of surfing and nightclubbing. While in Phuket, he injured his foot and was treated at a local hospital, where he met some medical tourists. He then registered 20 Yahoo Internet addresses (all variations on "medical tourism" names), where he offered to make arrangements for a $200 fee. The arrangement consists of putting the patient in touch with the hospital's international patient office, a matter of just sending an email to the client. The total cost of his investment? About $100 (Yahoo and other services will register your website for as little as $4.95, and they have free set-up programs). Now this enterprising beach bum has an impressive income even by Holland standards, owns a condo on the beach, and his work consists of an hour a day at a local Internet café.

If you don't get what you want, tough luck. Evidently, there are enough gullible people who will send money to these operators. The tragedy is that suffering individuals who get conned by these sites are often those who can least afford it.

Following are a few of the more popular referral sites, in alphabetical order:

- **Firefly Medical Corporation** (www.fireflymed.com) gives no address or direct phone number, just directions to send them an email. They claim that, "Firefly provides the only international directory and resource for medical procedures." Really! Have they tried a Google search? They may be surprised to discover the hundreds of others who provide the same information and much more. Firefly appears to operate by charging medical tourism providers a fee for inclusion in their listing. In other words, they seem to want to become the yellow pages of medical tourism. However, such listings can already be had for free on dozens of other Internet sites.

- **Lipotourism** (www.phudson.com/TOURISM/lipotourism.html) presents a large amount of useful information on cosmetic surgery. However, the website provides no information on medical tourism. Dr. Patrick Hudson, an Albuquerque-based plastic surgeon, claims to have coined the word lipotourism and often writes it Lipotourism©. However, his website just steers patients to his own practice. The website www.lipotourism.com is not related to the above site. It appears to be an Internet "phishing" site that tries to lure Internet readers with false information and collect information or direct readers to another service. This is misleading and has nothing to do with medical tourism (see further on for more on this practice).

- **Lipotourist** (www.lipotourist.com) is a referral site set up by a popular health writer, Michelle Boasten, to send people to Costa Rica for cosmetic surgery. Ms. Boasten has also developed a program to train medical tourism concierges — people who help facilitate the process, make arrangements, and even accompany medical tourists to and from their surgery (www.lipotourist.com/medicalconcierge.htm).

> **A Word of Caution:**
>
> While visiting some of the more shabby medical tourism hospitals in Asia, I met patients from the United States who had paid an Internet agent, and were only later told which hospital was selected for their surgery. It was the usual bait-and-switch tactic. Let the buyer beware!

- **medicaltourism.com** (www.medicaltourism.com) is far and away the best Internet source of objective medical tourism information. The breadth of coverage is astonishing! It will take you hours to read everything here. This is a good site to use once you have already decided where you want to go. Unlike virtually all the other websites, medicaltourism.com provides links directly to the hospitals or other facilities. It also has online forums for discussions, and many other interactive features.

- **Medical Tours International** (www.cmiregistration.com) appears to be a very ambitious and comprehensive site — until you get to their somewhat deceptive method of getting you to sign up. On the ambitious side, this site has a monthly publication entitled *The Traveling Patient* and offers a "Certified Medical Concierge Course." It all looks very impressive. However, closer inspection of the site reveals features that I warned about. The site states: "You will receive cost quotes for your procedures and travel that are the lowest you will find anywhere." Anyone making this claim should be suspect. Although the site claims to be a global referral agency, it appears that they mostly send their clients to selected clinics in Costa Rica. "In order to receive the lowest quotes and discounts you do need to contact us first. If you have already received a quote from a surgeon or dentist we are unable to offer you a lower price." In other words, they are warning you not to comparison shop. So much for the first claim! "When you have come to a decision and a date and have paid your surgical fees or deposit we will make all the arrangements and send you your receipts and your patient information packet with pre-operative instructions, a packing list, phone numbers and everything else you need." This is the most deceptive practice of such referral organizations: they are telling you to send them the money first, before telling you what arrangements they've made. I strongly discourage this sort of program. It is risky and you have no recourse once you've paid up front.

- **MediGoRound** (www.offshorexperts.com) is the website of the curiously named T MediGoRound Medical Tourism Pvt. Ltd, an overseas company that promises a lot but delivers little. You need to send them an email if you want to know more about their referrals, which, in my guess, are to lesser-known hospitals in India, since MediGoRound is based in Gurgaon, a town near New Delhi, India, and has no website of its own.

- **MediTour Asia** (www.meditour.com.sg) is a Singapore operation and not to be confused with another, also apparently "phishing" Internet site, www.meditour.com. Confusing? (Note that the first has the ".sg" extension.) This is typical of Internet scams that try to grab your attention and steer you to their own sites. MediTour Asia is rather evasive about its offerings, and probably is just a referral site to Singapore hospitals. If you want to know more about this "premier medical tourism specialist" you have to send them an email (there is no address). Otherwise, the website is just a bunch of blather about how great they are. The other address, www.meditour.com, is a travel site that has nothing to do with medical tourism.

- **Medorama** (www.medorama.com) is an informative and easy-to-use website, evidently with genuine concern about medical tourists: "We support patients and family members who find themselves at great distances from home, facing new people, new environments and complex medical procedures." This site provides information only on India and Thailand. Some of the international flavor comes across when they state: "we are a dedicated well experienced internationally qualified working in the state of the art hospitals group of doctors in the city of mumbai." I certainly hope their service is better than their grammar!

- **MedRetreat** (www.medretreat.com) is a U.S.-based company facilitating the health-care needs and travel desires of Americans. Their very impressive website promises medical tourism packages loaded with features, but you need to pay up front if you want any actual information. This is done by purchase of a "membership," which costs up to $195 and then allows you limited access to referrals. They also charge for telephone calls and even emails from their doctor! This site sounds like the worst of telephone solicitors and is clearly one to stay away from.

- **MedSolution** (www.medsolution.com) is located in Vancouver, Canada, and focuses on the Canadian market. They send patients to hospitals in France and India.

- **PlanetHospital** (www.planethospital.com) has a flat-rate charge of $200 plus the cost of the procedures for their referrals. In comparison to other websites, PlanetHospital is at least refreshingly honest about their billing. They feature a long list of procedures, but some of them sound a bit odd, and the overall operation evidently does not include any medical expertise. They also don't list the hospitals that they refer to — a warning sign — although my guess is that most of these hospitals are in India and probably reliable.

- **Travelers Digest** (www.travelersdigest.com/medical_tourism.htm) does not provide direct information, but functions as a gateway to other medical tourism referral sites.

- **Directory of the World's Healthiest Spas and Health Resorts** is an ambitious project headed by Joseph Levy of York University in Toronto, Canada. However, nothing had come of it by the time this book was being written. It is a good idea, but my guess is that it will be difficult to find funding for such a large project. The other choice is to accept "fees" from the spas and health facilities, which would undermine the objectivity of the project. If you want to find out how the project is coming along, send an email to Dr. Levy at joelevy@yorku.ca.

When you peruse the Internet for information on medical tourism, be very skeptical about sites that:

- Demand any information up front: they are using your information for "phishing" (selling your information to marketers, or even for the purpose of identity theft)
- Provide no physical address, just an email box
- Have no accredited physician on staff
- Want you to fill out a lengthy form
- Want you to pay any money up front
- Make grandiose or improbable claims
- Are vague about the actual hospitals to whom they refer (they don't want you to contact the hospital directly)

In addition to these Internet sites, there are dozens of websites that appear to involve medical tourism but actually have no relevance to the subject — they are just an attempt to get your attention so they can steer you to their website, which sells real estate, travel packages, and all manner of other commodities. For example, the Internet site www.medicaltrips.com has nothing to do with medical trips! Instead, the site has lengthy offerings of online degrees and such. The same is true of www.medicaltourmalaysia.com, and many others. This is an example of a proliferating activity on the Internet, where websites attract viewers by deceiving them.

Any information that you provide on the Internet, e.g. your name, email address, age, etc., will immediately be sold to others on the Internet and you will soon be deluged with junk email. If you provide your phone number, you may also get lots of calls from telephone solicitors for anything from "surveys" to real estate and investment scams.

Almost all referral sites get kickbacks from the medical tourism facilities to whom they refer. They are making money both from you and from the hospital. That is why they will not tell you the name of the hospital until you have already paid. If you argue with this deceptive practice, they might defend themselves by saying that they do so to prevent you from negotiating with the hospital directly. But they are ignoring the service they should be providing: the arrangement of all travel, accommodations, and other issues. A legitimate site such as PlanetHealth is justified in charging $200 because it is worth it for you to spend that to have them handle all the paperwork. Their service is similar to what a good travel agency provides. Getting a visa to go to India, for example, is a major hassle. In my opinion, it is worth spending a few

If you think you are getting objective information from any source — print, Internet, TV, etc. — ask yourself the time-honored question: Where is their money coming from?

Chances are that your "independent" source is getting some sort of payment in return for a referral. Medical tourism websites are almost entirely funded this way. In other words, their real customer is the hospital — and you are the bait.

---

dollars to save a lot of time and frustration — assuming the service is reliable, of course. A regular travel agency will help you with this, but usually only if you buy the ticket there. Otherwise, there are specialty visa and passport facilitators, but they can be quite expensive. An honest referral agency will help with these tasks, for a modest fee.

Website referral services that hold back information are trying to swindle you. It is as simple as that.

With this book, there is no need for these Internet referral sites. Scams on the Internet will unfortunately always be with us, and I hope this book will help you avoid them.

If you cannot trust the referral websites, how can you arrange a medical tourist trip? The simplest answer is to go straight to the hospital (or clinic, spa, etc.) website and work with them directly. These websites, addresses, phone and fax numbers, and other access information are provided in this book. The hospitals will be happy to answer your questions. In fact, you can usually even talk with the actual surgeon who will be doing your operation. There is no charge for any of this. Many of the larger medical tourism hospitals have international patient coordinators who will also arrange your airfare and accommodations — basically providing all of the services of the better websites, but at no charge. And best of all, if you are dissatisfied, you have an actual hospital and tourism director to whom you can bring your complaint, rather than just a website name. Some of these hospitals will completely refund your payment if you are not satisfied — you will certainly never get *that* from a medical tourism website!

Who Pays For What?

American hospitals are notorious for being deceptive about the true costs of medical care. Most medical referral agencies are not much better. This is partially due to a reluctance to quote a total cost, since you might go to a competitor who provides a lower quote, and partially because they simply do not want to be upfront about their fees. A reputable agent will tell you exactly what you can expect, breaking down the costs for each category: travel, accommodation, surgery, hospital stay, outpatient services, medications, and any additional fees, including expenses related to your care upon your return to the U.S. This is the sort of work they should be paid for, and a reasonable fee for their service is justifiable. Any evasiveness in this regard is a warning sign.

Health insurance rarely pays for medical tourism trips. This appears to be changing, and some major insurance plans are already setting up programs to allow their insureds to choose treatment overseas — after all, the insurance company is saving money, too. However, health insurance providers typically require you to obtain their approval before any benefit is paid, and they are unlikely to approve most of the procedures sought by medical tourists. The bottom line: Expect to pay for the travel and medical costs yourself.

A number of referral agents are now offering to extend credit to medical tourists, particularly if the total sum is large. Be very careful when evaluating these offers — they usually are not financially worthwhile. For example, PlanetHospital has financing available through third-party banks for its patients in the United States, United Kingdom, Australia, and New Zealand, and expects to make this offer soon in Canada. The interest rates are quite high, however — in the range of credit card interest or even those charged by pawn shops and other unscrupulous lenders. Medical tourism agents usually charge 12 to 20 percent interest — *if* you qualify by having good credit. This is far higher than a typical bank consumer loan (often called a "signature" loan), which is easily obtained if you have a decent credit score. A much better option is to get a secured loan, using your car or other property as collateral. The very best way to borrow is against your home. Not only are home loans at the lowest possible interest rate, but you can also deduct the interest paid from your taxes — which is not possible with other types of loans.

If you decide to arrange your own medical tourism trip, make an itemized list of all the anticipated expenses. Medications are typically a substantial item. In fact, it is not unusual for the medication to cost more than the travel. On the other hand, you can sometimes save more on the cost of medication than you have to pay for travel! Pharmaceuticals are almost always cheaper overseas. You should try to determine all

---

S ticker shock in medical care tends to be highest with the medication bill. In the hospital where I work, a single Tylenol tablet can be billed for $2.48. And that's actually trivial when it comes to major antibiotics, which can cost thousands of dollars.

Medications are much less expensive overseas. You are allowed to bring back personal medications with you. Buy a supply of everything you think you might need — including for the future. Your savings could be as much as your airline tickets!

---

possible medications needed and then arrange to get them overseas. Do *not* get them before your trip, or wait until you get back to the U.S. Hospitals overseas will generally include in their total bill all the medications you needed while you were in the hospital. Sometimes, they also include the medications you need as an outpatient. This is never done in the U.S., where medications are invariably billed separately, as is anesthesia, radiology, and just about every other service — right down to the cable TV channels.

The best arrangement is to buy all of your medications from the hospital or clinic where you have your procedure. That way, all medications are coordinated. In addition to the overseas discount, the hospital typically arranges a further discount with the pharmaceutical company, since they are buying in bulk. This saving is passed on to you. In India, several hospital chains are *owned* by the pharmaceutical company, which means an even greater saving on medication. (This could not take place in the U.S. because of anti-trust laws, and discounts given to an in-house pharmacy would run afoul of the Stark regulations, a set of anti-kickback laws).

The greatest concern about cost is the uncertainty of the actual amount of care you will need. Illnesses are not uniform, and people are not machines. When you need a new fuel pump in your car, your mechanic has a pretty good idea of the cost of the pump, the time it takes to install it, and the cost of the overhead for the service. A heart bypass operation is not so simple. Countless variables can result in enormous differences in almost every aspect of the surgery and recovery. This points to one major difference between U.S. and overseas hospitals: U.S. hospitals pass the extra costs on to you, while foreign hospitals are more likely to provide the additional treatment gratis. Because they want you to go away happy, they may even give you extra services free of charge, such as a free face-lift for people who have stomach-reduction surgery. I spoke with an elderly man in Thailand whose heart operation revealed much more serious disease than expected, and he ended up spending an additional three weeks in the hospital. There was no additional charge, despite his extensive intensive-care stays and need for expensive medications. He was so overcome by the thought that he did not deserve this largesse that he calculated the additional amount and gave it to the hospital's charity. He realized that he was already paying far less than he would have in the U.S., and did not think it was right to profit further from no fault of the hospital.

How Do I Determine Quality?

Americans are often told to shop for their healthcare with the same diligence they would use to buy a car or hire a contractor. Many people are beginning to do so. When you consider spending thousands of dollars at a hospital, it is a good practice to do a bit of homework and check on the hospital's quality, problem-solving, and overall patient satisfaction. There are many ways you can do this for U.S. hospitals. You can also go online and get a report of your physician's quality status.

Conventional wisdom about physician expertise generally holds that the longer a physician has been in practice, the better he or she is. But a new study at Harvard Medical School found that physicians who have been in practice longer may, in fact, provide lower quality of care.

It turns out that younger physicians are much more up to date. This is important for medical tourism, because overseas physicians — especially those working at high-end facilities in Singapore, Thailand, and India — tend to be younger and trained in state-of-the-art medicine.

The same ways of evaluating U.S.-based hospitals and physicians can be used overseas. In general, medical tourism facilities tend to be among the best, and their physicians are well qualified. For example, Bangkok's Bumrungrad hospital has more than 200 surgeons who are board-certified in the United States, and one of Singapore's major hospitals is a branch of the prestigious Johns Hopkins University in Baltimore. In a field where experience is as important as technology, Escorts Heart Institute and Research Center in Delhi, India, performs nearly 15,000 heart operations every year, and the death rate among patients during surgery is only 0.8 percent — less than half that of most major hospitals in the United States.

Conventional wisdom about physician expertise generally holds that the longer a physician has been in practice, the better he or she is. But a new study at Harvard Medical School found that physicians who have been in practice longer may, in fact, provide *lower* quality of care.

It turns out that younger physicians are much more up to date. This is important for medical tourism, because overseas physicians — especially those working at high-end facilities in Singapore, Thailand, and India — tend to be younger and trained in state-of-the-art medicine.

However, you are not being treated by a statistic — you will have your procedure done by a single individual. For cosmetic surgery, you might ask your surgeon the following questions:

- *Are you a member of the American Society of Plastic Surgeons (ASPS)?* Founded in 1931, the ASPS, despite its name, has an extensive international membership and is the largest plastic surgery specialty organization in the world. Membership in the ASPS should be expected of a highly qualified cosmetic surgeon. You can verify membership yourself by going to www.plasticsurgery.org. This website will also provide referrals to ASPS member surgeons in the country you are interested in visiting.

The doctors and facilities that do the most of a specific type of surgery also tend to have the best outcomes and fewest complications. For example, the renowned Shouldice Hospital in Toronto, Canada, does only indirect hernia repairs and uses just one procedure. Therefore, their surgeons have each done thousands of hernia operations and are extremely proficient at doing them. The result is that their complication rate is less than one hundredth that of hernia repairs in the United States In fact, it is so low that they provide care for any complications free of charge.

- *Do you have hospital privileges to perform this procedure?* If so, at which hospitals? Each hospital has its own credentialing board. Even if the surgeon operates out of a specialty clinic, being credentialed at one or more prestigious hospitals is a sign of competence.
- *How many procedures of this type have you performed?* As with every skill, the more you do it, the better you are. If you want breast augmentation, for example, it is best to have it done by someone who specializes in this procedure rather than just a general surgeon who does everything.
- *Am I a good candidate for this procedure?* The answer to this question is a bit tricky. Almost every surgeon will assure you that you are a good candidate for minor surgery, but the better ones will ask a lot of questions first. People with diabetes or certain skin, immunologic, or blood disorders should be evaluated very carefully for even the most minor surgery. The response to your question will indicate how thorough and careful the surgeon is.
- *What will be expected of me to get optimal results?* Be careful of surgeons who promise excellent results. The truth is, it is impossible to predict the outcome, and a good surgeon will give a lot of attention to instructing you in how to maximize your results.
- *Where and how will you perform my procedure?* Be careful of the "bait-and-switch" tactic. If the clinic features a highly regarded surgeon, make sure you will not be treated by a junior doctor instead, unless this is pre-arranged.
- *What are the risks involved with my procedure?* Every procedure has risks. You can expect a frank discussion here, and not just blanket reassurance that everything will be OK.
- *How long of a recovery period can I expect, and what kind of help will I need during my recovery?* This topic is particularly important for medical tourists, since they may be halfway across the world while recovering.
- *Will I need to take time off work? If so, how long?* This needs to be well determined, of course, since it will directly affect your travel and activity plans.

- *How are complications handled?* There should be a thorough plan for any foreseeable contingency. Without a plan, the risk of an adverse outcome increases enormously.
- *Is the surgical facility accredited?* There are two major forms of accreditation for healthcare facilities. The first involves general quality assurance. There are countless "quality" certifications that really mean nothing. In my opinion, having a wall full of certificates and awards is a bunch of baloney. In these days, you can get an award for anything. For that matter, you can print them off your computer. The most impressive distinction in general quality is certification by ISO 9001:2000 (in its latest version). ISO is the global standard of quality, based in Geneva, Switzerland. (ISO doesn't actually stand for anything, although many think it means International Standards Organization. The 9001 indicates quality management. You may see other codes, as well, for other services.) To obtain ISO certification, the establishment is reviewed and approved for every detail of its operations, ensuring excellent record-keeping and continual improvement in performance. Many medical tourism facilities, particularly in Asia, now proudly display their ISO 9001:2000 certification.

> ## What Exactly is Meant by "Risk?"
>
> - Very common means about 1 in 10
> - Common means about 1 in 100
> - Uncommon means about 1 in 1,000
> - Rare means about 1 in 10,000
> - Very rare means about 1 in 100,000

The second major type of quality certification applies only to inpatient hospitals: accreditation by Joint Commission International (JCI). This accreditation is difficult and time-consuming to achieve, but indicates a very high degree of quality. Only a few of the most prominent medical institutions around the world can boast of having achieved JCI accreditation. JCI is modeled on the Joint Commission Accreditation for Hospital Organizations (JCAHO, pronounced "Jake-oh"). This is the United States accreditation system for hospitals, and therefore you can be sure that any JCI facility will

---

Medicine As Business. **Every hospital has a mission statement,** usually some lofty goal of service to humanity. One Malaysian medical tourism hospital's mission statement reads: "To provide satisfactory return to shareholders." They certainly don't beat around the bush!

---

be at least the equivalent of U.S. hospitals in quality assurance. JCI accreditation does not come cheap: an already highly regarded hospital might expect to spend an additional $6 million to improve systems in order to satisfy the complex requirements.

In 2003, there were just 17 hospitals in all of Asia with JCI accreditation, out of a total of 57 in the world. Since then, dozens of Asian hospitals have entered the lengthy and rigorous process of applying for accreditation, and each year many more achieve the coveted certificate.

JCI accreditation is suitable only for major medical centers, being limited to in-patient facilities and out of reach for many smaller hospitals. This leaves a gap. With the tremendous growth in health tourism, an internationally recognized standard for clinics and other services would be very helpful. Several attempts have been made, but as of 2008, none has gained significant traction to be generally acknowledged or to draw sufficient attention from facilities. It is the chicken-and-egg dilemma. Overseas clinics see no reason to register with an organization that no one has heard of (or cares about), while any possible accrediting association can only succeed if a large number of clinics become members.

Another approach being floated is the certification of medical tourism providers. Indiana University is planning to offer a 22-credit health tourism certificate through their Department of Tourism, Conventions, and Event Management. (For more information, go to: www.iupui.edu/~indyhper) The director of the program, Sotiris Avgoustis, hopes that it will attract students to the Indianapolis campus to study issues related to medical tourism, such as the development and management of attractions, hospitality and tourism marketing, the tourism system, tourism internship, fundamentals of nutrition, introduction to exercise science, drug use in American society, and personal health. It will be interesting to see how successful it is.

In the meantime, your judgment of the quality of any medical tourism service is likely to be based on their promotional materials and, most importantly, others' personal experiences.

In addition to these questions, you might also ask where the doctor was trained and determine whether there might be a language barrier.

Top 10 Recommended Medical Tourism Centers

Early readers of this book all seemed to have the same comment: "There are an overwhelming number of great places! Can you just tell me which is the best?" I had thought that the country would be a deciding factor, but I was wrong. Many former travel agents jumping into medical tourism make the same error — they look at it as fundamentally a *travel* industry rather than a *healthcare* industry. Some people might decide to go to Thailand, and hey, while they're there, get some discount dental work. While this might have been the norm in the last few decades, the whole medical tourism industry has changed. Now people tend to go for major procedures — procedures that are too costly or otherwise less desirable to have done in the United States — and they are more interested in quality than location. If an advanced (and much less expensive) hip replacement is available in Singapore, so be it ... and where is Singapore anyway? The fact is: they want to be told where to go, and are less concerned about time on the beach.

The less satisfying answer to these questions is that there are now many excellent facilities, and more every year. There are easily two dozen excellent facilities for hip replacement, 200 for cosmetic surgery, and 2,000 for high-quality dental work. But putting the work on to the reader is not the purpose of this book. Therefore, while acknowledging that there are many superb facilities, I will describe a few of the best. By all means, browse through the country-by-country listings in the back of this book, check out the facilities and their websites, maybe call them or send an email. But if you feel overwhelmed by choices and just want a safe, inexpensive, and high-quality facility, you can't go wrong by choosing one of the following. I have visited most of these, and communicated with the senior management of all of them. I give them my personal recommendation, and feel free to contact me if you are disappointed.

Perhaps the most common request of medical tourists is cosmetic surgery. This type of procedure is ideally suited to be combined with travel:

Cosmetic alterations or enhancement are rather more personal than other types of surgery. If you break your arm, you might happily show off your cast and have it autographed. You might not be so happy to have people notice a post-operative facelift or hair transplant. Overseas, you have privacy, and — in places like the The Bodyline Retreat (see *Phuket, Thailand, page 302*) — you can even enjoy a wonderful resort without being self-conscious about looking like an accident victim swathed in post-operative dressings.

Because of many factors described in more detail in the next chapter, cosmetic surgery has advanced further in other countries, with newer and better procedures, and is far less expensive.

Having surgery can be a frightening and lonely experience. Wouldn't you like to be accompanied by your friend, spouse, or family — who can even stay in your hotel-like hospital suite — rather than recover in a bleakly clinical American hospital room? And your companions will surely appreciate the fun of a foreign country more than just watching TV with you.

There was a time when having cosmetic surgery was as denied as hair coloring and disparaged as a tattoo. Now cosmetic surgery is becoming mainstream. Where the sight of tattoos used to cause a lifting of eyebrows, people now are as likely to have eyebrow-lift surgery.

Deciding where to go is the next. But if you try the Internet, you will be swamped with thousands of locations — and probably swayed by who has the best website designer. Furthermore, chosing the facility is the easy part. What about personal counseling, travel arrangements, financing, and all the rest? There are some services that promise to handle all this for you. However, virtually all of them are funded primarily by commissions from the facilities they refer to, which is not necessarily the best facility for you. Instead, I strongly recommend that you contact the facility directly. They will help you with all the travel arrangements, or suggest someone to do this for you, if you prefer.

1. **Bumrungrad Hospital** (see *Bangkok, Thailand, page 289*)

Virtually every article on medical tourism mentions Bumrungrad — it is the global standard to which all other high-end medical tourism facilities are compared. Thailand originated the modern era of medical tourism and continues to feature some of the best facilities. While Bumrungrad seems to capture the headlines, other Bangkok and Phuket hospitals and services are equally impressive — especially BNH and the Bangkok Hospital chain.

Jinemed Medical Center in Istanbul has become a global center for assisted fertility and cosmetic surgery.

2. **Jinemed Medical Centers** (see *Istanbul, Turkey, page 309*)

Turkey is not often considered a center for medical tourism. Yet, its proximity to Europe (and indeed, eventual entry into the European Union) have made the beautiful city of Istanbul an attractive destination for discounted healthcare. Among the best of these is Jinemed — a world-renowned institution providing a wide variety of cosmetic surgery and other procedures, but especially known for infertility treatments and gynecology (www.ivfturkey.com). Jinemed accommodates just about every need related to infertility or gynecology, and has satellite facilities in Cyprus for some types of treatment that are difficult to find elsewhere. According to Ugur Camlibel, International Patient Director, about 80 percent of Jinemed's overseas patients come from the United Kingdom, but an increasing number are from the United States. There have long been close ties between Jinemed and top medical schools in the U.S., with doctors likely trained in both countries and fluent in English.

3. **Barbados Fertility Centre** (see *Barbados, page 139*)

Infertility affects one in six couples. While treatment is increasingly available, it is also horrendously expensive in the U.S., and most medical insurance will pay only part or none of the costs — which can easily run to $60,000, without any guarantee of success. The resulting emotional and financial strain is very demoralizing.

Barbados is a Caribbean island accessible by a short flight from the United States and just an hour ahead of Eastern Standard Time. This delightful tropical island, long a haven for upscale tourism, now is the location of the highly regarded Barbados Fertility Centre (www.barbadosivf.org). As Anna Hosford, the clinic director, explains, the Barbados Fertility Centre provides a unique approach to assisted-fertility procedures by combining treatment with a holiday and stress-reduction program. Many studies have shown that stress has a huge negative impact on both fertility and in vitro fertilization success rates. Perhaps because of its emphasis on stress reduction, the BFC has a very high success rate — in 2005, an astonishing 54 percent of their patients under age 38 achieved pregnancy. For older women, the BFC has consistently higher success rates than the United States.

The BFC, which recently attained JCI accreditation, tailors treatment options to the individual needs of the patient. Most couples arriving from the U.K., U.S., or Canada have already endured failed IVF cycles and looked to BFC as a last chance — and often a successful one. Combining world-class fertility treatment with a holistic approach, the BFC treats couples both mentally and physically, addressing infertility as the priority and using massage, reflexology, acupuncture, and counseling for support. The center's *Healthy Mind/Body* program is one of the contributing reasons for its success. Contact is usually made via telephone or email with an IVF nurse specialist who takes a detailed medical and fertility history from the patient. After this, an appointment is made for a telephone consultation between Dr. Skinner and the patient. Once the most appropriate treatment is decided upon, the couple will be asked to have some blood tests carried out in their home country, with a BFC nurse guiding the couple through the process. With an internationally trained team, the couple can be assured that they will receive the best possible care. Following their arrival on the island, the couple spends 10 days or so enjoying the lovely white sand beaches. Approximately every two days the couple will have scheduled sessions of massage, reflexology, acupuncture, and counseling, enveloping them in an environment that forces them to unwind and relax. The BFC offers a number of all-inclusive packages, including international air and local transportion and all services on the island.

4. Pana-Health (see *Panama, page 255*)

Dental care — particularly high-end cosmetic dentistry procedures — are another major incentive for medical tourists. Few dental insurance plans cover the more costly procedures, and often the payment out of pocket is exorbitant even for those with good dental insurance plans. Dental tourism is perhaps the fastest-growing sector of medical tourism because many dentists are already set up to do this sort of work and just need to roll out the carpet for international patients. Naturally, there is a wide variety of quality — while I was distinctly unimpressed by a highly touted dental clinic in Havana (see *Cuba*), I have been amazed by the sophistication of dental clinics in Thailand, for example, which rival the best in the United States. Pana-Health, in Panama City (see *Panama*), combines dental care with other medical care and offers

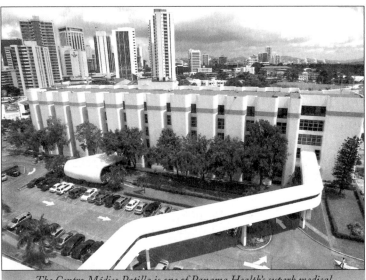

The Centro Médico Patilla is one of Panama Health's superb medical centers oriented to international patients.

a great service to people or families who want different types of healthcare. Having opened in 2003, Pana-Health has more than 100 specialists and is associated with the biggest hospitals in Panama City as well as renowned American centers such as the Cleveland Clinic, Miami Children's Hospital, Tulane University Health Sciences Center Hospital Clinic in New Orleans, Johns Hopkins in Baltimore, Harvard Medical School, and Beth Israel Deaconess Medical Center in Boston. Pana-Health is a personalized medical tourism facilitator, helping patients with all the needs they might require for their medical travel before, during, and after their treatment. Services include information exchange, matching of the appropriate physician(s)/hospitals, arrangement and confirmation of appointments, telephone consultation, travel and visa arrangements, hotel accommodations, expedition of medical information, in-country transportation, communication, pre-treatment (labs, x-rays), hospital pre-admission, post-treatment, hospital discharge, leisure activity arrangements, and after-care follow up. If needed, a personal assistant will accompany the patient every step of the way, to all medical appointments at the hospital and back to the hotel or resort selected by the patient. English-speaking doctors and nurses are available at all times. One of the nice features of Panama is that the country uses the U.S. dollar as its currency and is rated among the safest and most tourist-friendly nations in the world.

5. **Hip Resurfacing Center** (see *Bangalore and Coimbatore, India, page 206 and 211*)

When one of my nurses developed chronic pain from erosive arthritis in his hip, this is where I referred him. There are many superb hip-replacement, and the newer hip-resurfacing procedure, facilities around the world — especially in Asia, where some of the most sophisticated techniques have been pioneered. Entire hospitals are springing up in places like Bangalore, India, just to do hip repairs for international patients. It is an industry of astonishing growth. In the future, it may become as common to travel to India for surgery as it is to get a tan in the Bahamas. I've visited quite a few of the hospitals in Singapore, Thailand, and India, and have yet to find one that does not do top-quality orthopedic surgery — and I'm sure it is the same in many other countries. Given all these possibilities, it may be a bit difficult to choose. I recommend the Hip Resurfacing Center (www.hipresurfacingcenter.com) at Sri Ramakrishna Hospital in Coimbatore, or Columbia Asia in Bangalore, simply because they are good, very inexpensive, and have an excellent track record of satisfied patients. For the money, it is certainly among those offering the best value. The Manipal Hospital in Bangalore also looks to be an excellent value, but its orthopedic facility was still being built when I visited.

6. **PD Hinduja National Hospital & Medical Research Centre** (see *Mumbai, India, page 205*)

India has an amazing number of superb medical facilities — especially Wockhardt Hospital & Heart Institute, Apollo Hospital, Escorts Heart Institute and Research Centre, Fortis Healthcare, and Max Devki Devi Heart & Vascular Institute — all of which are very impressive and easily the equal of the best in the United States. Indeed, most of them are affiliated with major U.S. academic centers, such as PD Hinduja's association with Harvard University.

7. **Health Line India (Eye Surgery in India**) (see *India, page 205*)

For eye surgery, including cataract, glaucoma, LASIK, and many other procedures to improve vision or the appearance of your eyes, Health Line is located in India's capital, New Delhi. If you are not enthused about spending time in the nation's capital

— which is becoming increasingly crowded and polluted — an excellent alternative is the L V Prasad Eye Institute in the city of Hyderabad. At L V Prasad, you also rack up some good karma points since you're fees are going toward providing free eye care for impoverished people.

8. Gleneagles Intan Medical Centre (see *Malaysia, page 239*)

Medical tourism is a booming industry in Malaysia, and no facilities are more active than the Gleneagles medical centers — also located in nearby countries. They have comprehensive medical travel packages that not only offer something for just about everyone, but also provide an astonishing variety of travel and recreational activities.

9. Parkway (see *Singapore, page 269*)

The Parkway Group is one of the leading healthcare groups in Asia. Its subsidiaries include Parkway Group Healthcare, which owns a network of regional hospitals and medical centers in Malaysia, India, and Brunei; and Parkway Hospitals Singapore, which owns three hospitals in Singapore.

This is where presidents, emperors, and sultans from around the world go for treatment. The facilities rank among the best in the world, yet cost about half or less of what you would spend in the United States.

10. Singapore Health Services (see *Singapore, page 270*)

SingHealth, as it is more commonly called, is a vast network that is primarily devoted to the population of Singapore and Indonesia but also welcomes international patients. It has over 400 specialists, many of whom are among the world's best in plastic surgery and burn care. Another excellent Singapore facility is the Raffles International Patients Centre, associated with the landmark Raffles Hotel.

How Do I Prepare For My Trip?

Chapter 3

Putting Together Your "Flight Plan"

For any significant flight, pilots make a flight plan. This includes the details of all the legs of the journey, a list of information and numbers needed, including weather and airport advisories, and alternates for any segment of the trip in case there is a problem. A great deal of research has been done to improve airline safety. The research shows that the single greatest improvement in flying during the past century came down to one thing: checklists. In aviation now, all procedures are tracked by checklists — and the great majority of accidents are attributed to failing to follow these checklists.

Before you set out on your journey, you should make a checklist of every aspect of the trip. Then, for each aspect, you should make further checklists of the details. Finally, you should make a set of "plan B" alternates — and make checklists if necessary for those too. What if the flight is delayed? What if the hotel reservations are wrong, or the hotel is too noisy and uncomfortable? What if you lose your wallet? This sort of planning does two things: it helps you prepare for a possible catastrophe, and it gives you peace of mind if you are not a frequent traveler and have some anxiety about setting off on a long trip.

Charles Lindbergh attributed his successful flight across the Atlantic to his obsession with checklists.

As you are planning your trip, you might think that it is not necessary to write down every little detail of what you need. Most of them are obvious, right? How could you forget them? And yet, in the frenzy and distraction of the moment, it is so easy to lose track of things. I've learned the hard way that checklists are important. Once I flew across the country but forgot my wallet. Another time, I forgot my tickets (back when only paper tickets existed). Yet another time, I brought the wrong attaché case.

I'm embarrassed to admit how many times I've forgotten important paperwork. After a number of these silly errors, I started making checklists and a sort of flight plan for every trip. I discovered that not only does this prevent mistakes, but it helps me relax since I don't have to think about countless details, and I know that everything is under control.

"Getting Sorted"

I love this British phrase. As in, *Ra-iight. Let's get sorted, shall we?* While it is important to be organized and prepared for any travel, it is 10 times more important with a medical tourism trip. After all, in most cases you can pretty much rough it if you find yourself without the usual amenities, but it is no fun when you are having surgery.

There are three components to your preparations:

- Taking care of things at home (mail, pets, children, work, etc.)
- General travel preparations (flights, hotel, etc.)
- Getting ready for your health or medical procedure (list of medications you are on, etc.)

These are three completely different aspects of the trip and should be prepared separately, even if they overlap. If there is paperwork involved, it is a good idea to put the documents together into separate folders for each of these: one can include all your travel documents, with an envelope for receipts (it is a good idea to keep **all** receipts, not just for financial reasons but also because they make nice mementos for scrapbooks and such). Obviously, you do not want your medical record mixed in with your hotel reservations or phone lists and notes for your children with instructions for feeding the pets.

Travel Guides

Most people, especially those who do a lot of traveling, have a routine they go through before setting out on a trip. There are many helpful books, magazine articles, and Internet sites on this subject. They can show you what to take, how to pack, what you can carry aboard an airplane (this is continually changing, so make sure it is up to date), where to change money, and many other details.

For the specific destination, most people like to use a guidebook. It used to be that there were just a couple of choices — such as Fodor's or Thomas Cook — and they only covered the popular cities and countries. Guidebooks have become better and far more diverse over the years. Now they contain a lot of information that even local residents may not know. It is astonishing how many guidebook series there are. Let's Go has over

50 titles. The old stand-by, Michelin, and the newer Rough Guides both have about 200 titles. Frommer's has more than 330 titles at last count, and Lonely Planet has a staggering 650 different books describing 118 countries, with annual sales of $6 million — about one quarter of all English guidebooks sold.

Should you use a guidebook? I used to ignore them — I would rather get suggestions directly from local people than follow the recommendations in a book. However, there is no question that a useful guidebook makes travel and sightseeing less troublesome. But there are pitfalls. First of all, the accommodations and food services listed, especially those that are favored, are more likely to be chosen by fellow travelers who have read the guidebook. With this serendipitous popularity, the recommended hotel or restaurant is often full and may even have to turn people away, and it usually raises prices. Since the place no longer has to struggle for tourists, its hospitality diminishes. That eventually produces poorer service at a higher cost. When you think about it, it makes sense. Let's say a town has a dozen hotels. No guidebook, no matter how detailed, can list every hotel in every village, town, and city in the country — it would have to be the size of a phonebook. So the writer of the guidebook usually chooses a typical one in the town and lets it go at that. Major cities with thousands of hotels might have a couple of dozen listed. Now, these hotels probably all had rates that were roughly similar for their location, features, and other appeal. The staff was very hospitable in order to hang onto their customers and get positive word-of-mouth references — which are the best kind of advertising. In fact, the original Lonely Planet and other guides grew out of this word-of-mouth — a practice now continued in online discussion groups and blogs. But once a hotel is published in a guidebook — and recommended — it becomes the first one selected by the book's readers.

One Reason Your Guidebook May Not Be Complete . . .

I was traveling in France a few years ago. It was the time of the nouveau Beaujolais, a delightful late-harvest wine that is not nearly as good from a bottle as it is fresh from a carafe just days after it was made. Naturally, I relied on my guidebook to find inexpensive accommodations. The guidebook listed just one hotel for the small town I was in, although a few other hotels were nearby and looked about the same. How, I wondered, did the guidebook happen to choose to report this one? Since the listed one was full, I went to another one across the street, which turned out to be wonderful. I asked the owner why it was not in the guidebook. She retorted that representatives from various guidebooks came around every year or so, but they demanded 1,000 Euros to be included, and she refused to pay. "Surely not this one!" I said, holding up my favored guidebook — one with a reputation of fairness and honesty. She gave me a withering look. "They were here last month," she said. "Yes, they were nicer — they only asked for 600 Euros, plus a complimentary room and dinner."

Consequently, it gets the bookings. It becomes popular. If it has to turn people away, there is a strong temptation to increase room prices. I've found that prices are almost always higher by 20 percent or more than the book says. Service quality also tends to deteriorate as the place gets busy and staff get stressed or lose an incentive to attract customers. Amenities can be dropped since business is already good enough, so there is no need for costly or time-consuming extras. Meanwhile, nearby hotels that were not listed in the guide may be just as good, but they have to keep their usual prices and services, still working as hard — or harder — to attract customers as they did before.

How does a guidebook choose which hotel to feature? It is obviously impossible for the writer to stay in every hotel in a country. Even a quick visit to all of them could take years. The truth is that every guidebook has its own bias, and some of these inevitably come from financial kickbacks or other favors.

Cell Phone Coverage

Cell phone services are changing constantly. There are different international systems, and your phone may or may not work in a particular country. Even when a cell phone service promises coverage in a country, it may only be in selected areas, or at outrageous costs, such as $4 per minute. I learned the hard way about this when T-Mobile promised coverage in the Philippines and then charged me $261 for a few short calls I made. If I had done my homework, I would have bought a $2 phone card there good for dozens of calls. Phone cards are cheap and exist in every country. Unless you are sure that your service allows calls at reasonable rates, you should get a phone card. Even then, you have to be careful to avoid sneaky "roaming" charges. Sometimes it is better, safer, and cheaper just to buy a local throw-away cell phone with precharged minutes.

Skype is even cheaper than phone cards. This is a way of making calls through the Internet, referred to as voice over Internet protocol (VoIP). You simply open an account for $12, buy an Internet phone, plug it into your computer, and you can call just about everyone for 3 cents a minute. If the person you are calling also has Skype, the call is free! There are many other VoIP services, some of which offer more features but are also are more expensive. Some people say the quality on the Internet is not as good as by regular telephone. However, the phone cards use the Internet for their service, so the quality should be the same. In the countries section of this book, you will occasionally see that clinics and doctors list their Skype numbers so that you can call them for free.

You should also consider a webcam — a camera on your laptop computer — to see as well as speak to the person you are calling. This makes a big difference when a family member is going through surgery overseas.

Necessary Documents

All overseas travel requires a passport. If you don't have one, you should arrange this as soon as possible since the process can take longer than expected, and you cannot apply for a visa until you have the passport. Passports are generally valid for 10 years. Make sure that yours has not expired or is near the expiration. Most countries require passports to be valid for at least another six months before entry is allowed.

With an American passport, visas are generally not required for countries promoting tourism. An exception is India, which recently has become exceedingly onerous in its visa requirements (see *India, page 200*).

If you simply do not have the time or the patience to get a passport or other necessary documents, you can use a passport service for this. There are many such services around the country, and they can easily be found in the telephone yellow pages or on the Internet. A typical charge might be $50 (in addition to the passport fee) for an expedited passport. Rates go up for even faster service — as quickly as two days with FedEx overnight delivery. These services can also get a visa for you much more easily than you can do so yourself. Visa forms can be maddeningly complicated, incoherent, and slow to complete. If you don't do it exactly right, you'll get a rejection letter — perhaps more than a month later! That can put you into a panic when your trip is booked and paid for and the departure date is getting close. A benefit of visa services is that they know exactly what needs to be done and can get it done quickly. Services often specialize in certain countries, so make sure that the service is expert for the visa you need.

Some countries require vaccinations for infectious diseases. If so, you can get the necessary vaccination at a travel clinic, university hospital, or county public health clinic. You will be given a yellow booklet with a list of your vaccinations.

It is very useful to make two photocopies of all of your important documents, and a few extra passport-type pictures. Keep these in separate locations. It will make it far easier if you ever lose your documents. I also recommend taking a few dozen one-dollar bills. The American $1 note is the closest thing to a truly international currency — virtually everyone recognizes it and will accept it. You can use them for almost anything, from last-minute fees to tips to payments for little favors.

Passport and visa requirements are generally the same for Canadians. A notable exception is Cuba, which Canadians can visit easily, whereas Americans are technically breaking U.S. laws if they go there. I hope this half-century holdover from Cold-War politics will soon change.

Traveling with a Medical Condition

Traveling with an illness or infirmity can add complications. Increasingly, worries about transmittable diseases have resulted in airlines and immigration services being rather paranoid about travelers who appear ill. In the Philippines and some other countries, the airport departure areas have not only the usual x-ray control but also a body-temperature control: a sensor detects your body temperature and alarms the guards if you have a fever. If so, they can quarantine you for a week or more, and there is little you can do about it.

For any medical condition, I strongly recommend that you have prescriptions for all medications in your possession and perhaps a letter from your doctor stating your fitness to travel.

If you bring any medical equipment with you, especially aboard the aircraft, be sure to have a prescription or letter stating that you need this. Remember also that most other countries use 220 voltage rather than the U.S. 120 voltage outlets. This is the same as your oven or clothes dryer, and it packs quite a punch. The outlets used may also have a different configuration. It is helpful to find out what sort of outlets are used, and get a converter. Inexpensive converter kits have a collection of adapters and a list that shows which one is needed for a country. I also find it very helpful to bring an extension cord with multiple outlets, since outlets don't seem to be as common overseas.

Long flights can cause blood clots to form in the legs. If these clots break off and travel to the heart or lungs, you can have a serious problem. The risk is much higher after surgery. You should not fly until five to seven days after body surface procedures such as liposuction and breast augmentation; seven to 10 days after cosmetic procedures of the face including facelifts, eyelid surgery, nose jobs, and laser treatments; and sometimes even longer after deep surgery such as stomach reduction or heart operations. Your surgeon will tell you when it is safe to fly.

Avoiding Blood Clots on Long Flights

When I was working at the emergency department of Queen's Hospital in Honolulu, hardly a day went by without a newly arrived visitor with symptoms of blood clots. This is understandable, given that the shortest flight to Hawaii takes more than five hours, and others range up to 11 hours in duration. That's a long time to be sitting in a cramped seat.

The best way to avoid blood clots is to get up and walk every half hour or so (this is obviously much easier with an aisle seat). Do some squats and knee lifts. It is also helpful to wear compression stockings, which are now becoming more available as "travel stockings." And remember to drink a lot of water — dehydration contributes to blood clots.

Travel Insurance

Travel insurance involves both property and medical insurance to cover theft, injury, and illness while you are traveling outside of the country. It also provides trip insurance in case you get stranded. Your homeowner's or rental insurance may cover property loss while you are traveling. Travel medical insurance, which can be for as little as five days or as long as 12 months, is not the same as health insurance. If you have health insurance, it probably covers some emergency medical expenses overseas, but this is highly variable.

Why would you want travel medical insurance? The major reason is to fill in the gaps in your regular medical insurance. Read your medical insurance policy carefully. Often, there are geographic boundaries and exclusions based on activities, purpose of travel, or injuries sustained in political conflicts, etc. The exclusion of "participation in hazardous sports" is especially noteworthy. It really means just about any sport whatsoever, including skiing and bike riding! It also excludes any travel to participate in athletic events, no matter what sport is involved, so you will not be covered even if you are going to a bowling, badminton, or billiards competition. There may also be substantial deductibles and copays. Finally, there are typically limits to reimbursement for care — and if you need more expensive care, you will have to pay the difference.

However, any of these exclusions may also exist on the travel insurance, so it is important to read the policy carefully before purchasing.

A peculiar variant of travel medical insurance is provided by American Express to its Business Card holders. On the surface, the Travel Medical Protection program looks like a typical type of travel insurance: for an additional monthly premium ranging from $5.50 to $23.00 (in 2007), you have up to $100,000 in coverage. The program covers unexpected emergency medical or dental treatment expenses when you travel more than 150 miles from home anywhere in the world, for the first 45 days of your trip. Unlike traditional health insurance, it pays the benefits directly to the provider and carries no deductibles. The stated program also pays for emergency prescriptions and even a round trip for a visitor from home.

This sort of program seems rather open to abuse. How is it possible to clearly define "unexpected and emergency?" Let's say your arthritic hip has been bugging you for a while. When you happen to be visiting Bangalore, India, you slip on a cow patty in the street and fall over, hurting your hip badly. By remarkable convenience, you are near the Columbia Asia Medical Center, a premier institution in the world for hip resurfacing! You undergo the procedure — which is in some ways superior to a total hip replacement — and your hip problem is solved. Could you ask your Travel Medical Protection to pay for it? The plan excludes conditions that you have developed, or been treated for, within the 60 days prior to your trip. But that allows huge loopholes for exacerbations of earlier conditions, or long-standing chronic conditions. What if you need dental crowns, which you've been putting off for years? So much of pain and disability is subjective that it would seem difficult for the insurer to deny the coverage for your "unexpected and emergency" treatment.

Don't Skip Your Procedural Homework

If you are planning to have a medical procedure or other health treatment, you should be very clear about what it is that you are doing. I've talked to dozens of people who found themselves in Koh Samui, Thailand, and decided, on the spot, to get liposuction or dental work. They didn't appear to suffer terribly from their lack of preparation, but it seems like a risky way to go. A dozen things could have gone wrong, and the outcome could have been terrible or very costly. When you prepare for surgery, you don't want to depend on luck.

Proper arrangements for any kind of medical tourism should include:

A summary of your medical record. In these days of litigation, you practically have to beg and plead with your doctors to see your medical record, even though they must show it to you by law. As if to add further insult, many clinics will only show it to you briefly at the counter — hardly a place where you can go through a thick binder with sometimes hundreds of pages of information you barely understand. If you want a copy, you must submit a requisition, and you might be charged $3 or $4 per page for it. This sort of practice is unethical and frankly disgusting, in my opinion. A decent physician will prepare a proper summary for you, free of charge. At the minimum, you should describe your health problems and history on a sheet of paper and list any medications that you are on, as well as any bad reactions you have had from previous medications. Note that I don't say "medications that you are *allergic* to." This is a widely misunderstood term in medicine and has led to endless problems. Most of the time, a bad medication reaction is not a true allergy. That is why it is important to say what happened instead of "penicillin allergy," which can mean anything from stomachache to skin rash to full-blown shock.

Discuss your procedure with the overseas doctor who is going to do it, or at least have a pretty clear sense of who is doing it and what it will involve.

Review the sort of activities you have planned, and consider whether they fit in with your medical procedure. Even herbal treatments or acupuncture should not be combined with certain activities. And many medications are incompatible with alcohol or sun exposure.

Try to set out a schedule of anticipated appointments, hospital stays, nursing visits, or treatments at a spa, if that is the case. As much as possible, get names, addresses, and phone numbers of doctors and clinics or hospitals. These should be available at the facility's website, so you can just print it off.

There are many other items to consider depending on the specific procedure you're having done. For example, before you make arrangements for cosmetic surgery, you should do a little research on the procedure, along with its benefits and risks. With the Internet, this has become very easy. For the latest information on plastic surgery procedures, go to www.plasticsurgery.org

It is important to have realistic expectations. Don't be shy about asking questions. Medical tourism doctors tend to be very approachable and helpful. American doctors, in contrast, often subtly discourage questions. It is not that they are bad doctors; it is just the system in which they are forced to work. Questions rarely have a simple yes or no answer, and can involve a long discussion that often has to do more with reassurance and other psychosocial issues than factual information. In other words, it takes a huge amount of time — time that the U.S. doctor doesn't get paid for. So doctors tend to get impatient with patients who are "high maintenance" or "demanding." It is not entirely the doctors' fault, since the healthcare system makes it that way by rewarding doctors who are less personable. Next time you are blown off by a doctor, imagine how much advice you would get from a lawyer who was off the clock.

You should know what you can expect, especially for the recovery time and any possible side effects. One way to do this is to talk to patients who have had your procedure, gone to the same place, or were treated by the same doctor.

Medical Insurance

Many people who participate in medical tourism do so because they do not have medical insurance. It is a no-brainer: why pay the exorbitant costs of U.S. healthcare when you can have far cheaper and often more enjoyable care overseas?

As of 2007, 49 million Americans have no health insurance, and another 95 million are insured during only part of the year. Despite government hand-wringing and continual promises, the situation has only become worse every year. Until there is some sort of national health insurance (which is unlikely to happen, in my opinion), the number of uninsured will continue to climb. This failure is a major stimulus for medical tourism.

But having medical insurance does not solve the problems of access to healthcare. Before the insurance company will reimburse you for any procedure, the procedure must first be approved by the insurance company (unless it is an emergency). The decision is usually made not by a doctor but by an administrative clerk who refers to a list of conditions and knows little about the actual condition of the patient. Consequently, insurance plans routinely deny payment for a huge proportion of medical procedures. For example, a major study published in the New England Journal of Medicine looked at women with breast cancer who needed a bone marrow transplant. This is a very expensive procedure, and insurance companies are therefore reluctant to pay for it. Of the 533 instances of women who medically needed the treatment, only 77 percent were approved by their insurance. Some had to get a lawyer to sue the insurance company before their treatment was approved. The others had to pay for the treatment themselves. An estimated 60 to 80 percent of procedures recommended by doctors are denied coverage because the insurance administrator decides that they are not "medically necessary." Of those who are approved, insurance companies routinely refuse to pay an average of 15 percent, and as high as 50 percent, of the resulting reimbursement claims.

Even those *with* insurance may find medical tourism to be a bargain. This is because the cost of the annual deductible (typically $500, but ranging up to $2,500 or more) and copay (typically 20 percent) adds up to more than the cost of a trip and treatment overseas. Healthcare statistics show that patients pay, on average, about 30 percent of the total costs of surgical procedures covered by their insurance. The same procedure in Thailand would cost about one fifth as much, and in India, as little as one tenth as much. For example, say you need a hip replacement and luckily have health insurance that pays for it. After you've met the deductible, various copays and uncovered items on the $53,000 total bill, you are out of pocket about $15,000. But the total cost of the procedure in India, the flights, and a great vacation at a resort might add up to only $10,000. So you have saved $5,000 even though you — rather than the insurance company — paid for your procedure.

Canadian Health Insurance

Canadians have universal healthcare, but at the cost of sometimes lengthy delays for elective procedures. The government is sensitive to these complaints and more likely to approve reimbursement for healthcare obtained overseas. After all, the government may actually be saving money by this practice. In the United Kingdom, where the problem is even greater, the National Health Service actively encourages patients to get surgery overseas, even offering to pay their trips and expenses.

In order to be assured of full reimbursement, Canadians should obtain approval from the Ministry of Health beforehand. To obtain pre-approval for payment of out-of-country services, the attending medical specialist must submit either a written request or an Application for Approval of Insured Out of Country Medical Services, providing detailed information about the medical necessity for the referral and what options available within Canada have been investigated, in order to show that out-of-country medical care is necessary.

Health Saving Accounts

A new type of health insurance is starting to become available in the United States. The Health Saving Account (HSA) is an industry-based program in which the employer and patient pay into an account that can then be used for healthcare — *at the employee's discretion*. The big difference is that the employee can choose whether or not to spend the money in the account, and how to spend it. Employers like the concept because it costs less than traditional insurance. Employees like it because it gives them control over their health expenses, the account is tax-deductible, and it can be used for a great variety of healthcare not covered by standard health insurance.

The big question is: can you use your HSA to pay for overseas care? Because medical tourism is such a new phenomenon, the government has not yet addressed this issue. Instead, you have to carefully examine the list of qualified and disqualified expenses to see where medical tourism costs might fit in.

The following list, complete with spelling and grammatical errors, is taken from IRS Publication 502 - Qualified Medical and Dental Expenses:

Qualified Expenses

Acupuncture
Alcoholism treatment
Ambulance transportation
Autoette or Wheelchair
Birth-control pills
Blind persons services
Braces
Capital expenditures - home modifications for handicapped, primary purpose
    must be medical care
Car equipment - to accommodate wheelchair or handicapped controls
Childbirth preparation classes – mother
Chiropractors
Christian science treatment
Contact lenses
Crutches
Deaf persons - hearing aid and batteries, hearing aid animal and care, lip reading
    expenses, special education, modified telephone
Dental fees
Dentures
Diagnostic fees
Diapers (adult disposable) - used due to severe neurological disease
Doctor's fees
Domestic aid - rendered by nurse
Drug addiction Recovery
Drugs - prescription or over-the-counter

Dyslexia language training
Elevator for alleviation of cardiac condition
Eyeglasses and examination Fees
Fluoride device - on advice of dentist
Halfway house - adjustment to mental hospital
Healing services Fees
Health maintenance organization
Hearing aids
Hospital care
Insulin
Laboratory fees
Laetrile - by prescription
Lead paint removal
Lazer [sic] eye surgery
Lodging (treatment related, and with restrictions, up to $50 per person)
Medical conference fees (relating to chronic illness; no lodging or meals)
Medicare parts A and B
Legal expenses - authorizing treatment of mental illness
Lifetime medical care - prepaid; retirement home
Limbs - artificial
Mattress - prescribed for alleviation of arthritis
Membership fees - association furnishing medical services, hospitalization,
    clinical care
Nursing home - medical reasons
Nursing services - board and Social Security paid by taxpayers
Obstetrical expenses
Operations - legal
Optometrists
Orthodontia
Orthopedic shoes - excess costs
Oxygen / oxygen equipment
Prosthesis
Psychiatric care
Psychologists
Psychotherapists
Reclining chair - for cardiac patients
Remedial reading
Retarded person - costs for special home
Retirement home - lifetime medical care
Sanitarium rest home - medical, educational, rehabilitative services

Schools - special, relief, or handicapped
Sexual dysfunction treatment
Sterilization
Surgical fees
Swimming pool - treatment of polio or arthritis
Teeth - artificial
Television - closed-caption decoder
Therapy treatments - prescribed by a physician
Transportation - essentially and primarily for medical care
Weight-loss programs - as a treatment for the disease of obesity
X-rays
Mileage
Stop-smoking programs
Vasectomy
Vision correction

HSA Non-Qualified Expenses

Payment for services to be rendered next year
Athletic club membership
Automobile insurance premium allocable to medical coverage
Boarding school fees
Bottled water
Commuting expenses of a disabled person
Cosmetic surgery and procedures
Cosmetics, hygiene products and similar items
Diaper service
Domestic help
Health programs offered by resort hotels, health clubs, and gyms
Illegal operations and treatments
Illegally procured drugs
Maternity clothes
Premiums for life insurance, income protection, disability, loss of limbs, sight or
    similar benefits
Scientology counseling
Social activities
Special foods or beverages
Specially designed car for the handicapped other than an autoette or special
    equipment
Swimming pool

Travel for general health improvement
Tuition and travel expenses for a problem child to a particular school
Weight loss programs (subject to change under new IRS guidelines)

Note that qualified expenses include just about all aspects of medical tourism, and also "Transportation - essentially and primarily for medical care" — which implies that you can pay for your flight to Thailand with funds taken from your HSA account! Oddly, qualified expenses also include Laetrile treatment. Clearly, this is an example of a political lobby trumping medical science.

Notable exclusions include "Cosmetic surgery and procedures." This is a big gray area in medicine. When is a surgery "reconstructive" and when is it "cosmetic?" If you break your nose in an accident, surgery to fix the altered nose is reconstructive, but if you were born with a misshapen nose, the surgery is cosmetic — unless you have trouble breathing through your misshapen nose, in which case it is reconstructive. As you can see, there is a lot of judgment involved here. You and your surgeon may insist it is reconstructive procedure while the insurance may deny it as cosmetic. The outcome depends on many factors, including who is more clever and persuasive.

The bottom line is that HSAs are a tremendous boon to medical tourism by allowing employees to use healthcare funds as they see fit — whether at home or overseas. The increase in HSAs is likely to be followed by a great increase in medical tourism.

Borrowing Money

The United States is the country of credit. If Americans truly lived within their means, the economy would fall apart. Borrowing is the way to go when buying a house, a car, an education, and — increasingly — healthcare. With the high cost of specialty procedures, especially cosmetic or dental surgery, a number of lenders have popped up to provide loans for medical care at far better rates than credit card financing. Capital One healthcare finance (www.capitalonehealthcarefinance.com), for example, can provide approval in minutes for up to $25,000 loans.

Who Will Take Care of Me When I Return?

Concern about follow-up care is the major limitation of medical tourism. Those who lack insurance are the most likely to travel for care — and yet they are also the least likely to have a regular physician at home for follow-up. Others find that they are discriminated against or charged excessively for services. Some surgeons have refused to provide follow-up care for patients who had their surgery overseas. Others actively discourage people from medical tourism by threats of not treating them afterward, saying they would be liable for an overseas doctor's malpractice.

Follow-up care and monitoring is an important part of any surgery. Patients who have traveled outside the United States for cosmetic surgery and experienced a complication may find it hard to locate a qualified plastic surgeon to treat the problem or to provide revision surgeries. Local doctors may not know what surgical techniques the physician used in the initial operation, making treatment difficult or nearly impossible. Revision surgeries can be more complicated than the initial operation, and patients rarely get the desired results. Some return to the overseas facility for follow-up, but this is costly. Others try to stay as long as possible in the country after their surgery, since problems generally show up within a few days of the surgery.

MediCruiser

An innovative organization in the United States is planning to build a network of clinics specifically designed to facilitate medical tourism. In these clinics, highly qualified specialist physicians do pre-screening, give advice, and otherwise help guide a person seeking treatment overseas. The medical tourists are even placed in televideo-consultation with the overseas doctors and international patient offices. Upon their return, these patients are offered comprehensive and coordinated follow-up care, both locally and by consultation with the overseas physicians. MediCruiser is perhaps the most innovative and advanced health clinic yet devised, and appears to suit its tag line: "21st Century healthcare."

At the time of this writing, MediCruiser (www.medicruiser.com) is still in the formative stages. There is little doubt that MediCruiser would tremendously increase access to medical tourism, increase quality assurance, confidence and reliability, and play a major role in its expansion.

How Do I Handle Problems?

Countless problems can occur with any kind of trip. In medical tourism, however, most problems seem to involve just two: travel scams and poor medical treatment. The first is characteristic of most kinds of arranged travel. It matters more when you are going for medical treatment because there is more on the line. If you are just going for a vacation, you can always leave and go to an alternate location if things don't work out. But once you have arranged for a medical procedure and arrived, it is too late to choose an alternate. Moreover, you may not be feeling well, or you may simply have invested too much effort and money. Therefore, you should take care when you make your plans, and the best thing you can do is to talk to the surgeon or other care-givers *before* you put down any money and book your flight. This is a major reason why I discourage the use of Internet medical travel referral agencies — their assurances of quality are worth as much as the chance you'll get your money back if you are unsatisfied — basically zero.

> *Some of the work we've seen* that people have had done at bargain-basement prices is so substandard it can't be fixed."
>
> ~ Dr. Moelleken, a Beverly Hills plastic and reconstructive surgeon

The second kind of problem is even more worrisome. The possibility of a botched procedure frightens many people away from medical tourism. Here, again, it is important to contact the facility directly and get a sense of quality. If you are going to a prominent hospital or high-end clinic, your chances of a bad outcome are no different from in the U.S. That is not to say that it won't happen. According to U.S. statistics, about one in three stomach-reduction surgeries are followed by significant problems. The worst cases may require repeat surgery.

So, what can you do if a problem arises?

If it is a travel problem, you have better recourse if you made the arrangements yourself, especially if you use major airlines or hotels. They are eager to solve any difficulties. Major hotels also have concierge services that will help you with just about

A Real "Boob Job"

Toni Wildish, a former model, decided at age 28 to undergo breast enlargement. Working part-time in a shop, she could not afford the surgery. Then she discovered CTS Cosmetics, an Internet referral agency that promised much cheaper surgery in the Czech Republic. She flew to Prague for surgery, happy to combine her procedure with a holiday in the beautiful city. When she arrived at the clinic, she was dismayed to see that it was a dental clinic and that the surgeon spoke no English. Having paid her money, she went ahead with her plans. After the surgery, she had agonizing pain at the location of her new breast implants. Through an interpreter, the surgeon told her the pain was "completely normal."

Toni flew home, unable to enjoy her holiday. When the pain did not subside and she began bleeding, she went to a hospital, where she was diagnosed with septicemia — a potentially fatal infection from the surgery. Moreover, one of her breasts was a 32B and the other a 32E. She contacted a lawyer to sue the surgeon. "I feel like a freak — I've been left disfigured," she complained. The lawyer explained that it would be virtually impossible to sue the surgeon since the procedure had taken place abroad.

As for the referral agency, CTS Cosmetics? Their spokesman refused to give her any refund, but said, "As a gesture of goodwill, but without admission of liability," they would pay for a repeat surgery in the Czech Republic — with the same surgeon! Not surprisingly, she declined.

every issue. Medical tourism hospitals also often provide concierge services for the patient — someone to take you to your appointments, and even a personal nurse.

A reputable overseas hospital will go to great lengths to resolve any medical problem. In fact, they go much further than American hospitals. Medical tourism facilities generally treat any complications free of charge — even if they are not at fault.

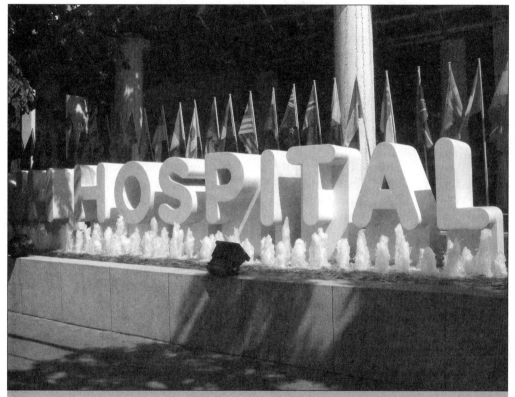

Medical tourism is rapidly becoming a major industry in Thailand. The flags accompanying this sign outside Bangkok's BNH hospital signal a welcome to patients from dozens of countries.

Chapter 4

Will Medical Tourism Solve America's Healthcare Crisis?

Medical tourism is fundamentally driven by the failure of the American healthcare system. If you have read this far, you already know all about medical tourism (in fact, more than almost all doctors, healthcare administrators, and politicians). This chapter is not about medical tourism in itself, but about its underlying causes and the effect it will have on U.S. healthcare. Do not read it if you are prone to depression, as it may make you feel discouraged, frightened, or outraged — and most of all, helpless. There is little you can do by yourself to change U.S. healthcare. But now, at least, you have an option not to participate in it: you can go elsewhere. When enough people do that, the healthcare system will change.

The American Medical Crisis

General Dwight D. Eisenhower was one of the greatest and most beloved presidents in American history. A hero in the Second World War, he presided over the build-up of the United States into the world's greatest military power. But the wise General also knew that the defense industry itself needed to be controlled.

On January 17, 1961, he gave the last speech of his presidency. "My fellow Americans," he began. "Three days from now, after half a century in the service of our country, I shall lay down the responsibilities of office." He went on to talk about the might of the United States as the new safeguard of world freedom. And then he described what has come to be known as one of the most astute warnings to the country:

"[The] conjunction of an immense military establishment and a large arms industry is new in the American experience. The total influence — economic, political, even spiritual — is felt in every city, every State house, every office of the Federal government. ... we must not fail to comprehend its grave implications. ... we must guard against the acquisition of unwarranted influence, whether sought or unsought, by the military industrial complex. The potential for the disastrous rise of misplaced power exists and will persist."

In short, this is what he said: The military industry is growing so large that it is almost out of control. If we are not careful to limit its power, this military-industrial complex is going to cripple us.

Forty-five years later, we are facing the same threat with the power of the medical establishment, except that the crippling of the American populace is already well underway. We now spend more than twice as much for medical care as any other industrial country — more than $14,000 per person per year, with the total rising faster than any other sector of the economy. And what do we get for that? In health terms, out of all industrialized nations, we are dead last. Some sectors of our citizenry have worse health and a lower life expectancy than many third-world countries. We are spending more and more to get less and less.

Just as the role of the military is to protect us from enemies, the role of the healthcare system is to protect us from illness. Both have the potential to get out of hand; therefore both must be limited in their power.

When Arnold Relman served as Editor of the prestigious *New England Journal of Medicine*, he wrote: "Increasingly, Wall Street and the interests of shareholders have replaced Main Street in shaping the organization of healthcare, the market, and even clinical decisions." He went on to describe how the American medical system had become so intertwined with profit-oriented industry that it had become a monster, gobbling up and putting out of business non-profit hospitals. This "medical-industrial complex," he warned, will cripple healthcare services and impoverish the population who are forced to use its services.

There is no question that his frightening scenario has turned out to be true.

Healthcare was once a mix of private practitioners and government-supported care (which still continues in the highly efficient Veterans' Administration hospitals), but it has now been replaced by ever larger and more profitable corporations whose only goal is profit. These medical corporations are *so* powerful, in fact, that they can hobble any attempt by the government to restrain them.

The brunt of this is borne by the patients — the general population that needs care, no matter what. In economic terms, healthcare is inelastic — the demand does not go down when prices go up. A person with a worn-out hip or an eye cataract simply has to pay the higher price or continue suffering. So these companies keep raising the price — healthcare costs have increased far beyond the consumer price index for almost every year of the past few decades — and profits follow. Meanwhile, the cost of this care is eating up an increasing share of the household budget, and now is the number one cause of personal bankruptcy. A health plan covering a family of four cost about $14,500 in 2006. One in three Americans has health insurance for only part of the year, and one in six has no insurance whatsoever. In 2003, uninsured people paid $230 billion out of pocket.

Even for those *with* health insurance, medical costs have become excessive. A recent survey by the Employee Benefit Research Institute of insured employees found that many are being forced to make sacrifices to meet their healthcare costs. Nearly a quarter said paying for healthcare made it difficult to meet other basic expenses such as food, heat and housing — 26 percent lowered their contributions to a retirement plan, and 45 percent put less money into savings. In order to cut medical expenses, more than one in five respondents said they didn't take prescribed medications, while 40 percent delayed doctor visits.

A 2005 survey by the Commonwealth Fund in 2005 showed that 34 percent of adults aged 19 to 64 had medical debt or problems paying their bills — even though 62 percent of them had health insurance! The hospitals pad their bills exorbitantly and justify the practice by saying that insurers are underpaying them. So they simply pass on the costs to the patients. For example, insurance normally does not pay for photocopying medical records. How much does a photocopy cost? Most copy centers charge about six to eight cents a page. Any decent clinic or hospital will have a powerful photocopy machine of their own, which would cost them maybe a penny a page, and they could add another penny for the few minutes it takes to copy a 100-page record (they should really be able to print it off on the computer without needing a photocopier, but many are so out of date that they still use paper medical records). By any reason, a copy of a medical record should cost no more than about $10. But when Loretta Dawson needed a photocopy of her husband's medical record at California Pacific Medical Center in 2007, the hospital billed her $1,030. And with the bill came a letter soliciting a donation to the hospital's foundation! The Commonwealth report stated that 26 percent of those with insurance nonetheless had to go into credit card debt to pay their medical bills, and another 11 percent had to take out a home mortgage.

The Impact of Healthcare Costs on Household Budgets

		Household Income		
	Total	Below $35,000	$35,000 – 74,999	$75,000+
Decreased savings	45%	52%	41%	38%
Have difficulty paying bills	34%	51%	25%	18%
Used up all or most of savings	29%	45%	21%	8%
Decreased retirement funds	26%	27%	32%	17%
Difficulty paying for basic needs	24%	38%	15%	7%
Had to borrow money	8%	29%	13%	6%

The changes have not been kind to doctors, either. In the past, most physicians were in private practice. Now, almost all new medical school graduates become employees of large firms, or join a group practice. They have lost the autonomy traditionally enjoyed by physicians, and especially the ability to give the best care for their patients without being ordered around by non-medical people. Many are so disgusted that they have quit medicine for another profession, and one of every two physicians has considering giving up practice. It is so bad that, in a 2003 survey by the American Medical Association, *70 percent* of doctors said they would not recommend a medical career to their children.

Some doctors opt out. They try to go back to a cash-based system, and some even do house calls. The medical establishment strikes back at these doctors by shutting them out of hospitals and other health networks, crippling their practice. Therefore, the few doctors who can make a decent living outside of the system are limited to those who do "concierge" medicine — charging a rather high fee for their private patients. This is great if you can afford it. Unfortunately, it does not, and will never, meet the needs of the majority of the population.

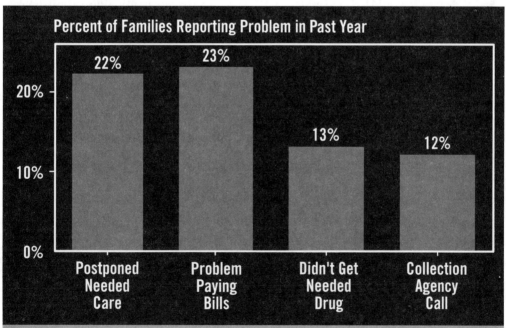

Medical costs are a major hardship for Americans — and becoming more excessive each year. This figure, from the Institute of the Future's Health and healthcare 2010, is a low estimate based on 2000 data. Healthcare is now the greatest cause of personal bankruptcy.

For-Profit Hospitals Take Over

Until recently, most hospitals in the United States were charitable institutions, supported by churches, or other non-profit facilities that charged only enough to keep the operation going. That began to change when investors saw the money-making potential of healthcare. They began to buy up community hospitals. Since these hospitals were non-profit or were actually losing money, the communities were happy to sell them. This was the result:

Community hospitals serve everyone, regardless of ability to pay. When they became investor-owned, for-profit hospitals, they began to minimize or completely exclude care for the poor.

For-profit hospitals spend much less on nurses and other clinical staff. In 1997, a national study of 5,201 hospitals found that for-profit hospitals paid 20 percent lower wages than not-for-profit hospitals.

For-profit hospitals spend much more on "administration" (especially executive compensation), marketing, and perks for upper management. Thirty percent of their income is diverted to such administrative fees, in comparison to about four percent for non-profit facilities.

For-profit hospitals charge patients more, for the same procedures, than do not-for-profit hospitals.

Despite their higher cost, for-profit hospitals provide worse quality of care. This is mainly because of cutbacks in nursing staff, which results in higher patient mortality. In a 1999 study, national death rates for Medicare patients were 25 percent higher in for-profit than not-for-profit hospitals. In another study in 2000, the mortality rate of 16.9 million surgery patients was 13 percent higher in for-profit hospitals compared with their not-for-profit counterparts.

Investor-owned hospitals lobby the government to skirt regulations about conflict-of-interest and other corporate safeguards.

These investors also bought up the rehabilitation, long-term care and psychiatric services, laboratories, and even the health insurance plans. Then they raised the prices of all of these.

Investor-owned hospitals are regularly implicated in fraudulent billing practices, overcharging Medicare, and giving illegal kickbacks to physicians for referrals. For example, in 2001, the for-profit Hospital Corporation of America (HCA), which owns 181 hospitals, was fined $840 million for Medicare fraud, and paid another $631 million to settle other fraud allegations.

Tenet Healthcare Corporation is one such investor-driven enterprise (NYSE: THC). Tenet bought up 70 hospitals, mostly in California and southern states. Tenet's hospitals charge an average of *10 times* the cost of drugs in other hospitals. One of its hospitals charges 18 times their normal cost.

The investors of for-profit hospitals have become very rich. While most businesses lost money in the recession of 2001, Tenet's profit increased by 45 percent and HCA's by 47 percent.

When for-profit hospitals do encounter financial difficulties (often because of fraud), their CEOs seldom suffer. For example, in 2002 Tenet's stock dropped 70 percent after the discovery of grossly inflated company earnings and other scandals. Just before the stock dropped, the CEO cashed in $111 million of his stock.

William McGuire, CEO since 1996 of UnitedHealth Group, Inc., was awarded illegally back-dated stock options worth $1.6 billion. He has now left the company, with $1.1 billion of that amount.

Richard Scrushy, CEO of HealthSouth Corp., was paid $300 million while his company went broke, and somehow managed to be acquitted of a $2.7 billion fraud by jurors who were convinced by his explanation that he "knew nothing about what was going on directly below him."

The problem is not that these for-profit hospitals are so much worse than the non-profit charitable, government, or teaching hospitals. The problem is that they are taking over. In many regions, investors have bought up *all* the hospitals so that patients no longer have a choice. Many healthcare authorities believe that non-profit hospitals will soon disappear altogether.

Treated for Illness, Then Lost in Labyrinth of Bills

Stacks of medical bills awaited Bracha Klausner when she came home from the hospital. Mrs. Klausner, 77, had suffered a ruptured intestine, but she expected that the combination of her private insurance and Medicare would pay for her treatment. Instead, she received bills of 15 pages or more, with lists of carefully detailed items and service codes, such as "Partial thrombo 2300214 102.00" and "KUB Flat 2651040 466.00," demanding immediate payment for amounts up to $77,858. Other statements, from her private insurance, included the notice: "This is not a bill," with explanations such as "G7 - Your benefit is based on the difference between Medicare's allowable expense and the amount Medicare paid" or "QN - Your claim may have been separated for processing purposes." Even her doctor could not make sense of the obscure codes. The whole system is set up to shift costs onto the patient, regardless of insurance, and to make the process almost impossible to figure out.

Dr. David Brailer, the National Coordinator for Health Information Technology, uses this analogy: "Suppose you walk into a restaurant and you don't get a menu, you don't get any choice of what food you'll eat, they don't tell you what it is when they're serving it to you, they don't tell you what it's going to cost. Then, weeks or months later, you get a bill that tells you all the food you ate and the drinks you had, some of which you remember and some you don't, and although you get the bill, you still can't figure out what you really owe."

Health Maintenance Organizations (HMOs)

The health maintenance organization (HMO) was invented to provide "managed care." The hope was to coordinate complete and more efficient care for the patient to reduce costs and confusion. It was pioneered by Kaiser Permanente to provide a type of socialized medicine for the working class. It was a noble idea, and it did help a lot of people. Like the old saying goes, however, the road to hell is paved with good intentions.

In practice, managed care quickly degenerated into managed cost. HMOs operate by collecting your premium up front and then trying to minimize their payout (and maximize profit) by "managing" your care. The original HMOs were non-profit — operating like a miniature version of the Canadian socialized healthcare system. Now, however, about two-thirds of HMOs are for-profit corporate organizations. They try to "cherry pick" the market by selecting only healthy and low-risk patients. Many will not even consider persons with chronic diseases such as asthma or diabetes. They set up all sorts of barriers to high-cost items like specialist referrals, sophisticated diagnostic tests, and expensive medications. They also do everything to keep a patient out of the hospital and, if that is unavoidable, send the beleaguered invalids home as soon as possible, sometimes pushing an IV pole still dripping medication into their arms. Doctors who minimize costs get bonuses; doctors who have high-cost patients, or don't comply with the HMO-restricted care, get fired.

How are HMOs different from other for-profit hospitals? The usual for-profit hospital skimps on labor and jacks up the cost to bilk Medicare and the insurance companies. But HMOs own both the hospital *and* the insurance company. They are one and the same. This results in a peculiar difference in their admitting practice. For-profit hospitals do everything to get a patient into the hospital, so they can bill the insurer or patient. They can bill insurance plans much higher amounts for an inpatient than for an outpatient. The average inpatient stays for six days and brings the hospital $10,000. These hospitals curry favor with primary care physicians such as family practitioners and internists, since they need a pipeline of patients referred to their facility. For every primary care physician in the hospital's network, the hospital gains an average $2.1 million per year from the referrals.

HMOs, on the other hand, *are* the insurance plan, so they try everything to keep the patient *out* of the hospital.

It all depends on the money. Actual concern for the patient is not a consideration. HMOs provide just enough care to avoid a lawsuit, since, by definition, anything more than that is subtracted from their profits. Not surprisingly, a national study of investor-owned HMOs in 1999 found that they scored worse on all 14 quality indicators than not-for-profit HMOs, sparking outrage and lawsuits from their patients. Meanwhile, these for-profit HMOs paid out 25 to 33 percent of their income to profits and astronomical salaries for their executives.

According to a report published in the Journal of the American Board of Family Practice, 2003, here are a few characteristics of our major for-profit HMOs:

The National Committee for Quality Assurance (NCQA) was set up to monitor hospital quality of care. Compliance is voluntary. For-profit HMOs usually manipulate or withdraw from the NCQA standards, and are over three times more likely to just stop reporting data to NCQA.

For-profit HMOs frequently deny medical necessity in an "arbitrary and capricious" manner. When challenged, they deny legal and ethical accountability.

For Well Point Health Networks of California (the parent of Blue Cross of California), $1 of every $5 dollars collected from patients is pure profit.

In 2000, the 23 top executives of investor-owned HMOs were each paid more than $63 million in salary plus $109 million in stock options.

HMOs don't like Medicare, although they exploit it as much as possible. After reaping short-term profits, many HMOs simply abandon Medicare patients, forcing them to find other coverage. Those who continue to accept Medicare increase premiums and reduce benefits.

In Missouri, a group of pediatricians serving inner-city patients won a $6 million judgment against Blue Cross and Blue Shield of Kansas City after the HMO diverted their non-profit earnings to a for-profit operation and then failed to honor their contract.

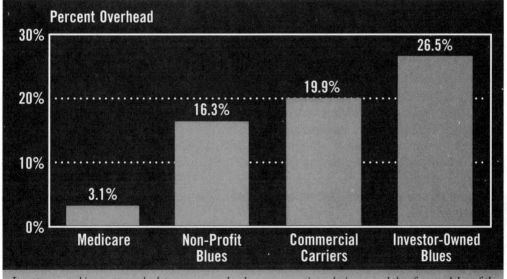

Investor-owned insurers spend a lot more on overhead — e.g. executive salaries — and therefore much less of the premium on actual healthcare. ("Blues" refers to the Blue Cross/Blue Shield health insurance providers)

Preventive care is a loss for HMOs, since the benefit to patients usually comes years or decades down the road.

How much preventive care do HMOs provide? A 2005 survey found that "managed-care providers managed to fall short in nearly every category of care — from adolescent immunization to cancer screenings to cholesterol control." Collectively, they failed to meet national health standards in 34 out of 39 areas. Cigna, one of the largest HMOs, failed to provide any information on preventive care in 17 categories.

Why, then, do HMOs survive? They provide a simple way to get care without the constant struggle to obtain insurance approval and other frustrating paperwork. When challenged about their practices, they respond with skillful manipulation of numbers and sophisticated marketing to make it look like they are providing a cost-effective service. Regardless, people know that healthcare is worse, and they are paying more for it.

Our Antiquated Medical System

In 1907, the Mayo brothers of Rochester, Minnesota, built the first clinic. They used equipment of the time: acoustic stethoscopes, handheld lights to look in the ears and eyes, and little rubber hammers to test reflexes. Patient notes were hand-written in paper charts. When patients arrived, they sat in a waiting room, along with all the other coughing and sniffling patients waiting to be seen.

Now, a century later, what does the typical clinic look like? Incredibly, it is just about the same. Doctors still use acoustic stethoscopes (even though far superior digital ones are available), a virtually unchanged ear and eye scope (even though much more accurate digital ones are available), and rubber reflex hammers (instead of far superior nerve conduction testing). With regard to the medical record system: 87 percent of current clinics and hospitals still record hand-written notes in paper charts! As for the waiting room and its exposure to infectious disease — that problem has actually become worse, to the point that patients have a one-in-five chance of picking up an infectious disease from other patients. Medication errors, misplaced charts, and lack of coordination among caregivers are a daily occurrence. Medication errors alone are estimated to cause 98,000 deaths per year in the United States and countless non-fatal outcomes.

It is interesting to compare the medical industry to the airline industry. Air transport also began in the early 1900s, with the very first paying passengers riding in open-cockpit biplanes. Needless to say, modern air travel has come a long way since then. You can now book and pay for your flight online and even select your seat assignment, indicate your meal preference, and make other special requests. A staggering amount of data on virtually every detail of airline flights is available to anyone with access to the Internet. You can find out instantly the location of every airplane in the air traffic control system in the U.S., along with its speed, altitude, direction, estimated time enroute, and estimated time of arrival. The system is superb — the best in the world. Every accident is exhaustively investigated by the Federal Aviation Administration, with mandatory modification of any equipment or procedure found to be at fault. Every incident, however minor, is also documented and studied for improvement in the future. Pilots are encouraged to file a report on the slightest incident, without penalty, even if they are at fault. In medical care, on the contrary, incidents are generally hushed up, doctors are terrified of malpractice lawsuits and rarely admit fault, and the most grievous errors generally come to light only after extensive malpractice investigations and then — nothing happens. A pilot who is responsible for an accident generally faces the end of his or her career. A doctor convicted of the most egregious malpractice can just move to another state and get right back into practice — and few people will know.

Most airlines have replaced paper tickets with e-tickets, and checking in at one of the new computer kiosks can be done in less than a minute. A couple of months before writing this book, I flew to Singapore for a business meeting. I counted all the steps I went through in the process of booking and paying for the ticket, checking in, going through security, and getting on the airplane. It was *one third* of the number of steps needed to check in at a medical clinic. When it becomes easier to fly halfway around the world than it is to see a doctor, we definitely have a problem.

In the modern hospitals in Asia, in contrast, everything is electronic. I was astonished at the efficiency of facilities such as Escorts and Max Devi in India, Raffles Hospital in Singapore, and Bangkok General in Thailand. As a medical tourist, you may not even see a waiting room, much less need to wait in one. (You will, however, see very comfortable lounges and the ubiquitous Starbucks.)

Why are we so far behind Asia? Or, more precisely, why are American medical systems so slow to change? The primary reason is lack of competition within the overly controlling medical-industrial complex that strangles innovation. When my colleague opened a new $5 million clinic, I was surprised to see that he used the same old paper-chart system, along with the rest of the traditional procedures. When I questioned him about this, he responded by saying that it was standard, everybody does it, and it is what the network expects. He didn't want to rock the boat by bringing in new practices. As long as everyone keeps to the old practices, there is no need to improve or innovate.

Until now. The new overseas facilities — no obsolete equipment, no waits, no paperwork, and no complex bills — are starting to rock our boat.

Globalization: A "Flattening" World

In *The World Is Flat: A Brief History of the Twenty-first Century* (revised edition, 2006), Thomas Friedman shows how economies, products, and services are becoming international. American jobs in manufacture or service can be outsourced to countries where labor is cheaper. This has been occurring for a long time; what is new is the incredible extent of outsourcing. It is one thing to have your running shoes made in Indonesia, but it is quite another to have your taxes done in India, your phone answered there, and even your drive-in hamburger request answered by someone 10,000 miles away. Outsourcing is beginning to penetrate almost all activities. Parents too busy to help their kids with homework can tell them to phone or go online to get help from tutors in India or Latin America. Too busy even to go to church? Catholics can have a mass said in their honor by a priest in India for a small donation.

When Friedman says the world is flat, he means that the peaks and valleys of the economic disparities in the world are changing; we are no longer at the top of the heap, leaving the crumbs for the poorer countries. Colonialism has run its course. Globalization is the new economy. Roughly, this means a leveling of the economic playing field — in other words, a "flattening" of the world.

Curiously, Friedman does not even mention medical tourism. Perhaps because the extent of outsourcing is so great, he would have to write an encyclopedia to look at all of its different aspects. However, the outsourcing of healthcare is a major phenomenon. The global healthcare market is estimated to be about $3 trillion. Medical tourism is now about $20 billion, therefore 1/150 of the global healthcare expenditure. However, it is growing at an estimated 30 percent per year, and will soon have an enormous effect on healthcare in industrialized countries — especially in the United States.

Medical tourism has come under the radar of both the World Health Organization (WHO) and the World Trade Organization (WTO). As far back as the early 1990s, the WHO commissioned Social Sector Development Strategies, Inc. (SSDS) to see whether the English-speaking Caribbean islands could provide health tourism. SSDS concluded that these islands would not be able to compete for medical tourists. They have since been proven wrong. Now, a number of Caribbean nations have a thriving medical tourism industry, especially in cosmetic surgery, dentistry, and fertility assistance (see *Barbados, Cuba, Dominica,* and *Dominican Republic*). Both WHO and WTO believe medical travel can improve the imbalance in global healthcare. Developed nations benefit as healthcare costs are reduced and access increased. Developing countries benefit as the new type of tourism provides income and builds the infrastructure for much improved medical care. Best of all, medical tourism has begun to reverse a brain drain of the most highly educated physicians from overseas countries. Now that they have the opportunity to stay home, they are much more likely to do so.

Each year, Bahrain hosts the International Health Tourism (IHT) exhibition, and every year it is much greater. In 2005, more than 150 exhibitors from 14 countries presented their services to over 7,000 visitors. These services are very competitive and have started to attract U.S. companies. Blue Ridge Paper Products of Canton, North Carolina, a manufacturing company, may soon offer employees a free trip overseas as a healthcare option. United Group Programs (UGP) of Boca Raton, Florida, a company that sells low-premium, bare-bones health insurance, is promoting Bumrungrad Hospital in Thailand as a preferred provider for its customers. Employees of self-insured businesses who use UGP will also be encouraged to go overseas for care. This means that UGP offers the option of partly or fully covered medical tourism to some 100,000 people. The UGP plan would cap reimbursement for surgery at $3,000 and hospital stays at $1,000 per day. That may not be enough for a U.S. hospital, but it's more than enough for the best overseas hospitals.

American retirees, especially snowbirds who winter in South Texas and Arizona, have turned Mexican border towns like Nuevo Progreso (9,125 population, 107 dentists) into dusty dental centers. Across the border from Yuma, Arizona, Los Algodones (15,000 population, 250 doctors and dentists) earns $150 million during the winter season from providing healthcare to Americans.

The founder of PlanetHospital, one of the largest medical tourism referral agencies, is Rupak "Rudy" Acharya. He has retained Mercer to help him develop an insurance plan for the uninsured that will combine primary and emergency care in the U.S. with surgery abroad. This plan, if it is successful, will do more to improve the American medical crisis than any proposal to date put forth by politicians.

Won't Medical Tourists Deplete Medical Resources in Other Countries?

A commonly heard criticism of medical tourism is that it will use up scarce medical resources in countries where healthcare is already insufficient. In 2006, a Philippine group of doctors vigorously opposed the government's "Philippine Medical Tourism" project, saying this would only further commercialize the country's healthcare system. According to Dr. Gene Nisperos, the Secretary General of the Health Alliance for Democracy (HEAD), the project is "more glitter than gold" and should be opposed. "Why is [Philippine President Arroyo] pushing for the commercial sale of our health services when it cannot even provide for the health needs of the vast majority of Filipinos?" he asked, and added that 50 percent of Filipinos die without receiving any form of healthcare. "Medical tourism will significantly decrease services available to charity patients, even as it opens up services to paying patients and foreigners or tourists. Such institutionalized privatization of healthcare will only further marginalize poor Filipino patients."

In fact, these fears have proved to be unfounded, and the opposite is the case. Wherever medical tourism has prospered, there has been a tremendous increase in the numbers of hospitals, clinics, doctors, healthcare staff, and ancillary services. Instead of losing skilled health professionals to emigration there is an influx of them, and local personnel have much more opportunity to stay at home. A single new hospital can employ 3,000 nurses and other ancillary medical personnel — all of whom would otherwise have been jobless.

The Philippines is an illustrative case. Despite Dr. Nisperos's concern, the problem with Philippine healthcare is not a shortage of doctors, but rather that there is no money to pay these doctors — so they are unemployed or forced to emigrate. Dr. Galvez Tan estimates that 80 percent of the Philippine's government doctors have re-educated themselves as nurses, or are enrolled in nursing programs, hoping for an American green card. It is better for these doctors to work as a nurse in the United States than to starve at home. But medical tourism reverses that. With demand — *paying* demand — from medical tourists, these doctors can now put their advanced training to use, not only for medical tourists but for locals, as well. The income from medical tourism serves to underwrite healthcare for the poor.

How Will Medical Tourism Affect U.S. Healthcare?

People in information technology, which is particularly affected by outsourcing, have a word for the loss of U.S.-based jobs: they say the job has been "Bangalored," meaning it was outsourced to Bangalore, India. Now, an increasing number of medical practices are going to be Bangalored.

This is bad news for the more lucrative parts of the U.S. healthcare industry, because it was long believed that healthcare was immune from such outsourcing. (Even Thomas Friedman writes that healthcare is one of the few service industries that cannot be outsourced.) The general wisdom has been that people would not trust overseas care, nor travel to get it. The general wisdom, as is so often the case, was wrong. Medical tourism is rapidly increasing as people become aware of the opportunity.

The medical establishment is not about to give up this lucrative industry. The one thing that American hospitals do not want to lose is surgical patients. Surgery and critical care account for a huge part of their income and the vast majority of their profits. It is not uncommon for a hospital to offer an $800,000 sign-up bonus to attract a prominent surgeon. They bring in the money, and everyone feeds at the trough. What happens when patients choose to go overseas for their surgery?

Organizations such as the American Medical Association and the American Dental Association have not yet adopted policies on medical tourism. Others, such as the American Society of Plastic Surgeons, have issued statements of caution. There is little they can do to stop it and protect their own industry from competition. The only recourse will be to adapt, to improve their services, make them more efficient, reduce frustrating and demeaning procedures, and generally provide more value for the price.

You may be wondering if medical tourism is going to put your family doctor out of business. Actually, it's quite the contrary. There will always be a need for a good primary care physician. If you have a migraine, an odd rash, a bad sunburn, if you wipe out on your mountain bike, or cut yourself with your new Ginza kitchen knife, you are not going to fly to Thailand for treatment. This level of medical care will not be affected.

The people who will lose income are the radiologists who charge $1,200 for an MRI and earn an average of $385,000 a year, and the ophthalmologists who earn over a million dollars a year doing LASIK or cataract surgery. These specialists should learn about medical tourism, because outsourcing may have a significant impact on their livelihood.

Will medical tourism hurt the American economy? Not at all. Going overseas for healthcare will have the same effect as the outsourcing of information technology — an actual increase in wealth. Let's look at the computer industry as an example. Many computer-programming jobs have been lost to Bangalore in India, Shanghai in China, and other emerging high-tech centers, where most basic software engineering is increasingly being done. The result of this trend is that jobs for computer programmers are disappearing. In the 1990s, computer science graduates fresh out of college could get jobs paying $100,000 a year. Now they have to get an advanced degree or become more specialized to make that kind of money. But this has not impoverished the U.S. The lower labor costs overseas have made software vastly cheaper for everyone. And the countries that supply the cheap labor, such as India and China, have seen growth in their economies and skyrocketing demand for American-made products. The end result is increased prosperity on both sides of the ocean. Medical tourism is part of the continuing evolution of international trade, improving overall health as well as the economy.

With competition from overseas hospitals, healthcare services in the United States will have to become more responsive to consumers. This is already happening in some areas. Not surprisingly, it started in Hollywood. Dr. Marc Mani, the Beverly Hills surgeon to the stars, is building a revolutionary Sunset Boulevard clinic with a sauna, a steam room, and a "serenity" room, where you can psych yourself up for liposuction and the operating room. "Our aim is to do everything from facials to face-lifts," says Mani. "Have a massage, get liposuction and be home the same day." These new "medispas" were modeled on similar services overseas. Dr. Stephen M. Krant's S K Sanctuary, in La Jolla, California, is an example of the new high-end clinic. A Tuscan resort with waterfalls, it has rooms named after Italian villages. The spa's director, Kelly Costa, says, "The best medical spa is a mixture of care and pampering. We specialize in pre-op skincare, from micro-dermabrasion to a good old-fashioned facial. If you're going to spend thousands of dollars on a face-lift and you break out in spots, you won't get the best results." Dozens of these spa-type surgical centers have opened across America, such as the MeSua Dermocosmetic Spa in Miami, the New York Skin and Spa Center, and Dr. Norman Leaf's Solutions Skincare Medical Clinic in Beverly Hills.

The transformation about to take place in U.S. medicine is not a one-way street. As Americans travel for cheaper and better care, U.S. facilities will respond and improve — and lure foreigners to the U.S. for care. The long-term solution, says Dr. Harpal Singh, Chairman of Fortis Healthcare, lies in partnerships. "It'll be mutually beneficial for both them and us." Adds Prathap C. Reddy, a physician who founded Apollo Hospitals, a 6,400-bed chain headquartered in Chennai, India: "If we do this right, we can heal the world."

Chapter 5

Cosmetic Surgery

It's Not Just Vanity

Cosmetic surgery has been done for thousands of years, but only in the last decade has it become widely available. Like so many other fashions, it first became popular in Hollywood and then spread throughout the population. Now, it is common for everyone from children to the elderly to have surgical adjustments made to parts of the body. It is not cheap, however. Medical tourism is likely to change that. For the cost of a ski lift ticket, you can get minor surgery done overseas — and banish forever an annoying or unsightly feature of your body.

Most people choose cosmetic surgery to reverse the signs of aging, such as wrinkly and sagging skin and pockets of fat. Others do so to enhance their appearance in order to meet the fashion of the day and place. In India, for example, a female plump face is considered attractive, whereas chin jowls are considered undesirable on American women. The same is true of noses — where Philippine women like the angular Western nose, women in the United States prefer the more petite nose. Dark people want lighter skin while light people tan and color their skin to look darker.

It is not only an issue of vanity. Throughout history, physical appearance has been linked to moral worth. People who are considered good-looking are more likely to get married or hired for a job. They get paid more and are promoted sooner. Strangers are more likely to assist good-looking people in distress. Attractive people are less likely to be reported, caught, accused, or punished for minor and major crimes. Is it unfair? Absolutely. But it is human nature.

Historically, physical appearance was a genetic lottery. Now, however, you can do something about it.

The most common types of cosmetic surgery are:
- Blepharoplasty (eyelid reshaping)
- Liposuction (removing fat from under the skin)
- Breast augmentation (enlarging breasts)
- Breast reduction (reducing overly large breasts)
- Breast lift (perking up sagging breasts)
- Face lift (tightening up the face and neck)
- Forehead or brow lift (tightening up the forehead)
- Rhinoplasty (nose reshaping)
- Abdominoplasty (belly reshaping)
- Ear pinning (ears pulled back)

In addition to these are countless very minor procedures to remove blemishes, tattoos, or damaged skin. According to *Time* magazine, cosmetic surgery increased 444 percent in U.S. from 1997 to 2005. In 2004, according to the American Society for Aesthetic Plastic Surgery, 9.2 million cosmetic surgeries were performed in the U.S., with patients spending $12.4 billion for the procedures. An estimated 455,000 liposuctions were done in 2005. Females account for 88 percent and males 12 percent of cosmetic surgery, but men are catching up, especially for liposuction and nose and eyelid reshaping. These U.S. figures do not account for those who have the surgery done overseas — a number that is likely to grow far larger.

Medical insurance has to pay for cosmetic surgery when it can be shown that the surgery is necessary for health reasons or as a consequence of illness or injury. However, there is a large gray area between "medically necessary" and "cosmetically preferable." The result is that insurers are having to pay out ever higher amounts as more

I had a little roll of fat hanging over the back of my jeans, like a spare bicycle tire in the back," said Dana Conte, 34, a bartender in Manhattan. It was so obvious that her mother constantly came up behind her and pulled her shirt down over it, Ms. Conte said. "When your mother is doing that, it means there's a problem."

She tried Weight Watchers and working out "like a lunatic," but couldn't get rid of her back fat. She ended up having liposuction on her lower back, and then again to remove "bra fat" — the bulges, she said, when her "bra pushes lumps of fat down my back and up over the bra fastening and to the sides right near my arms." The total cost was $10,000, but she thought it was well worth it.

Had she gone overseas, she might have paid just a fifth for the same procedures.

people find sympathetic physicians and avail themselves of the opportunity to improve their appearance. Some health insurers are requiring prospective patients to view graphic videos of surgery to try to dissuade them from having surgery. However, television shows like *Nip/Tuck* are doing the opposite — cosmetic surgery is increasingly seen as normal, routine, and even a nice indulgence for already attractive people.

A major benefit of medical tourism is privacy. With surgery done on vacation, out of sight of acquaintances and colleagues, the bandages are gone and the recovery well under way by the time you return.

According to the International Society of Aesthetic Plastic Surgery (ISAPS), five countries account for 47 percent of all plastic surgery procedures worldwide: the U.S. does 16 percent, Mexico 10 percent, Brazil 9 percent, Canada 6 percent, and Argentina 6 percent. The vast majority of these are residents of the country — medical tourism is just starting to proliferate. Because most cosmetic procedures involve same-day surgery with just local anesthesia, the cost of building such a clinic is not high. Therefore, many countries are starting to offer low-cost surgery. Mexico, Brazil, and Argentina already have a long tradition of high-quality care, so clinics in these countries are generally a safe bet. Newer on the horizon are hundreds of such clinics in Asia, particularly in Thailand. Many of them are associated with excellent hospitals and have doctors trained in the United States Eastern European countries also heavily advertise cosmetic surgery clinics, although most of their clientele appear to be from neighboring countries.

Liposuction

Fat in the body exists in two forms: that surrounding the organs and that under the skin. Although fat around the organs contributes to obesity, it is the under-skin fat that people usually find unsightly. The amount and distribution of fat under the skin contributes to the contours of the body and the shapeliness of form, as well as cushioning and insulating the body. Exercise and diet can shrink the overall amount, but not in targeted areas. For example, to remove "dinner-roll" waist fat, you need to reduce the overall fat percentage of the body. Sit-ups may target waist muscles, but not waist fat. Exercise can only remove fat indirectly, by changing the total body composition.

Liposuction is a direct procedure to remove fat in specific areas. A common misconception is that liposuction is done for weight loss. In fact, the majority of fat is deep and cannot be removed this way. The purpose of liposuction is for body contouring. It is usually done under local anesthesia. First, a numbing solution is injected to anesthetize the area. Small incisions are then made into the skin so that a tube can be inserted to suck out the fat tissue. Newer procedures make use of ultrasound machines to break up fat before it is extracted, allowing smaller, more precise cannulae — the blunt-tipped hollow tubes — to be inserted. After the surgery, patients may feel sore and look bruised for several days.

The old expressions for body fat — "love handles," "saddlebags," and "turkey wattle," — have expanded to describe more recent body shaping. Now, patients ask to get rid of a "buffalo hump" (upper back), "wings" (bulges around the bra area), "doughnut" (around the belly button), "banana fold" (below the buttocks), "piano legs" (calves), and the "chubb" (bulges around the kneecap).

Liposuction is a delicate procedure that needs the skill of a properly trained plastic surgeon. The techniques are becoming increasingly precise and sophisticated, with the best doctors able to remove as little as an ounce from areas such as the chins, necks, backs, upper arms, knees, ankles, and even toes! It is more a matter of art and aesthetics than medicine.

Dr. Luiz S. Toledo, a plastic surgeon in São Paulo, Brazil, who teaches this precise method to American surgeons, calls it: "liposuction for skinny people." Now, says Dr. Peter B. Fodor, a plastic surgeon in Los Angeles, "surgeons who a few years ago would not have touched areas like kneecaps, inner thighs, back rolls, calves, and ankles have extended their practices." Sometimes, the offending bit of fat is barely noticed by others. For example, Judy Goss, a former Ford model, has a very trim figure at 5 feet 10 inches and weighs 126 pounds. "By normal standards," she admits, "I'm pretty skinny. But my arms were getting a little flappy. I could feel it wiggle every time I shook hands." That was enough to convince her to get liposuction on her upper arms. For such small concerns, some plastic surgeons ask patients to wear their favorite jeans or bra right before surgery so they can mark the areas and reshape them more exactly.

Eyebag Removal, Facelift, and Tummy Tucks

When skin tone is lost with aging, parts of the body begin to sag. Eyebags are one of the earliest signs of aging, giving a person a stressed and fatigued appearance. Upper eyelid eyebags are due to thinning of the skin and the muscle underneath it. Lower eyelid eyebags are mainly due to bulging of the fat pad inside the eye socket. Blepharoplasty tightens skin and removes excess fat.

With aging, fat pads in the face slowly shift downward, pulling the skin with it and causing a noticeable sagging. Facelift surgery is a very delicate procedure that is best performed by a fully trained plastic surgeon. Poorly done, it can make the face look overly tight or misshapen, or worse.

The very popular "tummy tuck" (abdominoplasty) is requested for a number of reasons. It used to be done mostly to correct stretched and deformed skin after a pregnancy.

Now, it is becoming more popular among those who have lost weight rapidly (such as from stomach reduction surgery) and have excess skin. Tummy tucks are basically a two-step procedure. First, the underlying abdominal wall, along with its muscle and attachments, is tightened. Then, segments of the excess skin are removed. This procedure is more complex than other types of cosmetic surgery and also has a longer recovery period. With any kind of abdominal surgery, physical activities are restricted during the initial healing.

A Patient's Story of Transformation Through Cosmetic Surgery

Mike O'Keefe was not happy with his appearance. Since the surgery he needed was more than he could afford in his country, he decided to travel to Cape Town and have it done for a much lower cost. He was kind enough to share the following and gave me permission to print his before-and-after photos. Mike is an inspiration to countless people who are trying to work up the courage to improve their lives. Here is his story:

Well, I am a 38-year-old guy from Oxford, England, and single. I live and work on a farm looking after 200 dairy cows. I like to travel and do so every year for five weeks in February and to somewhere where it is hot! I have been all around the world many times!

I went for a nose job (rhinoplasty), ears (otoplasty), lipo (belly liposuction), jaw surgery, teeth (orthodontics) and Botox. I have never been very ill or ever been in a hospital before, which makes it more difficult to go into one when you are fit and well! I was very worried and nervous about going ahead with the surgery, but as you will see, all went really well.

Cheers,

Mike O'Keefe

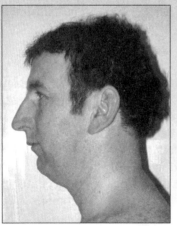 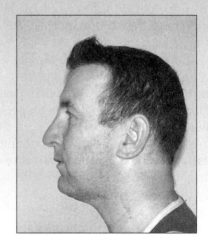

Mike O'Keefe before his surgery in South Africa ...   *... and after*

Breast Enlargement and Filler Injections

Just as body parts can be removed, they can also be added. Breast enlargement (augmentation mammoplasty) is a very common procedure for women who would like larger or fuller breasts. The enlargement is done through the use of either saline-filled or silicone gel-filled implants.

The two most common incentives for breast augmentation are aging breasts or having small breasts to begin with. The procedures are quite different.

As women age, breast tissue loses fat, and the breasts become more shallow. The excess skin results in droopy, or "ropy" breasts. Sagging breasts are often blamed on breastfeeding, although what has really happened is that milk-filled breasts had become that much larger, which resulted in a proportionately greater decline in volume afterward. Stretched skin generally resumes its earlier shape, but the degree to which it does so varies; some people end up with stretch marks or baggy, excess skin, while others don't seem to suffer as much from this problem. It is the same with weight-loss surgery: some people who lose weight from, for example, stomach banding, will gain a slimmer figure, while others will end up with flaps of extra abdominal skin. This is why many bariatric surgeons recommend a follow-up procedure to tighten the skin.

Slender or petite women often have relatively flat breasts. This can be a benefit to athletes and ballerinas, but some women prefer a fuller figure — and not just aspiring Hooters waitresses. Fashion has come full cycle from the 1950s, when prominent breasts were esteemed, to the 1960s when the thin model took over, to a resurgence of bigger breasts in the past decade. We now have the peculiar preference for women with skinny bodies but big breasts — which can usually only be achieved artificially.

There is a third reason for implants, less often discussed, which is when women have lost their breasts to breast cancer and opt for reconstructive surgery. Since these women have also lost the overlying skin, the common procedure is to pull the nearby skin together and tattoo a simulated nipple and areola. For more information, a particularly useful website is: www.implantinfo.com

Fat, collagen, and other materials may be injected to plump up other areas, such as the lips. The typical method of "filler injection" is to take fat from one part of the body (for example, the hip) and add it to another (e.g., the face). For very fine lines, an artificial material such as Dermalive™ may be used.

The "Mom Job"

Marina Plastic Surgery Associates, of Marina del Rey, California, is promoting what they call the "mommy makeover" (www.amommymakeover.com). It is a package of a breast lift with or without breast implants, a tummy tuck, and some liposuction to revise the typical ravages of motherhood. Although feminists don't like the notion that motherhood results in unattractive physical changes, the fact is that the new generation of American women is not so tolerant of the natural changes in the aging body. According to a 2007 article in the *New York Times*, doctors nationwide performed more than 325,000 "mommy makeover procedures" in the past year on women ages 20 to 39. These women may not have known that they could get the same procedure overseas at a far lower cost.

Hair Transplants

Forty million Americans are bald or well on their way toward it. Half of all men and over a third of all women will eventually experience a significant enough hair loss on their heads to be considered bald. Countless methods have been suggested to counteract baldness. By far the best involves transplanting hair follicles from the lower back of the head to the front and crown. The technique first was done in 1952 and has grown increasingly popular. Last year, 80,000 hair transplants were done. The majority were in the United States, with average prices about $7 per graft and a typical transplant requiring 1,000 to 3,000 grafts. That amounts to thousands of dollars for a hair transplant procedure — but the price is much lower in other countries.

An excellent online article on hair transplantation is available at: www.emedicine.com/derm/topic559.htm

Hair transplant is a detailed process that can take three to five hours, involving thousands of tiny incisions. Much of the work is done by technicians; the surgeon is primarily responsible for placing the puncture holes for the transplanted hairs. A typical scalp has 200 hairs per square centimeter, but only a 10th as many are needed to give the illusion of full coverage. The key is to create a natural appearance with clever spacing and slanting of the follicles. Poor-quality transplants look like corn rows and are obvious. This is why you want a skillful surgeon.

After surgery, semi-permeable dressings take care of blood seepage and tissue fluid. In the following 10 days, the dressings are changed at least daily, while virtually all of the transplanted hairs fall out. During this time, you must not shampoo and you must protect your head from the sun.

Within two to three months new hair will grow from the moved follicles and gradually thicken over the course of six months. Meanwhile, there may be further hair loss from other parts of the head. Some people have additional transplants as needed.

Since the equipment to do hair transplants is minimal, the service is offered in many places around the world. However, it is wise to choose carefully. Ask to see photos of previous work, and choose a clinic with a good reputation and a high volume. Also, it is a good idea to ensure that the surgeon you think is going to do the transplant is really the one who does it — and not a trainee or other doctor. Cyprus has developed a reputation as a good place for hair transplants. Although many heavily discounted services are advertised in India, keep in mind that hair of Asian people is much thicker and more oval than that from people of European ancestry, so transplanting skills developed on one type of hair may not be the same as on the other.

Hymenoplasty

Also referred to as "re-virgination," this is a minor operation that reconstructs the hymen — the thin membrane that partly covers the vagina and is typically torn during first sexual intercourse. It is possible only for women who have not had a vaginal delivery, and preferably have never been pregnant. Hymenoplasty is often done to assure virginity before marriage, or after marriage to revisit the experience of first intercourse. The surgery takes only a few minutes and is undetectable. The reconstructed hymen will tear and bleed again during sexual intercourse.

The hymen is a mythical symbol of chasteness in women, and its presence has been considered a guarantee of virginity in a society that places a high value on female chastity before marriage. However, the delicate hymen is easily ruptured even without sexual relations, such as during physical exercise, bike riding, gymnastics, or using tampons.

According to the American Society of Plastic Surgeons, vaginal surgery and hymenoplasty are the fastest-growing segments of cosmetic surgery. This is partly because of the influx of people from the Middle East and Latin America, where the bride-to-be may undergo inspection before marriage to ensure virginity. The procedure typically costs from $1,800 to $5,000 or more in the U.S. In Thailand and some other countries, it is as little as $200.

For her 17th wedding anniversary, Jeanette Yarborough, a 40-year-old medical assistant from San Antonio, wanted to do something special for her husband. She paid a surgeon $5,000 to reattach her hymen, making her appear to be a virgin again. "It's the ultimate gift for the man who has everything," she said. — reported in *Wall Street Journal*

Chapter 6

Dental Care

Dental tourism is one of the hottest sectors of medical tourism. Poland and Hungary offer cheap dental tours to residents of other European countries. India, Thailand, South Africa, Costa Rica, and many Caribbean nations advertise services for "orthodontal tourists." Although the basic attraction is less costly care, there are other reasons for getting dental work overseas.

Advanced care

Although American dentists are generally reliable, few of them are knowledgeable or equipped to provide the newest state-of-the-art care. If you want titanium implants, for example, your dentist will likely refer you to another specialized dentist, involving added complications of scheduling, travel, and coordination of treatment. Some of the overseas dental facilities that cater to medical tourists emphasize high-end care. These facilities often have several dentists together in one location, with multiple specialties, and continually re-educate their dentists to maintain state-of-the-art practices.

Comfort

Dental tourism services go all-out to make the experience as pleasant as possible. For example, American dentists may be stingy on pain medication — a trend called "opiophophobia" by pain specialists — because they are worried about drug-seeking patients. That doesn't do you much good when you are the one who is suffering through the after-effects of a root canal and have been given only a few low-strength codeine tablets to see you through the recovery. Overseas dentists tend to be sensitive to your pain — and you can call them in the middle of the night if you need to.

Access

Quality dentists are often very busy, and it may be difficult to arrange an appointment at a convenient time. According to an article in the *New York Times*, May

7, 2006, access to dentists in the United Kingdom has become such a problem that they now sell 6,000 do-it-yourself crown-and-cap replacement kits to frustrated consumers each week! The situation is not so bad in the U.S., but you can still expect a wait of many weeks to months in order to see a good dentist.

Types of Dental Treatment
Popular dental treatment available overseas includes:

- Bleaching
- Cosmetic dentistry
- Dental implant
- Gum treatment and grafts
- Metal-free ceramic crown
- Metal-free restoration
- Oral surgery
- Orthodontics
- Root canal
- Smile designing
- Veneers

When you travel for dental treatment, it is important to be as clear as possible about what you want and research the facility to make sure that they can provide it. The easiest way to do this is to email or call them. This is especially true if you want specialized treatment.

In addition to general dentistry, there are nine dental specialties recognized by the American Dental Association. Each of these requires two to six years of residency training after dental school. The specialties are:

- Endodontics (root canal therapy)
- Oral and Maxillofacial Pathology (diagnosis of diseases of the jaw, face, and mouth)
- Oral and Maxillofacial Radiology (imaging of the mouth region by x-ray, CT, MRI, etc.)
- Oral and Maxillofacial Surgery (extractions and facial surgery)
- Orthodontics and Dentofacial Orthopaedics (straightening of teeth)
- Pedodontics (dentistry for children)
- Periodontics (treatment of gum disease)
- Prosthodontics (dentures, bridges, and implants)
- Dental Public Health (dental epidemiology and social health)

Veneers

Tooth veneers are very thin pieces of specially shaped porcelain or plastic placed and glued over the front of your teeth. They can do wonders for your appearance — in fact, just about everyone in Hollywood or the entertainment business probably has them. Veneers can solve problems such as oddly shaped, discolored, chipped or crooked teeth. Or they may be used to improve appearance and create a pleasing smile. Veneers can be an excellent alternative to crowns. They need little or no anesthesia to apply, and, unlike crowns, veneers usually don't require removing much of the tooth itself. Veneers last from five to 15 years and brighten dark teeth without the worry of them changing color.

There are two types of veneers: composite and porcelain. Composite (direct) veneers are usually performed in a single visit to your cosmetic dentist. The veneer is color matched to the other teeth and then bonded directly to the tooth's surface. Composite veneers last about five to seven years. Porcelain (indirect) veneers are manufactured in a laboratory from a very thin porcelain material. They usually require two or more visits to the dentist; the first to make an impression of your tooth and color match the new veneer, and the second to apply it. The veneer is then bonded to the tooth. Porcelain veneers are more costly than composite veneers but last 10 years to 15 years or more.

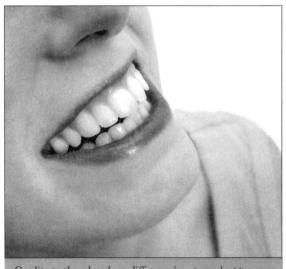

Quality teeth make a huge difference in a person's appearance and well-being. A complete makeover of the teeth is often referred to as a "new smile." Not only is it beautiful, but it also increases overall physical health by reducing tooth and gum disease and improving digestion.

There is only one problem with veneers: they're expensive. In the United States, they run about $600-$700 and up, per tooth. A complete, wide-smile restoration of 16 teeth therefore costs about $10,000. For models, actors, and television personalities, that's simply the cost of doing business — they can even deduct the cost on their taxes. For the rest of us, such dental work is considered cosmetic, and the IRS is not so understandable of its need. It is hard to justify spending so much money on personal appearance. Luckily, the dental tourism option now provides the same (or better) quality at a huge discount.

Step-by-Step Plan to Choose an Overseas Dentist

1. Determine the location and type of dentist you want.
2. Check the website of the clinic. This site should include a statement of the dentist's training and certifications. In some countries, such as India, there are dentists who do not have any qualifications or registration. These, of course, should be avoided.
3. Communicate with the dentist to be sure that you will feel comfortable. This can be done by telephone or email, or even by writing — most of them will be happy to send you a letter to answer your questions and brochures that describe their facility. A good clinic might ask you for x-rays or pictures of your teeth to help determine what is best for you and give a reliable estimate of the time and cost of the work.
4. Ask for the names and numbers or email addresses of others they have treated. Patients often don't mind giving out this information and commenting on their experiences. If you feel unsure about going, you can then call some of them to get their opinions.
5. If you prefer to use a referral service, make sure that you know who the dentist will be. If possible, try to talk to the dentist. If the service refuses to give you this information, find another service.

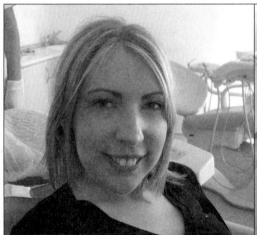 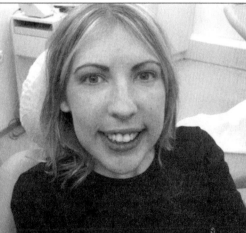

This young lady went to a clinic in Eastern Europe to have the extensive orthodontic surgery to change the position of her teeth.

She was so delighted with her new smile that she posted her before–and–after pictures on the Internet — and gave the author permission to copy them.

6. DO NOT pay anything up front, either to the dentist or to the service.
7. When you arrive at the dental clinic, look around and chat with people. Is it a clean, neat, and well-run clinic? If you feel uncomfortable, leave. Bad dental work is a lot worse than a bad haircut!
8. Before treatment begins, talk to the dentist directly to describe what you want and perhaps have an initial examination. Then discuss fees with the dentist or a staff person, and make sure that there is a good understanding of what the final fee will be. At this point, there may be a partial up-front payment. However, you should not pay the entire agreed-upon amount until the treatment is complete and to your satisfaction.
9. Confirm that confidentiality will be maintained in terms of your treatment records and health status disclosures.
10. Confirm that your approval must be obtained before any pictures are taken.
11. Be cautious of dentists who recommend extensive or elaborate treatment beyond that which you initially sought.
12. Be cautious of dentists who sell medicines or supplements.
13. Be cautious of dentists who recommend replacement of previous fillings that are still OK.
14. Make sure you get a copy of your dental record when treatment is complete.

Weight-Loss Surgery

Obesity is a global problem, largely a result of too little exercise and too much high-calorie food in a fast-paced world. And it seems to be the worst in the U.S., where fully two-thirds of the population is overweight. Fat is in the eye of the beholder. But there is a simple way of determining if you are overweight. It relies on the Body Mass Index (BMI), calculated as:

Weight (kilograms) divided by height (meters) squared, or kg/m^2.

The formula can be adapted to pounds and inches by multiplying by 703. In other words: lb/in^2 x 703.

For example, a person weighing 225 lbs and 5 foot 6 inches (66 inches) tall will have a BMI of 36, calculated as $225/66^2$ x 703 = 36.

According to the National Institutes of Health, your BMI falls into one of the following categories:

Less than 18.5 = Underweight
From 18.5 to 24.9 = Normal weight
From 25.0 to 29.9 = Overweight
30 and more = Obese

A simple pencil-and-paper way to calculate BMI:

1. Write down your weight in pounds
2. Multiply by 703
3. Divide by your height in inches
4. Divide again by your height in inches
Your BMI is over 25?   Uh oh, you are too fat (or too muscular!)

The BMI is not a perfect measurement of obesity, but it is generally useful for persons over age 20 (there is a different measurement for children). It is also not accurate for people who are excessively muscular, such as body-builders.

The dangers of obesity are well known: heart disease, diabetes, stroke, kidney failure, joint problems, and early death. But obesity also causes a lot of other problems that are less easy to measure, including:

- Social isolation
- Difficulty finding a husband or wife
- Difficulty getting a good job
- Preventing career enhancement
- Poor sex drive
- Marital problems
- Social and workplace discrimination
- Difficulty finding friends
- Medication problems
- High blood pressure
- High cholesterol
- Psychological stress, poor self-image, self-loathing, inhibition

Obesity is unattractive and associated with laziness. The good news is that obesity can be cured. By losing enough weight, health risks are greatly reduced, and social problems can essentially disappear. The problem is that losing weight is not as easy as it sounds. Diets simply don't work without accompanying exercise programs. And consistent exercise sufficient to lose weight is time-consuming and takes a lot of willpower. Most people fail — and the discouragement of failure often results in even more weight gain.

One solution is surgery. Remarkably, many of the health benefits from diet and exercise-induced weight loss — such as lowered blood pressure and improved blood sugar control — are also found with weight-loss surgery.

An Overview of Bariatric Surgery

Bariatric surgery involves the stapling, banding, excision, or rerouting of the stomach or intestines in order to reduce the number of calories that a person can consume and absorb. In the U.S. in 2005, doctors performed at least 175,000 stomach-reduction surgeries, according to the Nationwide Inpatient Sample, a database of in-patient operations at hospitals compiled by the federal Agency for Healthcare Research and Quality. The number for 2006 is over 200,000. Although this number might seem high, it represents less than 1 percent of those eligible for the surgery, according to Dr. Schauer, director of bariatric surgery at the Cleveland Clinic.

The problem is that bariatric surgery is usually not covered by insurance and is very expensive — a national average of $29,921 for uncomplicated surgery, $36,542 for those with complications, and a whopping $65,031 for those with complications that require readmission to the hospital. Considering that about 40 percent of patients have complications, that is a staggering cost for most people.

By now, you know the solution to this problem: medical tourism! In many countries, most notably India, Thailand, and Singapore, top-quality bariatric surgery can be obtained for as little as 1/10 of the cost in the U.S. Moreover, many overseas hospitals will have a single charge, with complications treated free of additional charges. In these countries, you can also get advanced types of surgery that are not yet commonly available in the United States, such as the highly effective lap-band surgery described below.

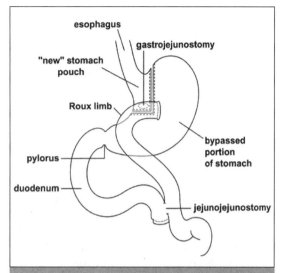

Conventional stomach-reduction surgery involves sewing shut the upper part of the stomach and then connecting it to the lower part of the small intestine. The result bypasses the majority of the stomach and the upper part of the small intestine, so that much less food is absorbed.

Is Bariatric Surgery Right For You?

Bariatric surgery is not the first choice for treating obesity. Most people consider it after years or decades of frustration. Others have such extreme obesity that they want to lose a lot of weight quickly, or feel unable to do enough exercise to achieve normal weight. In general, doctors will only consider those who are over 18 years of age, since younger people should be sufficiently able to lose weight from exercise instead. On the other end of the age range, many surgeons are reluctant to work on those who are over age 60 because of the increased risk from anesthesia and because most of these people have complicating conditions of heart disease, lung disease, and diabetes.

Sometimes, obesity is due to a metabolic imbalance such as thyroid disease. In that case, of course, the underlying problem should be treated first. Before bariatric surgery, you will undergo an extensive work-up to determine whether this operation is indicated and safe in your case. The pre-operative screening will consist of complete blood tests, imaging studies, endoscopy, and consultations with various specialists.

Surgery is a reasonable choice if:

- you have been overweight for at least five years, *and*
- you have tried repeatedly to lose weight without success, *and*
- your BMI is above 30.

This is especially true if you suffer from obesity-related health problems such as diabetes, hypertension, sleep apnea, or joint problems. These limitations are being waived, as even healthy, mildly overweight people increasingly elect surgery.

Surgery is not appropriate if you have any of the following:

- Unusually high risk of dying from surgery
- Severe inflammation of the esophagus
- Ulcer of the stomach or duodenum
- Bleeding from the stomach or intestine
- Inflammatory bowel disease
- Malformations of the bowel
- Pregnancy
- Alcohol or drug addiction
- Mental illness
- Eating disorder

If you are planning to become pregnant, you should wait at least a year and a half after surgery.

Possible Complications of Bariatric Surgery

Bariatric surgery is not for the faint-hearted. It is major surgery. Whether you have it in the U.S. or overseas, it is important to be aware of the risks. A federal government review of bariatric surgery in the United States reported that four of every 10 patients who undergo weight-loss surgery develop complications within six months. This brings up the question of whether the risk is higher in other countries. In general, the answer is no. Hospitals and surgeons who do this sort of surgery adhere to uniform standards and procedures. However, there is one way that you can ensure that you will get the very highest standard of treatment: check if the hospital is certified by JCI (see *Chapter 2*). Also, make sure that the place you choose has performed *many* of the procedure you want. That is probably the best guarantee of success.

The most common after-effect of the operation is sagging skin. If you lose a few pounds, or lose weight gradually, the skin can adjust. But the skin cannot keep up with the dramatic weight loss that occurs after bariatric surgery. Skin that has been stretched for a long time may not contract completely. As Dr. Robert B. Nemerofsky, a surgeon in Secaucus, New Jersey, describes it: "If you stretch a rubber band out for a second, it snaps back. But if you stretch it out and hold it for a week, the rubber band will not contract back to its original size." Therefore, many people who have bariatric surgery choose to undergo a second surgery after a couple of months to remove the excess skin. This is a much easier and simpler procedure. And if the weight is regained? The now-reduced skin simply stretches again to accommodate it, according to Dr. Jeffrey M. Kenkel, vice chairman of plastic surgery at the University of Texas Southwestern Medical Center in Dallas.

Post-surgical vomiting and diarrhea are also common. More worrisome are the risks of abdominal hernias, infections, pneumonia and respiratory failure, and the leaking of gastric juices caused by imperfect surgical connections between the stomach and the intestines.

Recovery Is Not Necessarily Smooth and Easy

Joanne Kayser, a 64-year-old retired New Hampshire state employee, weighed 320 pounds in 2003 when she had decided to have weight-loss surgery in Boston. She said, "The operation went well. It reduced my food intake. After the surgery, I lost 60 pounds." Even better, her diabetes improved to the point that she no longer needed to take diabetes medications.

Unfortunately, she developed complications during her recovery: "My incision did not heal for seven months. I could not exercise, and I stopped losing weight. The incision became infected, and I had to have surgery by a wound care specialist. In addition, after four months, I developed a hernia, a bulge in my tummy." Her complications required further surgeries to resolve.

Lap-Band Procedure

The latest improvement in bariatric surgery is the laparoscopic adjustable gastric band. This involves several small, about a quarter- to half-inch, incisions in the abdomen. A silicon band is slipped inside and tied around the upper part of the stomach to create a small pouch. This pouch is, in a sense, the new stomach. When the patient eats, the pouch fills up rapidly to create a sensation of fullness. As the pouch slowly empties, the patient does not feel hungry for several hours. The band has a balloon on the inside that can be expanded to prolong the period of fullness. Adjustments can also be made to the tightness of the band to regulate the long-term degree of weight loss.

Khaliah Ali, a daughter of Mohammad Ali, struggled with obesity most of her life. At one point, she reached 325 pounds, despite diet and exercise. She felt especially

---

embarrassed because of her renowned father and her supremely fit sister — also an accomplished boxer. Very pleased with her decision to have lap-band surgery, she describes her experience in her 2007 book: *Fighting Weight: How I Achieved Healthy Weight Loss with "Banding," a New Procedure That Eliminates Hunger — Forever.*

Although not every patient is suitable for the lap-band procedure, there are several advantages in comparison to the conventional stomach-reduction surgeries:

- No cutting or stapling of the stomach
- The size of the pouch and its opening can be individually calibrated
- The pouch can be adjusted after the initial surgery
- The lap-band is removable and the surgery fully reversible
- The hospital stay is typically just 1 — 2 days, much shorter than regular stomach-reduction surgery

Despite these clear benefits, the lap-band procedure is still not common in the U.S.; most doctors continue to prefer the older types of stomach stapling, cutting, and rerouting — primarily because that is the way they were trained. You are more likely to get state-of-the-art treatment in the newer medical centers in Thailand or Singapore.

After lap-band surgery, you can expect to lose about 2 pounds per week. For the first five weeks, you should stay on liquids and mashed foods to prevent the pouch from being stretched. After that, you are free to eat most foods, although some patients have complained that they do not digest meat well.

The band can be loosened during pregnancy, to permit eating more, and then retightened after delivery.

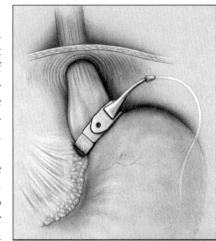

In the lap-band procedure, an inflatable collar is placed around the opening to the stomach, preventing more than a small amount of food from entering.

Joint Replacement

Joint repair and replacement has become one of the fastest-growing areas of medical tourism. The major draws are the much lower cost and, in some cases, the accessibility to procedures not yet available in the U.S. Three types of joint surgery account for almost all of the activity: hip replacement, knee replacement, and spinal surgery. Arthroscopy and repair of ligaments is less popular, partly because this is usually the result of trauma, and the injured person wants to have it done right away. But even in trauma situations, a savvy person can save a lot of money by going overseas. Consider, for example, a skier who wrenches her knee and needs an ACL repair. This type of sprain is very common in athletes, but total costs for the repair can easily be over $5,000. If she does not have insurance, she will have to pay the entire amount out of pocket. In many other countries, she could have this done for less than $1,000.

Hip replacements for medical tourists have become such big business in Thailand and India that many hospitals are now specializing in this.

Hip Resurfacing in India

Robert Vacca, of Sag Harbor, New York, had always been an athlete. As a young man, he was drafted by the Milwaukee Bucks and played with basketball star Kareem Abdul-Jabbar. But he had also experienced symptoms of a bone disease since he was 14, and doctors could not figure out the cause of his brittle bones. He underwent a series of six operations to remove bone chips from his joints, and eventually the disability forced his retirement. Even caddying at the Atlantic Golf Club in Bridgehampton eventually became too difficult. His hips deteriorated to the point where he was confined to a wheelchair and in constant pain. At age 55, his future looked dismal.

A friend at the Sag Harbor Gym told Mr. Vacca of a "60 Minutes" episode he had seen about new hip resurfacing treatment available in India. Unlike the standard hip replacement, in which the head and neck of the thighbone are removed, hip resurfacing does not remove bone. Instead, a metal cap is fitted over the end of the thighbone and

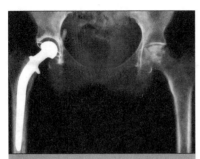

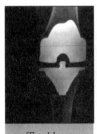
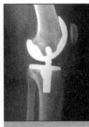

This X-ray shows a total hip replacement on the left. The newer hip-resurfacing procedure involves just a cap on the ball of the hip.

| *Total knee replacement, front view.* | *Total knee replacement, side view.* |

fitted into a metal socket in the hip. There are a number of advantages to this procedure. The usual hip replacement involves polyethylene, which produces wear particles that damage the surrounding bone, often requiring revision surgeries. With hip resurfacing, only metal is used, and the bone actually grows stronger, with no need for revision surgery. Hip resurfacing takes less than two hours and patients can resume strenuous physical activity in about three to six weeks. Range of motion is greater, and movement is not restricted as it is after conventional hip replacement, to prevent dislocation and excessive wear of the prosthesis. In fact, hip resurfacing patients are urged to be physically active after the surgery.

This innovative procedure has become popular in many countries but is still waiting for approval by the Food and Drug Administration in the United States. Vacca had the option of getting into an experimental clinical trial in the U.S. — at a cost of about $28,000 to $32,000. Or he could go to India, for a cost of about $6,000.

He read a *New York Times* article about Dr. Vijay Bose, at the Apollo Hospital in Chennai, who was considered one of the best resurfacing specialists in the world. So Vacca scheduled his own hip resurfacing with Dr. Bose, and after a 20-hour flight he arrived in Chennai.

Dr. Bose met with him for an hour before the first surgery to discuss his condition and the procedures, and after the surgery he checked on Vacca twice a day. Vacca then spent a week of additional recovery time at Fisherman's Cove, a lavish resort spa overlooking the Indian Ocean. Since he needed both hips resurfaced, the total cost amounted to $12,000 for his two surgeries, 14 days in the hospital and resort, anesthesia, and prescription drugs. A month later, his friend was astonished to see him walking and exercising — and because Vacca no longer stooped from pain, he appeared to be four inches taller.

> " *When I arrived, no one asked me if I had insurance, no one inquired as to my method of payment, and no one asked me to fill out one form. When I asked who should I give the bank draft to, I was told, 'That's not important right now. You have surgery in the morning. Take care of it when you feel settled.'*"

Heart Disease, Cancer, Transplants, and Stem-Cell Therapy

Heart Disease

Coronary artery bypass graft (CABG, pronounced "cabbage") is one of the most frequent open-heart surgeries in the United States. The medical costs, however, are not for the faint of heart. That may be a poor joke, but the reality is that people without adequate health insurance can face a tough choice: continue to suffer and risk a heart attack, or lose your savings and perhaps your home. At this time, it costs about $800 for a comprehensive physical examination that includes bloodwork and an exercise treadmill test. Everyone middle-aged or older should have one, especially those planning a fitness program. This sort of physical examination can be accomplished for as little as $50 overseas, although more typically about $150. And if the results show that you are a candidate for coronary artery bypass, meaning your heart arteries are partially blocked, well, that is where the real opportunity for saving appears. A CABG in the United States runs about $30,000 or more, and additional costs can push the total into six figures. At world-class facilities overseas, for example at Max Devi (see *India, page 201*), it can be done for as little as a 10th of that cost.

Cancer

There are at least 120 different types of cancer — all of them frightening, worthy of serious attention, and often demanding expensive treatment. Although modern medicine has greatly improved survival, there is still a general fear of even discussing cancer, and facilities providing cancer treatment tend not to feature such care in their promotions. If you would like more information on cancer treatment, look for facilities that offer "general" care — especially the large hospital systems in Asia. They also commonly include a broad variety of alternative and complementary medicine in the same facility.

In India, for example, you can have not only state-of-the-art western medicine, but also ayurvedic treatment, with practitioners working well together as a team.

Organ Transplants

Dr. Thomas Starzl is often referred to as "the father of modern transplantation." This incredibly prolific physician and researcher, who often worked three days nonstop on a particular procedure, managed to author four books, 292 book chapters, and 2,130 scientific articles. His accomplishments in surgery, immunology, and many other medical fields are legendary. He is considered the most cited physician in the world. The renowned Thomas E. Starzl Transplantation Institute was named in his honor.

I was quite impressed, therefore, when Dr. Starzl came to the University of California, Davis, where I was a medical student. His lecture was held in the largest hall, and it was standing room only. After the lecture, I found myself in the crowded lobby near the dean of the medical school. Next to him, almost hidden by the dean, was the diminutive Dr. Starzl — who caught my eye and gestured hello. The dean noticed and introduced me as a somewhat outspoken medical student. "So," Dr. Starzl asked me. "What do think of transplant medicine?"

"Really impressive," I replied, "but I think it's a gimmick."

The dean's face hardened and turned ashen. Starzl was slightly taken aback. "Why do you say that?"

"Well, no matter how good it gets," I said, "the number of available organs will never meet the need, and in the end, a few thousand transplants won't make any difference in the overall public health." At that point, the dean quickly introduced a couple of other people to the famous surgeon, and the attention turned away from me. (Weeks later, I apologized for embarrassing him, but he laughed and said he privately agreed with me.)

Many years have passed since then. Transplant surgery is much improved and commonplace throughout the world. But it is still horrifically expensive, and medical insurance is understandably reluctant to pay for it. A liver transplant is about $350,000 and up. The fact is: Organ transplants are still available only to the wealthy and the fortunate.

Some poorer countries have entered this rather exotic type of medical tourism. Because of ethical issues, they have shied away from publicity. Patients who desperately need a transplant, and are losing hope, might learn informally about kidneys available in India for about $40,000. Regardless of what the official line is, most people suspect the truth; these kidneys are purchased from poverty-stricken beggars, of which India has tens of millions. Most people are disgusted by the thought of people resorting to selling their organs for cash. In fact, this is illegal in the United States Those who need the organs, however, often find a way to rationalize this activity.

The transplant business in China is much more insidious and therefore officially denied. However, a December 2005 article in a British financial magazine revealed the truth in its headline: "China's death-row kidneys get U.K. buyers." It appears that executed prisoners in China had "voluntarily donated" their organs for transplant to foreigners. The price charged to the U.K. patients — about $30,000 for a kidney — included a month-long hospital stay. In Chinese prisons, inmates have a blood sample taken for type and matching. Every year, about 5,000 prisoners are executed, typically with a bullet to the back of the head. Official government policy allows the "harvesting" of organs if the prisoner or prisoner's family has given written consent, or if the body is not claimed after execution. The actual practice is slightly different. According to confidential reports, the transplant service simply puts out an order for a prisoner with the medical tourist's blood type. Professor Nadey Hakim, head of transplantation surgery at Hammersmith Hospital, United Kingdom, believes that the prisoner's organs are then harvested *before* execution, in order to ensure quality. (In October 2007, the Chinese government officially denied further harvesting of prisoner's organs for foreign transplants; but I suspect this denial may join a long list of other official denials — such as not having political prisoners, not forbidding religion, not destroying Tibetan monasteries, etc. — which are all rather unconvincing when you look at the evidence.)

For the near future, organ transplant will continue to be the only recourse for some patients. But another therapy is on the horizon, which will ultimately make transplants a relic of history. It is a way of regenerating organs that will be available to everyone, at a much cheaper cost, and truly has the potential to transform the public health. This is stem-cell technology.

What Are Stem Cells?

The life of a human begins at conception. At that moment, a single cell, the egg, is fertilized. Soon after, it begins to divide — into two, four, eight, 16 cells and so on, with each division doubling the number of cells. After just 20 divisions, there are over a million cells. These first cells are all the same. Gradually, with successive divisions, the daughter cells become more specialized. The process of increasing specialization eventually leads to the highly specific tissues of the body. The early, not yet specialized cells are called stem cells — they have the capacity to produce cells that become specialized into any kind of tissue.

Stem cells are remarkable. They can divide many times to create a large number. After receiving certain chemical signals, they can produce directed specialized cells, such as a heart cell or nerve cell. If these cells could be produced and transformed at will, they could create new heart and nerve tissue. Actor Christopher Reeve, who suffered neck-down paralysis after a horseback riding accident, had hoped before his untimely death that stem-cell therapy could eventually restore his spinal cord. With new tissues from stem cells, organ replacements would no longer be necessary. Each person could replace any damaged tissue — endlessly. The potential of stem cells can barely be imagined.

During the 20th century, the discovery and development of antibiotics transformed medicine. In the 21st century, I am convinced that stem cells will do the same.

Types of Stem Cells

- *Totipotent* stem cells can differentiate into any cell type in the body plus the placenta, which nourishes the embryo. A fertilized egg is a type of totipotent stem cell, as are the first few divisions.
- *Pluripotent* stem cells are descendants of the totipotent stem cells of the embryo, developing about four days after fertilization. They can differentiate into any cell type, except for totipotent stem cells and the cells of the placenta.
- *Multipotent* stem cells are descendents of pluripotent stem cells. They are partly specialized. The hematopoietic (blood) stem cells, for example, can differentiate into the dozens of different types of blood cells. Neural stem cells can differentiate into all the different nerve cells.
- *Unipotent* or *progenitor* stem cells can produce only one cell type. But they can reproduce these cells endlessly.

Where Do Stem Cells Come From?

There are three sources of stem cells: embryos, fetal germ cells, and adult peripheral stem cells. When a particular stem cell is grown in the laboratory to produce a colony for later use, the colony is called a stem-cell line. In the U.S., the National Stem Cell Bank distributes these lines for researchers. In other countries, many private companies do so.

Embryonic stem cells (ESCs) are derived from four- to five-day-old embryos, which contain about 30 pluripotent cells. The embryos are generally taken from excess embryos from fertility clinics. Each time a woman has in-vitro fertility treatment, about a half dozen embryos are created. If the extra ones are not frozen for later use, they are destroyed. Currently, there are over 400,000 unused frozen embryos in U.S. fertility clinics. Since the rest would be destroyed anyway, it is considered ethical to use them for scientific research. ESCs are pluripotent and relatively easy to grow. However, the use of embryonic stem cells has run into tremendous opposition in the United States Religious organizations, in particular, feel that embryos or fetuses should have the same rights as humans do after birth. In their view, killing an embryo to use its tissue is equivalent to murder. (They are also against IVF, because that typically involves discarding unused embryos; in other words, killing them.) President Bush has faced this dispute by trying an awkward compromise: to allow the use of current stem-cell lines (which numbered just 25 useful lines at the time of his order) but prohibit development of more embryonic stem-cell lines. He also sharply restricted further research. Other countries — notably Israel, Singapore, South Korea, and India — have no such qualms and are forging ahead in research. It is estimated that the U.S. now lags three to four years behind these countries in stem cell research.

Fetal (or embryonic) germ cells are derived from so-called primordial germ cells, the cells that go on to produce sperm and eggs in adults. Germ cells are pluripotent stem cells. Less research has been performed on fetal germ cells, mainly because they are taken from fetuses that are deliberately aborted — an even more contentious issue in the U.S. Other countries are less interested in fetal germ cells because they are difficult to grow, and the differentiation into specialized tissue is much harder to control.

Adults also have stem cells, which allow continued production and specialization of new cells. They are multipotent cells, although recent research shows that some may be pluripotent. These cells would be the ideal stem cells. However, they are extremely difficult to identify. At this time, there are two major ways of getting adult stem cells: from bone marrow and from umbilical cord blood.

Bone-marrow transplants are really a sort of stem-cell therapy. Since the stem cells cannot be identified, a tube of marrow is extracted from a donor and put into the patient — hoping that it contains sufficient stem cells and that they will be accepted. The procedure is complex and expensive. Some types of health insurance will pay for it; otherwise, the patient has to pay upwards of $100,000 for the treatment. Bone-marrow transplants can be had for much less in other countries — it is a growing part of medical tourism — but it is still expensive.

Since the fetus has a large number of stem cells, it makes sense that the placenta and umbilical cord would have some as well. These birth products used to be discarded. Now, some of the blood from the placenta and umbilical cord after birth is often kept as a rich source of hematopoietic (blood-forming) stem cells. Many people are banking umbilical cord blood for a supply of stem cells that could be used throughout the baby's life should the need arise. For-profit private storage cord blood banks will store

Sheep Stem Cells?

A number of border clinics in Mexico and elsewhere offer stem-cell therapy at a huge discount. Closer inspection of their claims reveals that they inject, or administer orally, so-called "stem cells" from sheep. This is total fraud. Even if the cells were verified stem cells, injected sheep cells would be quickly destroyed by the human immune system. Any such cells taken orally would be quickly destroyed by stomach acids. These clinics are operated by charlatans, and their claims are highly suspect.

a baby's cord blood for use by that individual or a designated family member. The fee for private storage varies but averages about $1,500 initially plus $100 per year. This is also considerably cheaper overseas.

Stem-Cell Therapy

The body has about three trillion cells, creating and destroying millions every second. There are several thousand different types of cells, like the leaves of a tree. All of them get their start from stem cells. Therefore, stem-cell therapy has the potential of replacing any tissue. People with neurological diseases, such as Parkinson's and Lou Gehrig's Disease, and spinal-cord injuries have few options, and their illnesses are generally regarded as incurable. Stem cells promise to change that. Already, people with certain kinds of cancer can be cured by being given a bone marrow transplant to provide the stem cells needed to restore healthy blood cells. In a few years, it will be possible for persons with diabetes to have stem cells injected into the pancreas, enabling it to once again produce insulin. Already, stem cells are being used in racehorses to replace worn-out knee cartilage — a technique that has tremendous potential for football players and other athletes whose knees are often destroyed before they reach middle age.

Currently, stem-cell therapy is not available on a commercial basis in the United States Largely because of ethical concerns, it is unlikely to be approved for many years to come. On the other hand, several countries are now actively promoting stem cell therapy. India leads the way, with many state-of-the-art facilities that operate with American physicians, and some are even guided by U.S. university research centers that are not allowed to pursue this practice at home. An entire hospital devoted to stem cells is being built in Chennai. LifeCell, a pioneer company in cord-blood stem-cell banking in India and Sri Ramachandra Medical Centre, a tertiary care multi-specialty university hospital, have entered into a joint venture to create a facility that is "exclusively for stem-cell transplants and will be conducted by experienced and renowned stem-cell transplant specialists from around the world."

Theravitae is a multinational company with facilities in the United States, Israel, and Thailand. It claims to have found a way to extract stem cells from the peripheral blood of a person — the blood is routinely taken from the arm or elsewhere. It is already treating medical tourists in Bangkok (see *Thailand*).

Assisted Reproduction

Chapter 10

Types of Assisted Reproduction

World population has gone through remarkable changes in the last century. It has quadrupled in size — from about 1.6 billion in 1900 to 6.5 billion today — leading many to fear the effects of overpopulation. However, looking at world population as a whole obscures the real picture: while growth continues in the poorest countries, the industrialized countries of Europe, North America, and elsewhere have shown much less growth. In fact, many European countries have a *negative* growth rate, and actually depend on immigrants to maintain the work force. The reason for this disparity is, of course, the many career options open to empowered and educated women. In industrialized countries, women tend to have many fewer children — often just a single child — and to postpone childbearing into their 30s and often into their 40s. However, this postponement means that many, when they do decide to have a child, face difficulty in conceiving.

Assisted reproductive technology (ART) is a relatively new field of medicine in response to the tremendous demand from women who need medical help to conceive a child. There are many such technologies. The one factor they have in common is that they are all expensive. This is a natural industry for medical tourism. Many countries now offer not only all the ART available in the U.S., but also a few additional techniques that are not available outside of experimental settings in American universities.

Because of ever-newer technology, this sort of medical tourism is not a one-way flow. The U.S. continues to hold a certain cachet around the world, attracting many "reproductive tourists" from overseas, especially to the high-status clinics of Beverly Hills, Los Angeles, where some 2,400 doctors reap a windfall for the local tax base. For example, these women can select sperm or eggs based on the donor's appearance — from height, hair and eye color, right down to the shape of the mouth and eyes, IQ, talent for sports or music, and so on. Those who don't want to travel to the U.S. can order sperm on the Internet. Donated, frozen human sperm has become an American export trade product.

Women can also purchase eggs from a donor. Attractive and academically accomplished American college students — especially if they are also gifted in sports, music, or other arts — are being offered $10,000 and more for a single extraction of ovarian eggs. This is also happening, to some extent, in other countries.

By far the most common ART service desired by medical tourists is in vitro fertilization. Cost is the primary reason: Each attempt at IVF costs about $10,000 to $12,000 in the U.S., and it is generally not covered by health insurance. Data from the National Center for Health Statistics shows that IVF is successful only 17 percent of the time. That means a woman can expect an *average* of six cycles to conceive. The final cost can therefore easily approach $100,000. In contrast, overseas clinics are far cheaper and usually offer further substantial discounts on multiple cycles.

Additional popular ART services include:

Transvaginal ovum retrieval

In this procedure, a small needle is inserted through the back of the vagina and guided via ultrasound into the ovarian follicles to collect the fluid that contains the egg.

Assisted hatching

Sometimes, the fertilized egg is perfectly healthy but has an abnormally thick wall and cannot implant into the uterus. This procedure is done during IVF, after the egg is fertilized but before it is inserted. It involves cutting a small opening in the outer layer surrounding the egg.

Gamete intrafallopian tubal transfer (GIFT)

In this procedure, a mixture of sperm and an egg is placed directly into a woman's fallopian tubes. It is a surgical procedure, following transvaginal ovum retrieval. When the egg is fertilized before the placement, it is *zygote intrafallopian tubal transfer (ZIFT)*.

Autologous endometrial coculture

For patients who have failed previous IVF attempts, or who have poor embryo quality, this procedure involves placing the fertilized eggs on top of a layer of cells taken from the patient's own uterine lining, creating a more natural environment for embryo development.

Gestational carrier and surrogacy

This is the final option for a woman who simply cannot achieve and complete a pregnancy, but still wishes to have a child with her DNA. There are many reasons for this: A woman may have a medical condition that does not allow a safe pregnancy, or has no uterus, or any number of other conditions. A "surrogate" woman is found who agrees to have the fertilized egg implanted and then carry the pregnancy to delivery, after which she hands over the baby to the genetic mother. In the U.S., this process is fraught with legal and ethical concerns, and therefore strongly discouraged. Even when the most clear-cut agreement is made, problems arise when the birth mother decides to keep the infant rather than give it up. It is also, naturally, extremely expensive. These factors combine to make such an arrangement far easier to accomplish overseas, particularly in poorer countries.

Several procedures are also possible when it is the man who is the cause of infertility: *Epididymal sperm aspiration (ESA)* and *testicular sperm extraction (TESE)*

These are types of *surgical sperm retrieval (SSR)*, in which the reproductive urologist (a specialized surgeon) extracts sperm from testis, vas deferens, or epididymis. It is a short outpatient procedure, which often can overcome cases of extreme male infertility.

Intra-cytoplasmic sperm insertion (ICSI)

Also called intra-cytoplasmic sperm *injection*, it involves the injection of a single sperm into an egg, which is then further managed as IVF. This involves an astonishingly fine needle and dexterity to accomplish the maneuver under microscopic visualization. ICSI is a very useful technique when the sperm count is low. Even if the sperm count is zero, ICSI can be performed with the use of ESE or TESA. Remarkably, ICSI allows the use of even malformed or immotile sperm, since even non-functional sperm may still carry the genetic material.

Overseas ART clinics also offer pre-implantation genetic diagnosis (PGD). This involves the use of fluorescent in situ hybridization (FISH) or polymerase chain reaction (PCR). DNA amplification is then used to help identify genetically abnormal embryos and improve healthy outcomes. The idea, in short, is to identify undesirable traits *before* implanting the embryo. The undesired embryos are destroyed.

In-Vitro Fertilization (IVF)

In vitro literally means "in glass." The act of conception — the entry of a sperm into an egg — takes place in a dish in the laboratory. Any assisted conception procedure where fertilization takes place outside the body is a form of IVF.

IVF was originally intended to overcome infertility caused by blocked or absent fallopian tubes. In recent years, IVF has become increasingly popular for women who have other reproductive problems such as irregular ovulation and a host of other poorly understood causes associated with older age.

Before considering IVF, you should have failed attempts to achieve pregnancy for at least a year or two, have ruled out infertility due to the male, and be thoroughly educated about the procedure. Once you have decided on IVF, you should have a complete gynecological check-up with breast examination and PAP smear. You should also make sure that you are immune to rubella (German measles), and it is wise to start taking a dietary supplement of folic acid.

A Typical IVF Cycle

IVF takes place in a series of steps. For medical tourists whose time is limited, some of these steps can be done before and after traveling in order to save time. The most costly parts of the treatment are steps 2-5. The remaining steps can be performed by your primary care doctor.

1. About one week before your cycle, you will be given fertility medications to stimulate egg production.
2. Eggs are then extracted from your ovaries, by use of a long needle guided by ultrasound.
3. The eggs are fertilized in the laboratory with sperm.
4. The embryos are allowed to develop for 2-5 days.
5. The highest-grade embryos are selected and transferred into the womb by use of a special catheter.
6. Further medications are given to encourage pregnancy.
7. Ultrasound and hormone tests are done once a week.

Side Effects and Complications

The most immediate side effect of IVF treatment is from the hormones used to stimulate the ovaries at the beginning of the cycle, causing moodiness, headaches, bloating, tiredness, and tender breasts.

Also related to the hormones is the risk of hyperstimulation of the ovaries. Ovarian hyperstimulation syndrome (OHSS) is characterized by painful enlargement of the ovaries, collection of fluid in the abdomen (and sometimes the chest), nausea, vomiting, dehydration, and a risk of blot clots. If OHSS happens, it is usually in the last week of the cycle, after the eggs have been collected and a few days after the embryos have been transferred.

Comparative Cost of IVF

Bulgaria $1,433	Greece $2,500	South Africa $3,500
Russia.....................$1,500	India $2,500	Argentina................$3,865
Iran........................$1,800	Israel......................$2,560	Canada $4,800
Cyprus $1,900	Poland $2,750	Barbados.................$6,000
Thailand..................$2,125	Egypt......................$3,000	Australia..................$7,000
Malaysia..................$2,250	Czech Republic $3,300	United States $10,000
Brazil......................$2,500	Dubai......................$3,400	

Possible complications with pregnancy are less immediate. Multiple pregnancy is much more common with IVF, and the more fetuses there are to share the womb, the riskier the pregnancy. Even with just one fetus after IVF, there is a slightly increased risk of premature delivery, low birth weight, or miscarriage. However, birth defects are no more common with IVF that after natural conception.

Single vs Multiple Embryos

In order to increase the chances of pregnancy, most ART providers transfer several embryos into the womb. However, this practice has resulted in a lot of twins, triplets, and even higher numbers of fetuses — greatly increasing the risk of miscarriage and numerous other problems. Now there is a trend toward transferring just one embryo. It is also possible to have an IVF cycle without having any hormone treatment. This is called a "natural cycle," and just one egg is collected for fertilization in the laboratory.

The use of multiple embryos is common, especially for older women, who are thought to have less chance of becoming pregnant during IVF. However, a recent study in Finland of 2,000 IVF treatments found that single embryo transfer was as effective for older women as for younger women. Nonetheless, most women still prefer to have two embryos transferred to enhance the likelihood of pregnancy.

With more sophisticated technology, higher-quality eggs and embryos can be selected. This has raised the success rate per cycle to 25 percent, or more. Be very skeptical, however, of clinics that claim more than 30 percent overall success.

Abortion

The medical termination of pregnancy is one kind of medical tourism that is not promoted. Many religions forbid abortion, it is illegal in many countries, and almost everywhere there is extreme social stigma or opprobrium attached to the procedure. Therefore, the typical motivations to have an abortion overseas are because they are available, inexpensive, and, most of all, anonymous.

Islam, for example, forbids abortion. Consequently, India has a thriving business of providing abortions for Muslim women, especially from Arabic countries where abortion is strictly illegal.

The procedure itself is quite simple, particularly if it is very early in the pregnancy. After an ultrasound examination to confirm pregnancy, the surgery takes about six to seven minutes. The cost in India is about $150 to $250.

Many clinics have restrictions on who they will accept for abortion. Some limit patients to women who already have at least two children, or are in a precarious state of health such that pregnancy would result in a great risk, or those who have been raped, or are very young. At a quality clinic, there will be an interview to make sure the procedure is appropriate before it is carried out.

Alternative Medicine

Chapter 11

What is Alternative Medicine?

Modern, scientific medicine developed from laboratory research, clinical trials, and complex statistical analyses of large populations (the science of epidemiology). Because of its evident success it has become the standard medical system throughout the world. But not everyone is satisfied by it. There are still many chronic diseases for which scientific medicine does not have good options. There are also many conditions of poor well-being that standard medicine does not even recognize as illnesses. Therefore, people are increasingly turning to other medical traditions, folk remedies, and countless newer therapies ranging from herbs to massage and other types of "bodywork."

To distinguish the enormous variety of these types of healthcare from standard medicine, they are referred to as alternative medicine. The terms "naturopathic" and "complementary" medicine are also used, especially for well-established practices such as homeopathy, acupuncture, and ayurvedic therapies. Finally, there is a growing interest in "integrative medicine," as espoused by Andrew Weil and others, that emphasizes general well-being and is very eclectic in its use of therapies.

Over 500 systems of alternative medicine have been identified; there are well over 150 types of massage therapy alone. The most extensive are those that originated in India (especially ayurveda and panchakarma) and China (acupuncture and traditional Chinese herbal treatments). Most of these are now available in the United Staes However, there is a big difference between an ayurvedic treatment from an American young adult who has taken a (perhaps mail-order) course in ayurveda, and a middle-aged or elderly healer in India who has a six-year degree in ayurvedic medicine from an established university, often followed by many years of apprenticeship under renowned masters, and has been practicing for 30 years. There is also a big difference in price. For the cost of 10 sessions in the U.S., you could probably pay for a ticket to

India to get the real thing. The same is true for acupuncture. Why pay $100 for a treatment session in the U.S. from someone who doesn't speak Chinese and therefore cannot read the original texts, and has spent anywhere from a few months to a couple of years studying acupuncture, when you can go to China, get acupuncture from a master who has studied intensely for a decade or more, and pay just $1 for a treatment?

What is Laetrile?

Amygdalin is a chemical found mostly in the pits of peaches, apricots, and bitter almonds. Ernest T. Krebs, Sr., a California physician, was the first to try apricot pits as a cancer treatment in 1920. But the substance he used was highly toxic. Still convinced of its value, he and his son extracted the amygdalin, marketed as Laetrile, and called it "Vitamin B17." Cancer, they claimed, was caused by a deficiency of this vitamin. Although medical research showed that Laetrile had no value in treating disease, clinics in Mexico continued to promote it. Most famously, actor Steve McQueen spent enormous sums of money on Laetrile injections from cross-border clinics before his death from cancer. Medical tourists continue to seek Laetrile treatments in Mexico and other countries.

Alternative medicine was historically available from specialized clinics or individual practitioners in the countries where the therapies originated. They were popularized mostly by word-of-mouth. Now, medical tourists have a much better and more consistent way of finding these services — at spas. The spa phenomenon is mostly associated with recreation and soaking in hot springs, but it has evolved throughout the world to provide an astonishing variety of alternative health treatments, and even minor cosmetic surgery.

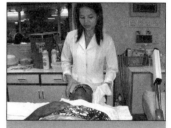

An American enjoys a relaxing Thai facial massage in Bangkok.

Spa Tourism

The word spa comes from the Latin phrase "*solus per aqua*," meaning "health by water." It is an ancient phenomenon, not only in Europe, but everywhere in the world. For much of the past millennium, spa was synonymous with healthcare. Towns grew up around renowned hot mineral-water baths. Consider, for example, the towns and cities in Germany designated specifically as a place of the bath (*bad* in German):

- Alexisbad
- Bad Berka
- Bad Doberan

- Bad Abbach
- Bad Bevensen
- Bad Elster

- Bad Aibling
- Bad Cannstatt (Stuttgart)
- Bad Ems

- Bad Endorf
- Bad Klosterlausnitz
- Bad Kösen
- Bad Marienberg
- Bad Neuenahr
- Bad Pyrmont
- Bad Salzuflen
- Bad Segeberg
- Bad Tölz
- Bad Wildbad
- Baden-Baden
- Wildbad Kreuth

- Bad Godesberg
- Bad König
- Bad Kreuznach
- Bad Mergentheim
- Bad Oeynhausen
- Bad Reichenhall
- Bad Salzungen
- Bad Sulza
- Bad Vilbel
- Bad Wildungen
- Heilbad

- Bad Honne
- Bad Königshofen
- Bad Lausick
- Bad Nauheim
- Bad Orb
- Bad Säckingen
- Bad Schwartau
- Bad Sülze
- Bad Wiessee
- Bad Wörishofen
- Wiesbaden

The city of Bath, in England, is named after a prominent spa established by the Romans. In Wales, the term wells is used, with resulting towns named:

- Builth Wells
- Llandrindod Wells
- Llangammarch Wells
- Llanwrtyd Wells

The Medispa

Spas lost a great deal of their role as a place of healing with the advent of modern medicine. In recent years they seem to have come full circle and are once again a popular provider of healthcare. The spa industry is booming. According to a recent survey by PriceWaterhouseCoopers, it has doubled in size since 1999. The International Spa Association (I/SPA), which sets the standards for the spa industry, states:

A spa serves as an educational and cultural institution that promotes and integrates individual wellness, health and fitness as well as social well-being, harmony and balance through wellness, prevention, therapy and rehabilitation of body, mind and soul.

But many spas are delving much further into general medical care. The greatest trend is for medical spas — sometimes called medispas — to offer a wide variety of plastic surgery procedures, including Botox and collagen injection, blepharoplasty (eyelid surgery), breast augmentation, lipoplasty (liposuction and liposculpture), rhinoplasty (nose surgery), breast reduction, facelift, and abdominoplasty. Many also offer LASIK eye surgery and dental procedures such as teeth whitening and even root canals. Resorts and sanitaria in former communist countries in eastern Europe are being turned into medical tourism destinations.

Medical spas are able to offer plastic surgery in a relaxed, vacation-like atmosphere of luxury and pampering. Patients don't worry about having to hide their surgery bruises and pain from family and friends at home. Instead, they can relax and be waited on. According to the International Medical Spa Association, medical spas currently earn $450 million in annual revenues and are growing rapidly, at a rate of 11 to 14 percent annually.

Ayurvedic Medicine

India is the birthplace of the ayurvedic system of medicine. The fundamentals of this system include balancing the three main "doshas" — *kapha*, *pita*, and *vata* — which are believed to be imbalanced in illness. The three doshas (tridoshas) are analogous to the two cosmic forces in traditional Chinese medicine (yin and yang), and the four "humors" of ancient Greek medicine (blood, yellow bile, black bile, phlegm). Kapha is considered heavy and wet, pita is light and fiery, and vata is changing and airy. The body needs each of these doshas — kapha for body fluids, pita for energy, and vata for impulse — but illnesses result when the doshas are out of balance. This imbalance can be restored by certain foods, types of exercise (particularly yoga), medications, and, especially, types of massage. This system is thousands of years old and complex enough to demand many years of study by those wishing to master it. Some of the therapeutic claims of ayurveda may seem a bit hard to believe, as you can see in the following list, but over a billion people are convinced it works. In any case, many of the therapies are pleasant and relaxing and worth trying on that account alone.

Q: Why do health tourists swarm to Kerala, in southern India, during the monsoons, when it rains constantly day and night?

A: They believe that Ayurvedic therapy works best at that time.

Abhyanga

A whole-body massage with specific herbal oils to nourish and revitalize the body tissues (Dhatus) and to allow the toxins to be removed from the cells. Abhyanga has much deeper and more far-reaching effects than an ordinary massage using mineral oils and lotions. Abhyanga achieves deepest healing effects by naturally harmonizing the body with the mind and spirit. This massage is performed symmetrically by two therapists for one hour and is usually followed by a medicated steam bath (Sweda). It is one of the most rejuvenating treatments of Ayurveda.

Treatment: 75 minutes with two therapists

Touted benefits: increases tissue strength; improves blood circulation; rejuvenates the whole body; removes cellulite; beautifies the skin; delays aging; induces sound sleep; promotes vitality; pacifies vata imbalance; reduces stress, and removes toxins.

Chakra Basti

The Basti, a warm oil, is applied to the umbilical region. It acts on the solar plexus and balances the digestive fire.

Treatment: 60 minutes with one therapist

Touted benefits: helps alleviate indigestion and constipation.

Greeva Basti

Bathing the back of the neck using warm medicated oil or herbal decoction.

Treatment: 45 minutes with one therapist

Touted benefits: relieves pain from cervical spondylosis, chronic pain in the neck region and compression fractures.

Hrid Basti

This procedure is applied over the heart using warm medicated oils or herbal decoctions.

Treatment: 45 minutes with one therapist

Touted benefits: strengthens the heart; relieves deep-seated anger and sadness; relieves cardiomyopathy.

Janu Basti

In this treatment the knee is bathed in warm medicated oils or herbal decoctions.

Treatment: 45 minutes with one therapist

Touted benefits: eases pain of knee joint; reduces symptoms of osteoarthritis of the knee joint; promotes the strength of the knee joint by improving the circulation.

Kashayasekha

This revitalizing treatment is given immediately after Abhyanga. A continuous pouring of a warm herbal decoction all over the body and simultaneous massaging by four therapists is performed, with Shirodhara given at the same time. This therapy removes kapha and vata toxins.

Treatment: 60 minutes with six therapists

Touted benefits: eases rheumatoid arthritis, osteoarthritis, and varicose veins; improves circulation; improves skin complexion; relieves body pain.

Kati Basti

A special technique aimed at providing relief to the lower back using warm medicated oils or herbal decoctions when bathing the lower back.
Treatment: 45 minutes with one therapist
Touted benefits: relieves chronic and acute backaches; eases pain of prolapsed disc, lumbar spondylosis, osteoporosis, and sciatica.

Navarakizhi

Considered a highly effective rejuvenation technique, Navarakizhi uses a special type of rice that is cooked, tied into boluses and dipped into an herbal decoction and warm milk, then skillfully massaged into the body by two therapists simultaneously for one hour, after the Abhyanga.
Treatment: 90 minutes with two therapists
Touted benefits: aids patients who have had paralytic strokes; is anti-aging and rejuvenating; strengthens tissues; eases body ache; benefits patients who have emaciation, debility, monoplegia, osteoarthritis, and rheumatoid arthritis.

Netradhara

A special cleansing technique of pouring herbal decoctions in a continuous stream over the eyes.
Treatment: 20 minutes with two therapists
Touted benefits: relaxes strained eyes; delays cataract formation; treats chronic conjunctivitis; improves eyesight; makes the eyes sparkle.

Netra Tarpana

This is a special treatment in which the eyes are bathed in pure medicated cow's milk ghee (butter in which milk solids have been removed).
Treatment: 30 minutes with two therapists
Touted benefits: relieves eye strain due to glare from computer and TV screens; improves refractive errors of the eyes, chronic conjunctivitis, corneal ulcer, dry eye syndrome, eye diseases due to aggravation of vata and pita toxins, glaucoma; helps prevent formation of cataracts; improves improper coordination and loss of movement of the eyeballs; eases pain and burning sensation in the eyes.

Pada-abhyanga

A very stimulating massage of the lower legs and the feet to activate the acupressure points.

Treatment: 30 minutes with two therapists
Touted benefits: improves eyesight; soothes and cools the eyes; alleviates burning of the eyes; induces deep sleep; improves luster of the skin; helps smooth cracked skin of the feet; relieves hypertension and tiredness of the feet.

Padaghata

This is a very unique whole-body massage using feet instead of hands.
Treatment: 60 minutes with two therapists
Touted benefits: removes deep-seated pain in the joints and bones; is deeply relaxing; helps in removing toxins from deeper tissues; removes excess fat.

Patra Pinda Sweda (PPS)

A highly rejuvenating treatment in which fresh plants are fried with several other herbal ingredients and tied into boluses, dipped into warm medicated oil and simultaneously massaged by four therapists all over the body for one hour. It is applied after Abhyanga.
Treatment: 60 minutes with four therapists
Touted benefits: lessens chronic back pain; helps regain lost function of a part or whole limb; eases joint stiffness, swellings, and muscular pain; is anti-aging and rejuvenating; relieves pain of sciatica, spondylosis, sprains, and cramps.

Sarvangadhara

Medicated oil or medicated milk is poured onto the body in continuous streams while being gently massaged by four therapists for one hour. It is extremely soothing and relaxing. It acts as a free radical scavenger, toning, strengthening and deeply rejuvenating the whole body. It is given after Abhyanga.
Treatment: 60 minutes with six therapists
Touted benefits: relieves chronic fatigue syndrome; increases immunity; is anti-aging and rejuvenating; alleviates the burning sensation in the body; ensures better circulation; helps to recover from paralysis; and promotes healing of fractures.

Shirobasti

A special technique of bathing the head in medicated oils using a special apparatus.
Treatment: 45 minutes with one therapist
Touted benefits: eases anxiety, facial paralysis, insomnia, neurological disorders, psychological disorders, and skin disorders such as eczema and psoriasis; relieves stress.

Shirobhyanga

A soothing massage of the head, neck, and shoulder using warm herbal oils.
Treatment: 15 minutes with one therapist
Touted benefits: brings sound sleep; cools the eyes; relieves headache; removes dandruff; wards off premature graying and hair loss; is profoundly soothing and relaxing.

Shirodhara

A continuous stream of medicated warm oil and herb decoctions with medicated milk or buttermilk is poured onto the forehead for 20 to 40 minutes. This procedure often induces a mental state similar to a trance, which creates profound relaxation of the mind and body. It is deeply relaxing and revitalizes the central nervous system. Shirodhara gives the best results when taken after an Abhyanga.
Treatment: 45 minutes with two therapists
Touted benefits: relieves anxiety, depression, epilepsy, hypertension, diabetic neuropathy, central nervous system problems, hemiplegia, paraplegia, and insomnia; wards off premature graying of the hair and hair loss; beneficial to those with mental retardation, paralysis or stress, and strengthens the sensory organs.

Shiropichu

Medicated oil is applied to the head in a ritual manner.
Treatment: 45 minutes with two therapists
Touted benefits: eases facial palsy, headache, and insomnia; improves memory; relieves dermatitis of the scalp, dandruff, other neurological disorders; helpful for paralysis and skin disorders such as eczema.

Sweda

By using special herbs specific to the patient's doshas and ailments, an herbal steam bath is administered, which opens the pores and flushes and cleanses the system through the skin. Its effect is enhanced when taken after Abhyanga.
Treatment: 20 minutes with one therapist
Touted benefits: reduces pain in the body; eliminates toxins; promotes a feeling of lightness in the body; reduces stiffness; beautifies the skin; removes cellulite.

Talam

An herbal paste with oil is applied to the head.
Treatment: 15 minutes with one therapist
Touted benefits: relieves insomnia; gives a cooling effect to the head and relieves

burning sensation of the scalp; improves eyesight; relieves skin disorders and headache.

Talapodichil
An herbal paste is applied to the entire head.
Treatment: 45 minutes with two therapists
Touted benefits: eases headache, depression, and hyperactive conditions; relieves burning sensation in the eyes; helps improve insomnia and skin disorders.

Udvartana
This is a specialized herbal treatment for weight reduction. An herbal paste or powder is applied all over the body and deeply massaged with specific movements by two therapists for one hour.
Treatment: 60 minutes with two therapists
Touted benefits: tones the skin and muscles after child birth or weight loss; removes cellulite; treats obesity by facilitating weight reduction; imparts good complexion to the skin; revitalizes the sense of touch; and removes kapha toxins from the body.

Panch Karma

Panch karma (also called Panchakarma) is a purifying therapy to enhance the metabolic process through food and herbal medicines. It is used in deep-rooted chronic disease as well as seasonal imbalance of *tridoshas* — in other words, all the doshas. As the wastes are eliminated from the body, the person becomes healthy. Literally *panch* means five, and *karma* means action. So panch karma means five types of actions or techniques or treatment. These types of therapeutics are based on elimination therapy.

Doshas and waste materials accumulate in the body as a result of following an improper diet and lifestyle. Various panch karma treatments are used to eliminate these excess doshas or impurities from the body. The five techniques are:

- *Vamana*: Use of emetics
- *Virecana*: Use of laxatives
- *Basti*: Medicated enemas
- *Nasya*: Nasal administration
- *Rakta Mokshana*: Blood letting

Before actually doing the panch karma, some preparatory treatments are done. These *purva karma* include:

Snehan

This is olation (oil) therapy.

Internal Snehan uses medicated oils or ghee (clarified butter) for internal use. External Snehan comprises different kinds of massage. Medicated oils are applied to the body, and different methods are used to rub them in.

Swedana

This refers to fomentation or heating therapy. Different types of fomentations, such as steam baths and poultices, are used on specific parts of the body. Many kinds of warm medicated oils, water, milk, and herbal decoctions are also used. They are either used in a bathtub or poured on the body.

Panch Karma is normally followed by *paschat karma*, which includes:

Samsarjan Karma

A special diet and lifestyle are prescribed for about two weeks. The patient need not be admitted for this karma.

Shamana

An internal medicinal treatment is given for the disease for which panch karma was done. This is to give permanent relief from the disease.

Rasayana

This means rejuvenating therapy.

PART II

A Global Guide to
Medical Tourism Facilities

Captain Renault: What in heaven's name brought you to Casablanca?
Rick: My health. I came to Casablanca for the waters.
Captain Renault: The waters? What waters? We're in the desert.
Rick: I was misinformed.
~ from the 1942 film, *Casablanca*

If you start with Internet medical tourism referrals, you may end up being sold on a watery paradise in the Sahara Desert.

The following chapters describe medical tourism services in 45 countries that actively promote the industry. Use these descriptions as a starting point. For further information, it is best to contact the facilities directly.

Keep in mind that overseas calls from the United States are preceded by 011, after which you enter the country code and other phone numbers, as listed. Each country has an international dialing code for calls to the country and a different code to make a call from that country. For example, if you want to call Thailand from the United States, you would enter 011 (to call overseas from the U.S.) and then 66 (the Thailand country code) followed by the telephone number in Thailand. On the other hand, say you bought a cheap phone card in Thailand and want to call the United States. You would enter 001 (to call overseas from the Thailand) and then 1 (the U.S. country code) followed by the 10-digit telephone number (area code and local number). Confusing? Here is a website to make it easy: www.countrycallingcodes.com

Space limitations prevent an exhaustive listing of every service, and in any case, new ones are appearing continually. Those listed here are generally the most prominent and long-standing.

Prices, which are based on figures reported in 2006, are given in U.S. dollars. This is because many hospitals, physicians, and facilities now prefer being paid that way — or indeed, demand it — and because local currencies can be unstable. Most facilities accept credit card payment. Some, especially the larger hospitals, will help arrange payment plans if necessary.

Argentina

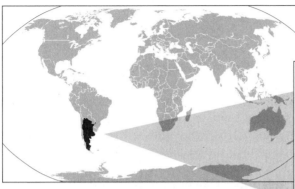

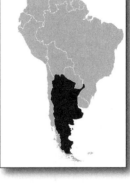

Argentina Politics:

Along with a strong presence of Italian culture, Argentina seems to have inherited Italy's habit of short-lived governments. After seemingly endless turmoil, the government and economy are now relatively stable, and foreigners are welcomed with the warmest hospitality. A slightly testy subject, however, is the Falkland Islands, which Argentines call Las Malvinas and consider to be part of their country even though the islands have been inhabited only by British sheepherders throughout their history.

Argentina Travel Requirements:

A valid passport is required. U.S. citizens do not need a visa.

República Argentina is the second largest country of South America and the eighth largest country in the world — a vast land ranging from the tropics to the southern tip of the continent and jumping off point for Antarctica. The strong Italian and German influence flavors the Spanish dialect and gives the country a very European feel. There is a long tradition of advanced education and international medical research, with major hospitals and medical centers simply named British Hospital, French Hospital, German Hospital, Italian Hospital, and Swiss Hospital. It is therefore no surprise that Argentina has taken a lead in the development of medical tourism in Latin America. The entire range of healthcare is included — from state-of-the-art surgery in the university hospitals of Buenos Aires to volcanic spas with thermal waters next to the highest mountains in the Americas. This combination draws both medical and health tourists. Perhaps the ultimate experience is a combination of surgery in the capital followed by a rejuvenating stay in one of the rural resorts.

For Americans, healthcare in Argentina is a bargain. The overall cost of living was described in the *New York Times* (April 2006) as "shockingly inexpensive." However, few Americans seem to be aware of this except for Argentine expatriates. At this time, the majority of Argentina's medical tourists are from Europe.

In summary: Argentina is bold. Think tango and beef, gauchos and Patagonia, and the exuberance of Buenos Aires, one of the world's greatest cities. There is nothing shy about this country. The result is a potential for excellent and inexpensive healthcare along with a great vacation. Argentines take pride in their education and culture, and their doctors tend to be very personable. A medical tourism blog of Argentina had the following comment:

What can be better than having a qualified doctor come to your house and arrange to have medicine delivered to your house? I know of several expats who have relatives on chemo come here to do their cycles because it is a more gentle and human approach to treatment. I have a child with Type 1 diabetes and the care is comparable to what we were receiving at Yale; and I have the doctor's home phone number.

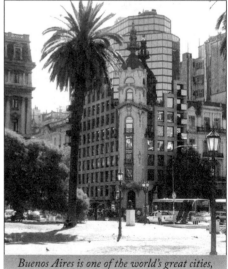

For more personal questions on medical tourism in Argentina, please send an e-mail to gaelle33j@yahoo.com.

Buenos Aires

Plenitas

Plenitas is a collective medical tourism agency that offers care through alliance agreements with 17 leading medical clinics, hospitals, and centers with access to hundreds of board-certified doctors and specialists. Medical tourists have access to more than 20 medical specialties such as cardiology, dentistry, ophthalmology, and plastic surgery, including the most popular procedures of breast

Buenos Aires is one of the world's great cities, combining European and tropical, old and new, in its culture and architecture.

augmentation and liposuction. The website, in both English and Spanish, provides information for all clinics, doctors' *curriculum vitae,* and the procedures available.

Once you arrange treatment with Plenitas, you are set up with:

- A 24/7 personal assistant
- Pre-travel consultations with your doctor
- Post-surgery consultations with your doctor
- Post-treatment recovery

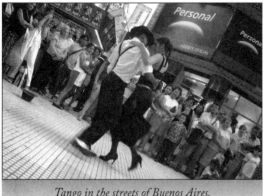

Tango in the streets of Buenos Aires.
This is the place to take a few lessons from the best.

After flying to Buenos Aires, you will arrive at the Ezeiza International Airport (EZE). One of the Plenitas personal assistants will welcome you at the airport and take you to the hotel. The representative will confirm with you all the details of your trip. Your assistant will be your personal interpreter, accompany you to every medical consultation, and answer your questions regarding medical treatments.

Plenitas specializes in breast implants, liposuction, nose surgery, gastric banding, dental implants, hair transplant, and angioplasty. The most popular package at Plenitas is the "Breast Implants & Tango Package," a seven-day experience that combines private tango dance lessons with FDA-approved silicone implants. The highlight of this package is a tango dinner-dance show at the world-famous *La Esquina de Carlos Gardel.* Plenitas also offers tours to Buenos Aries, Iguazú Falls, Patagonia, Mendoza, Ushuaia and Tierra del Fuego, which can be coordinated with your medical procedure.

Plenitas requires an up-front charge of 30 percent of the package's total cost in order to make the reservations, with the remaining 70 percent due at least 15 days before the trip. Payments must be made by a bank transfer or via Western Union. In my opinion, such stringent payment demands indicate that you should be very sure that you want to proceed, and get a detailed written agreement on the services provided. In general, when you pay up front with wired funds, you have virtually no recourse if things do not turn out as you expected.

☎ Roberto Gawianski 54-11-6771-9097 (Argentina)

☎ Alec J. Rosen 786-457-6680 (Florida)

🌐 www.plenitas.com

British Hospital (Hospital Británico)

This hospital was started in 1844 by English immigrants as a non-profit hospital to serve the public. It has since grown into a major medical complex. The curious thing about the British Hospital is that few of the doctors speak English, although translators are provided. This hospital does not focus on the usual medical tourism procedures such as plastic surgery, but offers standard medical and surgical services.

- Hospital Británico
- Perdriel 74
  Ciudad Autónoma de Buenos Aires - C1280AEB Argentina
- 54-11-4309-6400
- www.hospitalbritanico.org.ar

German Hospital (Hospital Alemán)

Perhaps the largest complex in Buenos Aires to encourage medical tourism, the German Hospital provides all standard services, including an extensive organ transplant facility. Virtually all the doctors here speak English, although sometimes slowly.

- Hospital Alemán
- Av. Pueyrredón 1640 1118
  Ciudad Autónoma de Buenos Aires Argentina
- 54-11-4827-7000
- 54-11-4805-6087
- www.hospitalaleman.com.ar

Italian Hospital (Hospital Italiano)

This facility emphasizes pediatrics among the comprehensive services it offers. Most of the doctors here speak at least some English.

- Hospital Italiano
- Gascon 450
  Ciudad Autónoma de Buenos Aires - C1181ACH Argentina
- 54-11-4959-0200
- www.hospitalitaliano.org.ar

Robles Clinic of Plastic Surgery (Clinica Robles)

The Robles Clinic was established in 1983 by the highly regarded Dr. Marcelo Robles, who is a specialist in reconstructive and plastic surgery and a member of the International Society of Aesthetic Plastic Surgery.

- Clinica Robles
- Virrey del Pino 2530
  Buenos Aires C1426EGT Argentina

☎ 54-11-4781-7147

✆ 54-11-4786-0560

@ info@clinicarobles.com

Swiss Medical Center
A high-quality hospital with comprehensive services.

🏥 Swiss Medical Center

✉ Av Puerredón 1414
Buenos Aires Argentina

☎ 54-81-0333-8876

🌐 www.swissmedical.com.ar

Hair Recovery Argentina (Centro médico de microtrasplante capilar)
This is a chain of seven clinics throughout Argentina and one in Madrid, Spain.

🏥 Centro médico de microtrasplante capilar

✉ Avenue Córdoba 827, Pisos 1ro y 2do
Buenos Aires Argentina

☎ 54-11-4311-1025

@ info@hairrecovery.com.ar

Kaufer Eye Clinic
All eye surgeries with particular specialty in cataract removal.

🏥 Kaufer Eye Clinic

✉ Carlos Pellegrini 2266
Martínez B1640BNT Prov. de Buenos
Aires Argentina

☎ 54-11-4733-4563

@ info@kaufer.com

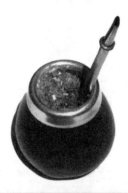

The national drink is Yerba maté. Its supposedly healthful ingredient is mateine — don't tell them it is really just caffeine.

Barbados

A top destination choice for:
assisted reproduction, fertility assistance, and
in-vitro fertilization.

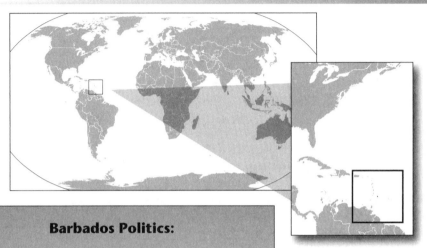

Barbados Politics:

Stable. It is always fun to be in a tiny country, where you might find that your hotel manager is also the Minister of Transportation and the bar owner is the Minister of Health. In these "micro-states," everyone knows just about everyone else, which adds to the sense of community and isolation from the problems of the greater world.

Barbados Travel Requirements:

A valid passport is required. U.S. citizens do not need a visa.

Sun, sand, and romance are the reasons so many tourists go to the tropical islands of the Caribbean. Now add to that in-vitro fertilization (IVF) treatments. Maybe this is no surprise. For decades, young vacationing couples worried about preventing pregnancy. As the youngest of the baby-boomers become middle-aged, many of them now worry that they *won't* become pregnant. Delayed marriages, careers, and busy modern lives have pushed back the desire to have children, and then, when the time finally seems right, it is nature's turn to be reluctant. In the past, adoption was the only other choice. Today, IVF and its many variations provide new options for women to conceive. In fact, many do so without waiting for Mr. Right to come along, or even — like the group Single Mothers By Choice — prefer to go it alone.

The problem is that IVF is expensive. In the United States, the procedure typically costs about $10,000 for each cycle. Given that it takes half a dozen or more cycles for success, the total cost is staggering to prospective parents on a modest budget. It is far cheaper overseas.

IVF was a natural opportunity for the tiny island nation of Barbados since it already was a major tourist destination for young urban professional couples — the greatest market for IVF. Located in the Lesser Antilles between St. Lucia and St. Vincent, about 270 miles northeast of Venezuela, the 166-square-mile island is mostly low-lying coral and limestone and mangrove swamps. Cooled by constant trade winds, it has a colorful history of sugarcane plantations — some of which still exist — and now boasts one of the highest standards of living and literacy rates in the world.

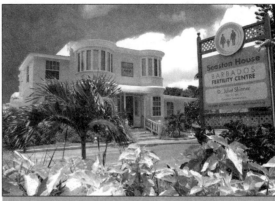

The ornate Seaston House, in Christ Church, underwent extensive renovation to become the highly sophisticated Barbados Fertility Centre, while still retaining its old world charm.

The island's single major airport, Sir Grantley Adams International Airport (GAIA; IATA identifier BGI), receives daily flights by several major airlines from points around the globe, as well as several smaller regional commercial airlines and charters. The airport serves as the main air-transportation hub for the Eastern Caribbean and is currently undergoing a $100 million upgrade and expansion.

Barbados Fertility Centre

According to Dr. Joy St. John, the island's chief medical officer of health, "the IVF procedure is turning out to be a godsend for Barbados." She feels that the procedure's value is not fully recognized by those who have not experienced infertility first-hand. "Infertile women experience distress levels equivalent to those of women who are diagnosed with cancer, heart disease, or HIV." By coming to Barbados, she says, women are given a chance to conceive that might be far beyond their budget at home.

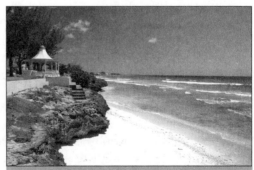

The Barbados Fertility Centre offers a beautiful view of the adjacent beach.

The major facility is the Barbados Fertility Centre (BFC), which has now moved to a new location with a commanding view of the South Coast. The BFC is equipped with ultra-modern laboratories, egg retrieval operating theatre, a four-bed recovery room as well as consultation suites and ultrasound rooms. The medical director is the highly accomplished Dr. Juliet Skinner, MRCOG, MRCPI. Despite her intimidating qualifications, she hasn't lost the characteristic Caribbean charm and hospitality and will personally ensure that your experience is enjoyable.

   📷 Barbados Fertility Centre
   ✉ Seaston House
      Hastings Christ Church Barbados
   ☎ 246-435-7467
   ✆ 246-436-7467
   🌍 www.barbadosivf.org/clinic.htm
   @ info@barbadosivf.org

Consultation Costs
Initial Consultation $125
Follow-up Consultation (Review) $100

Treatment Costs for International Patients (U.S. dollars)
IVF (inc. embryo freezing for 1 year if required) $6,000
ICSI (inc. embryo freezing for 1 year if required) $7,000
Embryo storage (per additional year) $400
Embryo thawing and transfer (including assisted hatching) $1000
Laboratory fee (sperm preparation and cryopreservation) $400
Assisted hatching $250
Refund for failed ovarian stimulation (IVF) $3,750
Refund for failed ovarian stimulation (ICSI) $4,750
Refund (if no ET) $750
Blastocyst fee $250
Testicular biopsy sperm extraction (TESE) $500
IVF with known donor eggs (incl. embryo freezing for 1 year) $6,750
ICSI with known donor eggs (incl. embryo freezing for 1 year) $7,750
IVF with anonymous donor eggs (incl. embryo freezing for 1 year) $7,500
ICSI with anonymous donor eggs (incl. embryo freezing for 1 year) $8,500

All of the above charges include in-cycle blood tests, ultrasounds, theatre charges, anaesthetic charges, doctors' fees, and one day in recovery lasting up to four hours. The costs of medication, pre-cycle tests, and counselors fees are not included.

BCF also offers complete packages including roundtrip flights from major North American cities, accommodation, and other amenities.

Belgium

A top destination choice for: breast augmentation, buttock implants, cancer treatment, cardiac bypass surgery, plastic surgery, reconstructive surgery

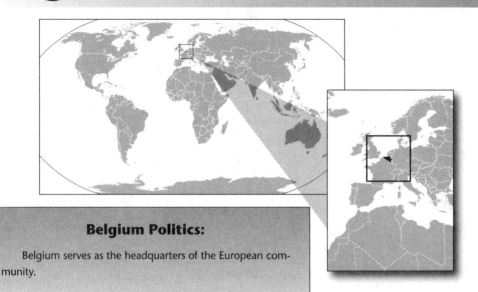

Belgium Politics:

Belgium serves as the headquarters of the European community.

Belgium Travel Requirements:

A valid passport is required. U.S. citizens do not need a visa.

The Kingdom of Belgium has a population of about 10 million, divided into distinct linguistic and cultural groups: the Dutch (unofficially called Flemish) to the north, the French to the south, German to the east — and just about every educated person can speak English. So it is perhaps no surprise that Belgium serves as the capital of the "new Europe," as well as the headquarters for NATO and many other international organizations.

As such a cosmopolitan country, it is also becoming well known for international healthcare and is becoming an attractive alternative for everything from minor cosmetic procedures to high-level surgery.

Belgium tends to be low-key, overshadowed by the much more prominent France. Yet the culture and cuisine are equal to those of its more famous neighbor. Belgium has more castles per square mile than anywhere else in the world, and in the early 20th century it created the Art Nouveau movement, which spread to Paris, Barcelona, and Glasgow. Agatha Christie's shrewd detective, Hercule Poirot, was Belgian, as was the comic strip character, Tintin. And with regard to enjoying a cool drink, Belgium produces more beer than any other country. Belgians don't take themselves too seriously and are typically warm and welcoming people. Think France, without the attitude.

Belgium has long been renowned for its healthcare. All doctors are trained for a minimum of seven years and specialists for 12 years. According to a European Heart Journal analysis of 24 European countries, Belgium ranks at the top of the list for best heart treatment in Europe. The large number of

> ### Reflecting its cosmopolitan status, Belgium has three official names:
>
> In Dutch it is *Koninkrijk België*
> In French it is *Royaume de Belgique*
> In German it is *Königreich Belgien*

private hospitals and the independent status of its hospitals mean that revenues and profit are plowed back into new equipment and technology. In a recent study by The World Markets Research Centre (a leading provider of independent business and industry intelligence), Belgium ranked top for medical care out of 175 countries.

Belgian law states that all cosmetic surgery must be carried out as same-day surgery. Therefore most surgery is done under a local anesthetic.

Prices for surgery average less than half the price in the U.S. For example, a total hip replacement is about $16,700, gastric bypass is about $16,000, a tummy tuck runs about $2,800, and liposuction is just $1,800.

Brussels

Clinic BeauCare

Located just outside Brussels at Vilvoorde, Clinic BeauCare specializes in cosmetic surgery. The staff consists of:

- Dr. Luc Vrambout, medical director
- Dr. Plovier, plastic, reconstructive and aesthetic surgery
- Dr. Berbinschi, a specialist in liposuction for over 7 years
- Dr. Carine Wijnen, a specialist in wrinkle reduction with Botox and other non-surgical modalities.

As they like to say: "The patient only has this done once; we do this all the time, and it's our duty to get it right."

- Clinic BeauCare
- Peutiesesteenweg 111
  B-1830 Machelen – Brussels Belgium
- 32-2-756-04-03
- 32-2-756-04-05
- www.clinicbeaucare.com
- @ contact@kliniekbeaucare.com

Some all-inclusive prices (please contact the clinic for up-to-date prices)

Bodycontouring
- Lifting inner thigh $2,940
- Lifting buttock..$2,220
- Armlift $1,860

Breast enlargement
- Salt-water implants $2,352
- Gel silicone implants $2,520
- Anatomical (teardrop) implants..$3,264
- Breast uplift without implant $3,000
- Breast uplift with implant..$3,720
- Breast reduction $3,120

Buttock implants $3,420
Chin enlargement with implant $1,860
Ear reshaping $1,080
Eyelid, both upper and lower...$1,920
Mini facelift (S-lift) $2,280
Mini facelift and upper eyelids $3,060
Mini facelift and lower eyelids..$3,180
Mini facelift and both eyelids $3,540
Neck correction...$1,980
Mini facelift and neck correction $3,540
Mini facelift, neck correction & both eyelids $4,260
Endoscopic forehead brow lift $2,340
Brow lift..$984
Labia reduction...$1,536
Lip enhancement...$780
Liposuction..$840
Lipostructure...$780
Male chest reduction $1,860
Areola reduction $840
Inverted nipple $840
Nose reshaping (rhinoplasty) $2,640
Nose tip reshaping..$1,260
Mini abdominoplasty...$1,680
Full tummy tuck $2,400

Brazil

A top destination choice for:
cosmetic surgery, facelift, plastic surgery,
reconstructive surgery, rhinoplasty

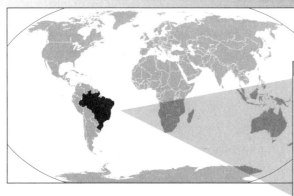

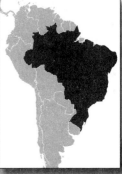

Brazil Politics:

Such a gigantic, largely undeveloped country is bound to suffer some political turmoil. While some tourists are charmed by the cultural exuberance, others are horrified by the poverty and crime. Brazil has a difficult stewardship of the world's most extensive rain forests, creating a constant conflict between those who wish to exploit them for industrial gain and those who wish to preserve this region, which truly serves as the "lungs of the earth."

Brazil Travel Requirements:

Passport with minimum validity of six months and visa required. Tourist visas are issued within two business days if the application is submitted in person. First entry into Brazil must be within 90 days of visa issuance. Submit one application form, one passport-sized photo, and proof of onward/return transportation. Travelers who have recently visited certain countries, including most other Latin American countries (check with the Brazilian Embassy), may be required to present an inoculation card indicating they had a yellow fever immunization. Children ages three months to six years require an international polio vaccination certificate. Minors under the age of 18, if not traveling with both parents, must provide a notarized letter of consent signed by the non-accompanying parent(s) or guardian authorizing the consulate to issue a visa. There is a processing fee of $100 for tourists. An additional $10 fee is charged for applications sent by mail, or by anyone other than the applicant. Provide SASE for return of passport by mail.

Brazilian Embassy (Consular Section)
3009 Whitehaven St. NW, Washington,
DC 20008
ph 202-238-2828
Internet: www.brasilemb.org
or nearest Consulate:

California ph 323-651-2664 or 415-981-8170
Florida ph 305-285-6200
Illinois ph 312-464-0244
Massachusetts ph 617-542-4000
New York ph 917-777-7777
Texas ph 713-961-3063

The Federative Republic of Brazil (*República Federativa do Brasil*) is the largest and most populous country in Latin America, and the fifth largest country in the world. As a former colony of Portugal, Brazil's official language is Portuguese. With over 4,500 miles of tropical coastline and its seemingly endless sandy beaches, blue skies, hot sun, and warm, azure waves, the usual draw for tourists is the beach. But inexpensive cosmetic surgery and dentistry are also becoming a big draw for international travelers.

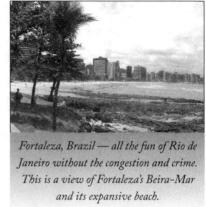

Fortaleza, Brazil — all the fun of Rio de Janeiro without the congestion and crime. This is a view of Fortaleza's Beira–Mar and its expansive beach.

Fortaleza

The magnificent beaches, warm water, clean air, and its more than 300 days of sunshine a year have combined to make Fortaleza the number-one tourist destination in Brazil. This northeast city of 2.5 million is known for its nightlife with bars, restaurants, and shows, and having the "wildest Monday nights in the world."

Bionexus International
Bionexus is a large clinic specializing in cosmetic surgery and dentistry. All of their cosmetic surgeons and dentists have completed a three-year residency at the renowned Ivo Pitanguy Institute.

Bionexus has no up-front charges. Sample costs:
Rhinoplasty (nose reshaping)..$1,860
Breast augmentation...$2,814
Upper and lower eyelids...$1,860
Facelift $2,338

     Bionexus International
     Av. Abolição, 2111, Ste. 1605
     Fortaleza, CE, Brazil
     55-85-3219-2857
     55-85-9905-0032
     55-85-3248-1931
     www.bionexus.biz
     bionexus@bionexus.biz
     Skype bionexus

Brunei

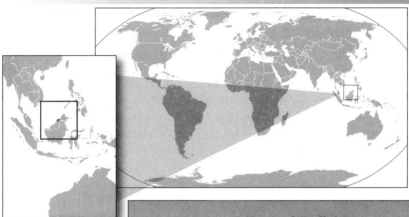

Brunei Politics:

Brunei is Muslim and has a strict authoritarian government ruled by the Sultan. Crime is minimal, and the generous oil income seems to keep everyone happy.

Brunei Travel Requirements:

Passport with minimum validity of six months and onward or return ticket required. Visa not required for stay of up to 90 days.

Formally entitled the Sultanate of Brunei (*Negara Brunei Darussalam*), this isolated country is little more than a patch of mangrove swamp on the north coast of the island of Borneo. On my first visit there, some 30 years ago, a friend translated a huge billboard for me. It read: One Purpose, One Nation, One God. "It might as well add," my friend said, "One Oil." And that is the key to this peculiar country. Southeast Asia is known more for its technological prowess than petroleum, but by luck, this tiny Sultanate has enormous reserves just off its coast in the South China Sea. The result is more money than the government seems to know what to do with. The capital — really the only town in a country with no road contact with the rest of Borneo and just a single airport — is Bandar Seri Begawan, with about 46,000 inhabitants. Its hospitality industry and medical services are probably more a matter of prestige than a need for tourism income. When I was there, I was the only guest in an enormous and lavish hotel. Since nobody knew quite what to charge me, they decided not to bother with this technicality — and my stay was free!

Gleneagles JPMC

Part of the prestigious Singapore Parkway Group of medical centers, this full-service hospital maintains Singapore-level quality in an unusual location. Prices are about the same as those of Singapore (see Parkway in Singapore), but the cost of living is lower than Singapore's, and the city is much more tranquil.

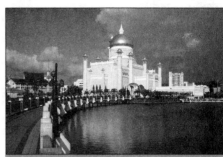

Brunei's Omar Ali Saifuddin Mosque is a sight to behold, exquisitely crafted of pure marble.

For the international visitor, there may not appear to be much to do in this rather isolated city, and tourist sites are minimal. Bring your own entertainment. But remember — this is an Islamic country. When my friend wanted a beer, he was told he risked 18 months in prison!

- 🏥 Gleneagles JPMC
- ✉ Jerudong Park, BG 3122
  Brunei Darussalam
- ☎ 673-2-261-1883
- ℘ 673-2-261-1886
- 🌍 www.gleneaglesjpmc.com.bn
- @ glenjpmc@brunet.bn

Bulgaria

A top destination choice for:
balneotherapy, Botox treatment, cosmetic surgery,
dental care

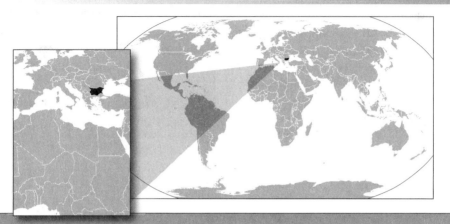

Bulgaria Politics:

Bulgaria has historically struggled to maintain its independence between shifting Eastern and Western empires. During the Second World War, it was the only country that saved its entire Jewish population (around 50,000) from the Nazis by refusing a demand to deport them to Auschwitz. The following decades brought control by the Soviet Union. Ironically, this probably preserved the country from western development and maintained its bucolic appeal. Bulgaria joined the European Union in January 2007.

Bulgaria Travel Requirements:

Passport required. A visa is not required for stays of up to 30 days. Persons staying more than 30 days should obtain a visa in advance. Visas are free of charge for U.S. citizens with regular passports; the processing fee is $25. All visitors must be able to, upon request, show proof of valid medical insurance or equivalent funds covering the duration of their stay.

For more information, contact:	or
Consular Section	Bulgarian Consulate in New York,
Embassy of the Republic of Bulgaria	ph 212-935-4646
1621 22nd St., NW, Washington, DC 20008	Consulate General of Bulgaria in Chicago,
ph 202-387-7969 or 387-0174	ph 312-867 1904
Internet: www.bulgaria-embassy.org	Consulate General of Bulgaria in Los Angeles,
	ph 310-478 6700

The Republic of Bulgaria is a small country in the southeast of Europe. Historically, it served as a crossroads of Europe and Asia. Like other countries that came under the Russian influence, it uses the Cyrillic script in its language.

This sleepy country has a long tradition of tourism, mainly Europeans coming to ski or relax among the ancient castles without the hustle of modern-day Europe. Health tourism goes back even further — as long ago as the 5th century BC. Roman Emperors used to come and stay for treatment in the healing waters of Augusta and Pautalia. Many present-day spas were built on the sites of ancient Roman *thermae* or Turkish baths. The best-known are Pavel Banya, Hisar, Velingrad, Narechen, Vurshets, Kyustendil, and Momin Prohod (near Kostenets), each of which has waters with a distinctive palate of minerals and therefore specializes in the treatment of different ailments. For example, Narechen specializes in neurological disorders, Pavel Banya in orthopedic illnesses and traumas, and Sandanski in pulmonary diseases, while Hisar, located among the impressive ruins of an ancient Roman fortress, is recommended for kidney and gastrointestinal illnesses. Sapareva Banya sprang up around the hottest water spring in Bulgaria. Two large seaside resorts, Albena and Pomorie, focus on mud-bath treatment.

Taking advantage of this history, the Bulgarian government has decided to develop health tourism in a big way, declaring in 2004 that health and medical tourism will be a leading priority. It began a campaign to push European countries to allow pension and health insurance funds to be used for care at Bulgarian resorts. The campaign worked. Now Europeans have discovered that dental care and cosmetic surgery are much cheaper in Bulgaria, with friendly service and English-speaking doctors who are happy to cater to foreigners.

Balneotherapy — A New Name For Mineral Water Treatment

Bulgaria is one of the richest countries in mineral water sources, with about 1,600 mineral springs scattered throughout the country. The quality is similar to those in world-renowned spas like Baden-Baden and Vichy. Curative mineral water for drinking, baths and mud treatment is called balneotherapy — probably, in my opinion, to make it easier to get health insurance to pay for it.

Most of the spas also offer professional rehabilitation and toning programs with a variety of modalities. For example, a 10-day anti-stress program with aromatherapy, massage, and iontophoresis in addition to the standard spa facilities costs about $120 per day. Accommodation ranges from $24 to $85 a day, including meals.

Bulgarian spa hotels work at full capacity on weekends, but typically average half capacity during the week, with corresponding discounts. If such a discount is not readily offered, it is worth inquiring about.

Slimming Centers

The most popular clinic for non-medicinal treatment of obesity is located in the Black Sea resort of Sts. Constantine and Helena. There, you have the opportunity to undergo a "mild form of medical starvation" under constant medical supervision. You

---

are generally allowed to eat one kilogram of raw fruit per day. Packages include accommodation in a four-star hotel, daily doctor's rounds, personal consultation with the head physician, medical examinations, and your own personal dieting and nutrition schedule. The stay in the sanatorium usually lasts 10 to 20 days, and costs about $600 to $2,400, depending on the package chosen.

Plastic Surgery

In the 1990s, Bulgaria experienced a proliferation of clinics providing plastic and cosmetic surgery, largely in response to demand from residents of nearby countries where such services were less available. Competition among these clinics has brought excellent quality and low prices. The owners vie with one another to get the best specialists, have the most modern equipment, and provide an increasing range of amenities for patients. All this has been a boon for medical tourists looking for quality and value. Expect to pay about $1,500 for a face-lift, $550 for reshaped lips, and $360 for liposuction.

Dental Services

The easiest entrée for a country promoting medical tourism is to start with spa and health resorts, followed by dental care. Bulgaria has taken the same path and is heavily promoting inexpensive dental care. Prices in Sofia, Burgas, Varna, and Plovdiv are relatively the same: from $12 to $18 for an initial examination, from $18 to $24 for cleaning and a photo polymer filling, and from $24 to $36 for the treatment of gum disease.

Sofia

Sofia is a very pleasant small city with many dental and cosmetic services. Most of these do little advertising, but are of generally excellent quality. Ask the hotel manager and other tourists for the latest in advice, recommendations, and offerings. Many medical tourists stay at the comfortable Castle Hrankov Hotel, which has a close familiarity with the clinics and makes arrangements for medical tourists.

🏨 Castle Hrankov Hotel
✉ 53, "Krusheva gradina" St.
Dragalevtzi
Sofia – 1415
Bulgaria
☎ 359-2-967-29-29
📠 359-2-967-29-45
🌐 http://clients.ttm.bg/hrankov/office@hrankov.com

Medstom

The Medical and Dental Clinic, known as Medstom, was founded in 2002 to provide full-service medical and dental care, ranging form ear-nose-and-throat surgery to urology.

A sample of procedures ....Price (U.S. dollars)
Amalgam filling ....$24–$36
Composite resin filling ....$54–$96
Veneer (per tooth) $132
Porcelain inlay...$180
Tooth extraction ....$96–$156
Prophylaxis and fluoride therapy..$18
Sealant (per tooth)..$24
Deciduous tooth extraction..$12
Pulpotomy $42
Partial denture (plastic framework)......................................$240
Complete denture (plastic framework) $300
Partial denture (metal framework) $500
Complete denture (metal framework)......................................$510
Fixed dental prostheses $72
Dental implant...$510–$1080
🏨 Medstom
✉ 26 "Dondukov" Blvd.
Sofia – 1000
Bulgaria
☎ 359-2-981-00-00
📠 359-2-988-31-80
@ medstom@abv.bg

Velingrad

Velingrad is the most beautiful and most famous of the Bulgarian balneological resorts. It lies at the western end of Chepino Valley, in the Rhodopean Mountains of southern Bulgaria. There, mineral waters from about 70 springs vary considerably in temperature, mineralization, radon, silicic acid, and fluorine content, and are suitable for treatment of a wide range of illnesses. The town is surrounded by ancient pine forests, which locals believe provide a beneficial influence on pulmonary emphysema, chronic bronchitis, post-bronchial pneumonia, and other lung diseases.

One of the most attractive places for spa and beauty tourism now is Hotel Dvoretsa ("The Palace"). It was thoroughly renovated two years ago and is now a five-star hotel famous for its mineral outdoor and indoor swimming pools. The spa center offers more than 100 different treatments and prophylactic procedures for wellness and beauty, including thalassotherapy, pearl therapy, whirlpool and contrast baths with mineral water, herbs, lye or medical preparations, manual and underwater massage with bio-products and lotions, and aromatherapy.

☎ 359-359-56-200
✆ 359-359-5-10-98
🌐 www.dvoretsa.com
@ reservations@dvoretsa.com

China

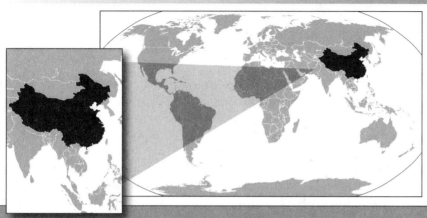

China Politics:

After the horrendous failures of communism and the "cultural revolution" of the 1960s, during which much of the nation's business and intellectual capital was destroyed, China has emerged to embrace international trade and domestic entrepreneurship. The result is a growing financial power that seeks to excel in every industry and service — including healthcare.

China Travel Requirements:

Passport and visa required. Due to a tightened visa policy, travelers may be required to undergo a personal interview. Transit visas are required for any stop in China — even if you do not exit the plane or train. Tourist visas are issued only after receipt of a confirmation letter from a Chinese tour agency or letter of invitation from a relative in China. Single-entry visas require a $50 processing fee; double-entry visa fees are $75 (no personal checks), $100 for a 6-month multi-entry, and $150 for a 12-month to 24-month multi-entry visa. Allow at least four business days for processing. Visas are valid 90 days from date of issue. If the traveler is HIV positive, entry is not permitted for any purpose. Previous visits to Taiwan can complicate matters: China considers Taiwan a "renegade" province, and therefore travel to Taiwan without Chinese permission is viewed as illegal!

For more detailed information, contact the Visa Section of the Chinese Embassy, 2201 Wisconsin Ave., NW, Washington, DC 20007 (202-338-6688) or nearest Consulate General: Chicago (312-573-3070), Houston (713-521-9859), Los Angeles (213-807-8006), New York (212-868-2078) or San Francisco (415-674-2940). Internet: www.china-embassy.org

With over one-fifth of the world's population, the People's Republic of China is rapidly turning into a global powerhouse. Its civilization has gone through countless

> *Doctors in China are more understanding and kind* *and with more patience. It doesn't matter how many patients are waiting to see the doctor, the doctor will take his time with each patient, as much time as he needs."*
>
> *~ Sylvia, who has traveled to China seven times for healthcare*

upheavals over 4,000 years. The nation is now gradually, hesitantly, and sometimes awkwardly shifting toward capitalism and unleashing its enormous manufacturing potential. This is obvious from a stroll through Wal-Mart or just about any major retailer, where the apparent majority of the products carry a "Made in China" sticker.

China has not yet made the same push into medical services, but the trend has already started, with many people choosing to go to Shanghai and Hong Kong for medical and dental care that is far less expensive than in the United States At this time, China lags far behind other Asian countries as a medical tourism destination — in fact, it is better known as a source of tourists traveling to these other countries for care. However, there are plans to change that. Sun Jishan, editor-in-chief of *china international business* magazine, estimates that medical tourism in China will be a $10 billion industry within a decade.

Traditional Chinese Medicine

At this time, China offers little in medical tourism other than traditional Chinese medicine (TCM). This name is commonly given to a range of ethnic medical practices that have developed over the course of several thousand years. TCM is very different from scientific, "western" medicine, by focusing on the whole person rather than a mechanical view of the parts, and by using non-invasive diagnostic measures such as meticulous examination of pulses, the coating of the tongue, and the appearance of the eyes and hair. TCM is very complex, taking as long to study as scientific medicine. Chinese medicine is based on ancient principles, such as the Theory of the Five Elements, human body energy meridians, principles of yin-yang, the flow of qi (chi), and Taoist and Confucian philosophy.

While scientific medicine tends to treat symptoms one at a time as they arise, TCM seeks to treat the entire body for imbalances that affect not only health but also overall psychological and social well-being. This method is believed to be superior because symptoms will continue to accumulate, in a deceptive variety of forms, until the underlying malady is addressed.

Acupuncture is the most common form of TCM in the United States, with treatments typically costing about $75 per session. In China, the same treatment, often in the hands of a far more experienced practitioner, will cost less than $2!

Organ Transplants

On the opposite extreme from traditional Chinese medicine is the highly controversial area of organ transplants. Because transplant services in China are often accused of procuring organs from executed prisoners, international medical associations have complained of human rights abuses and have strongly discouraged foreigners from seeking transplants. The services are not advertised and operate with a great deal of discretion. Nonetheless, it is well known that desperate individuals can obtain a kidney transplant for the right amount of cash — perhaps as little as $20,000 — and there is no doubt that other organs are also available.

"Transplant tourism" is the dark side of medical tourism. Yet it reveals a tremendous need by people who have little other recourse. As long as there is money involved, it is likely to proliferate.

Guangzhou

While there are countless TCM facilities that will gladly take foreign patients, it is a safer bet to go to the very best: the Guangzhou University of Traditional Chinese Medicine. This is one of oldest medical institutions in China. It is affiliated with 18 hospitals and treats about 3 million people per year. An advantage to travelers is its proximity to Hong Kong, making travel easier than to other Chinese cities.

Guangzhou University of Traditional Chinese Medicine

  Guangzhou University of Traditional Chinese Medicine
  10 Jichang Road, Sanyunli
  Guangzhou 510407
  P.R. China
  ☎ 359-8659-1233
  359-8659-4735
  www.acupuncture.edu

Costa Rica

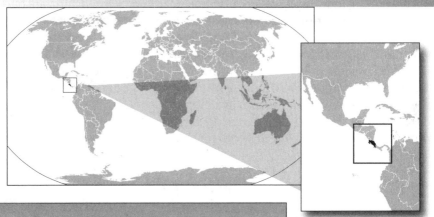

Costa Rica Politics:

Costa Rica is one of the most peaceful and prosperous countries in Latin America, with global recognition for its preservation of the tropical forests. It is the first country in the world to constitutionally abolish its army — a model other countries in the region would do well to emulate.

Costa Rica Travel Requirements:

Passport and onward or return ticket required. U.S.citizens do not need a visa.

The Republic of Costa Rica (*República de Costa Rica*) lies between the Pacific and the Caribbean, south of Nicaragua and north of Panama. Central America is a region of astonishing beauty — tropical forests, volcanoes, and white sand beaches — with activities such as deep sea fishing, swimming, surfing, sailing, scuba diving, river rafting, waterfalls, and steamy rainforest treks where you are likely to cross paths with monkeys, jaguars, deer, countless reptiles and amphibians, and about 500 species of birds. Not to mention ruins of the Mayan civilization. Despite this natural wealth, most of these countries have become agricultural exporters ruled by dictators and rapacious feudal landlords — the typical "banana republics." Costa Rica is the exception. Through brilliant leadership, its government actually *abolished* the army, created enormous nature preserves, and developed one of the best healthcare systems in the world. The result is a flourishing tourism industry, of which an increasing part is medical tourism. In 1995, the World Health Organization ranked Costa Rica in the top 20 of the best medical systems, right next to the U.S. and Canada.

Most physicians in Costa Rica have government jobs in the national health system and maintain private practices on the side, where they offer low-cost care to foreigners. A private office visit to a specialist usually costs about $30 to $50.

Major surgery is done at the large medical centers, also by private arrangement with the surgeons. One patient reported that his heart valve replacement, done with the same equipment and expertise as in the United States, cost around $15,000, including pre- and post-operative care. In the U.S., he was quoted over $50,000 for the procedure. A facelift, one of the most common requests from medical tourists, costs about $3,000 to $4,000, including clinic stay, medicines, nursing care and the surgery, in comparison to $6,000 to $12,000 in the United States. On average, medical treatments typically are about 20 percent of the cost in the U.S.

The Health Tourism Corporation of Costa Rica coordinates medical tourism efforts and provides an excellent information service.

Health Tourism Corporation, Inc.
📠 Corporación Turismo Salud, S.A.
✉ Apartado 56-2070
   Sabanilla, Montes de Oca
   San José, Costa Rica
☎ 506-229-4498
@ hlthtour@sol.racsa.co.cr

Costa Rica Health Gateways
This referral center specializes in cosmetic and dental treatment. The bilingual staff refers to CIMA Hospital, Hospital Clinica Catolica, Peralta Clinic of Plastic and Aesthetic Surgery, Gil Clinic San Pedro, and Gil Clinic Escazu.
📠 Costa Rica Health Gateways
✉ Apartado 293-Plaza Colonial
   Sabanilla, Montes de Oca
   Escazu, Costa Rica
☎ 506-203-0145
@ feelgood@costaricahealthgateways.com

San José

Prisma Cosmetic Dentistry
- ⚒ PRISMA Cosmetic Dentistry
- ✉ Banco Uno, 3rd floor
  Rhomoser Boulevard
  San José
  Costa Rica
- ☎ 506-291-5151
- ☎ 506-291-5252
- ℡ 506-291-5454
- @ dental@cosmetics-dentistry.com

Approximate costs for dental treatment at Prisma:
Root canal	$250
Post	$190
Metal crown	$250-$450
Resin filling	$75
Laser bleaching	$250

Meza Dental Care
This modern, expansive clinic was established in 1990. It provides comprehensive dental services, has fully bilingual staff, and is located 25 minutes from the San José airport. A representative shuttles medical tourists around and facilitates their stay.
- ⚒ Clinica Hospital Santa Catalina
- ✉ Banco Uno, 3rd floor
  Rhomoser Boulevard
  San José
  Costa Rica
- ☎ 506-291-5151
- ☎ 506-291-5252
- ℡ 506-291-5454
- 🌐 www.mezadentalcare.com
- @ info@mezadentalcare.com

Las Cumbres Inn Surgical Retreat
This resort is specially targeted to recuperating medical tourists. It offers a private and intimate way to recover from plastic surgery, cosmetic dentistry, and eye surgery. Located about 15 minutes from San José, the resort offers views of the city, the Cen-

tral Valley Mountains, and the Irazu, Poas and Barva volcanoes. The resort has licensed nurses and staff who have been specifically trained to meet the special needs of surgical patients and your comfort and well-being. They are coordinated with local surgeons and will provide the specifically prescribed medical aftercare, pick up prescriptions, and prepare fresh daily meals that meet specific dietary needs.

The daily resort charge covers nursing assistance, transportation to and from the airport, transport to and from surgery, guest computer with free high-speed Internet service, and three meals and afternoon tea. A $10 round-trip surcharge is added for additional doctor's appointments.

🏨 Las Cumbres Inn Surgical Retreat

✉ P.O. Box 1335-1200
Pavas
Costa Rica

☎ 506-228-1011

☎ 506 291-5252

📱 506 228-1011 ext. 215

🌐 www.surgery-retreat.com

Croatia

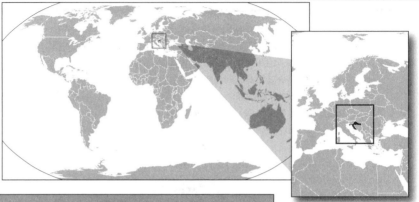

Croatia Politics:

After a horrific civil war in the 1980s, Croatia achieved independence from Yugoslavia in 1991. It is now peaceful and rapidly redeveloping its flourishing tourism industry. It is expected to join the European Union soon.

Croatia Travel Requirements:

Passport and onward or return ticket required. Visa not required for stay of up to 90 days.

The Republic of Croatia is a crescent-shaped country along the Adriatic coast of the Mediterranean. The combination of crystal-clear blue water, pebble beaches, vineyards, olive groves, and endless fields of lavender have long made it a destination for travelers seeking health and recuperation. In fact, the very first mention of "health tourism" occurred with formation of the Hygienic Society in 1868 — which also happened to be the first organized tourist society.

Today, Croatia leaves most hospital-based medical tourism to other countries but continues to excel in spas and health resorts, and its specialty — the healing mud.

Magic Mud

During the days of the Roman Empire, it was well known that you could travel across the Adriatic to a place where the ground itself would heal your ailments. They called it *peloid*, the healing mud. This mud is actually a type of silt, composed of microscopic plant pollens that settled over millions of years to form a thick deposit on ground that was once under water. The deepest concentration can be found in Morinj Bay (*Morinjski zaljev*), which now attracts people from all over the world to be treated for countless health problems. The Academy of Medical Science of Croatia has issued a certificate that confirms the benefit of this pollen for treatment of cardiovascular, neurological, rheumatic, and skin diseases, as well as disorders of metabolic, kidney, digestive, urinary, and respiratory systems.

It is believed that *peloid* heals by a combination of physical, mechanical, and chemical effects.

Thermal Springs

South from Zagreb on the river Glina lies Topusko, a spectacularly beautiful hot spring discovered in prehistoric times and founded by the colony of Ad Fines in the 1st century. Topusko's waters have been credited for curing the following illnesses:

- rheumatoid arthritis
- sterility
- skin diseases
- post-traumatic stress syndrome
- mental illness
- allergies
- degenerative rheumatism
- myofibrositis
- periarthritis
- gout
- neuropathy

Too Many Resorts to Mention ...

The number of healing resorts and the variety of treatments available in Croatia is astonishing. Evidently, 2,000 years of visitors seeking cures have produced some very imaginative treatments, including such peculiar therapies as:

- balneotherapy
- kinesiotherapy (individual and group)
- electrotherapy, with a variety of electrical currents
- thermotherapy, using infrared light and paraffin
- hydromassage
- magnetotherapy
- spinal traction

- cryotherapy (cold compresses and cryomassage)
- ultrasonic therapy and sonophoresis
- aromatherapy
- fangotherapy
- algaetherapy
- hypobaric therapy

It is not clear what most of these involve, and perhaps it is pretty much up to the individual practitioner to develop a distinctive type of therapy. Many have been created out of centuries of tradition blended with modern innovations, producing admirable results in treating chronic disease.

Croatia also has a number of more conventional cosmetic surgeons, especially in Dubrovnik and the country's capital, Zagreb.

Average prices are:
Rhinoplasty (nose reshaping) $1,860
Breast augmentation $2,700
Upper and lower eyelids $1,680
Facelift $3,420

Hrvatsko Zagorje
The Tuheljske toplice Spa and Resort is located less than 30 minutes northwest of Zagreb, within easy reach of Zagreb International Airport, and is therefore a favored destination for visitors.

Tuheljske toplice
📠 "Mihanovi " d.d.
✉ TUHELJSKE TOPLICE
LJ.GAJA 4
TUHELJ 49215
Croatia
☎ 385 49 556-224
📱 385 49 556-216
🌍 www.hupi.hr/tuhelj
@ tuhelj@hupi.net

Opatija

Antiaging Adriatic Program
The Anti-Aging Center's Fasting

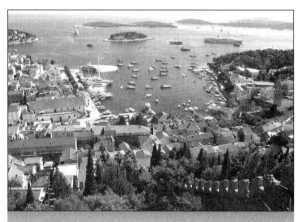

Hvar, off the coast of Croatia, was declared one of the 10 most beautiful islands in the world by Traveller Magazine, *1997.*

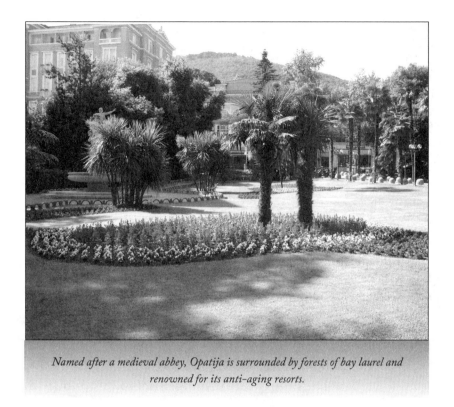

Named after a medieval abbey, Opatija is surrounded by forests of bay laurel and renowned for its anti-aging resorts.

Program consists of a seven- to 60-day program (with one to 10 days of fasting), of a variety of therapies under the supervision of an experienced fasting doctor. Their claims of cures are a bit hard to believe, but here is what previous visitors had to say about it:

> *"My goal was to regain my health, and I feel as though I have actually been given my life back; this is said with NO exaggeration! My back pain, sleep disorder, fibromyalgia, high blood pressure, excess weight, and depression are completely gone. I'm 'in love' with life again, and my entire family is delighted."*
> ~ Amy Thompson

> *"According to my wife, the whites of my eyes have also become whiter. Prefast, I also had traumatic arthritis in my hips, but during the fast and since, I've had virtually no pain in my hips."*
> ~ Tim Sheffield

☏ Antiaging Adriatic Program
✉ ul. Marsala Tita 87
51410 Opatija
Croatia
☎ 3670-202-3142
☎ 3630-612-5826
✆ 361-302-3548
🌐 www.antiaging-europe.com
@ service@antiaging-europe.com

Rovinj

The Clinic for Esthetic and Implant Dentistry
The picturesque town of Rovinj does a brisk business in medical tourism, mainly because of its well-known cosmetic and dental services.
☏ Clinic for Esthetic and Implant Dentistry
Dr. Zeljko Popadic
✉ M Benussi 5
Rovinj 52210
Croatia
☎ 385-52-830-830
@ dr.popadic@pu.htnet.hr

Terme Selce

Vlasta Brozi evi , M.D. is a specialist in physical medicine and rehabilitation at the health resort of Crikvenica resort fostering programs for preservation and promotion of health.
Crikvenica
☏ Crikvenica
✉ 1. prilaz I.L.Ribara 8
51266 Selce
Croatia
☎ 385-0-51-76-40-55
✆ 385-0-51-76-83-10
@ info@terme-selce.hr

Cuba

A top destination choice for:
abdominoplasty, cosmetic surgery, dental care

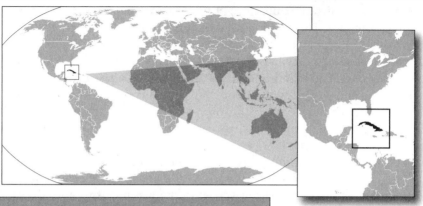

Cuba Politics:

Cuba continues to be caught in a political stand-off with the United States, in which neither side is willing to lose face by backing down. This is all due to one man: Fidel Castro. A nuisance to every American president since Eisenhower, the Cuban revolutionary leader was notorious for his preposterously long speeches — one of them lasting seven hours! As this book was going to press, Castro gave the leadership to his younger brother Raúl, who is widely expected to introduce more friendly relations with the United States.

Cuba Travel Requirements:

Passport and visa required. For specific requirements, consult the Cuban Interests Section, 2630 16th St., NW, Washington, DC 20009 (202/797-8518). Attention: U.S. citizens need a U.S. Treasury Department license in order to engage in any transactions related to travel to and within Cuba (this includes the use of U.S. currency). Before planning any travel to Cuba, U.S. citizens should contact the Licensing Division, Office of Foreign Assets Control, US Department of Treasury, (202-622-2480) or www.treas.gov/ofac

"This is the most beautiful land human eyes have ever seen!"
~ *Christopher Columbus, arriving in Cuba, October 27, 1492*

The Republic of Cuba (*República de Cuba*) is just 90 miles from the Florida Keys, but for most Americans it might as well be on the other side of the earth. Until the U.S. releases travel and trade embargos with Cuba, it is unlikely that many Americans will go there for treatment. Medical tourists from other countries, especially Canada, have no such restrictions, and Cuba is rapidly developing a significant medical tourism industry. Many Italians now couple their annual vacations to Cuba with their dental work, while others come for discounted knee replacements or eye surgery. But perhaps Cuba's most popular medical service, and the one it heavily promotes to tourists abroad, is cosmetic surgery. Cuban doctors have become expert at breast implants, tummy tucks, liposuction, and nose jobs.

The rise of Cuba as a medical tourism destination is an example of the odd and completely unpredictable outcomes of history. In 1959, Fidel Castro installed a communist government. This was followed by the U.S. trade embargo, forcing Cuba to rely on the Soviet Union for economic assistance. One of the promises of communism had been universal healthcare. This is perhaps the only promise that Castro delivered: before he took over, Cuba had one physician per 960 people and medical care was no better than in most third-world countries, which is to say, terrible. After the revolution, Cuba — with huge Soviet subsidies — built a healthcare system which became the envy of Latin America, producing one doctor for every 170 people (in comparison to one for every 188 in the U.S.), and Havana became a prominent medical center with special flights from 10 Caribbean countries and more than 15 Latin American nations.

When the Soviet Union fell apart in 1991, Cuba had to develop new revenue-producing industries — fast. The answer was obvious: tourism, and especially medical tourism. Special hospitals were built, and floors set aside in others, for exclusive use by foreigners who paid in hard currency. By 1996 more than 7,000 "health tourists" paid Cuba $25 million for medical services. Further investment flooded in, most of it from 17 international hotel chains, which now operate more than half of Cuba's hotels. By 1999, more than $3.5 billion was invested in the tourist industry, increasing hotel capacity to 35,000 rooms, and further resources were devoted to infrastructure such as airports, causeways connecting the keys, and other tourist facilities. At the beginning of the 1990s, the sugar industry provided about 70 percent of foreign income, and the tourist sector accounted for 6 percent. By the end of the decade, these numbers were reversed. In the Caribbean, Cuba is now the second most popular tourist destination.

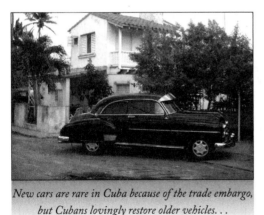

New cars are rare in Cuba because of the trade embargo, but Cubans lovingly restore older vehicles. . .

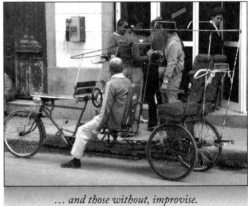

. . . and those without, improvise.

It is interesting to compare Cuba with another fiercely nationalistic country that has made tourism, and especially medical tourism, the new locomotive of its economy: Thailand. But the contrast is also quite distinctive. While Thailand emphasizes a hedonistic vacation with a dubious reputation for sex tourism (in Bangkok, it seems every middle-aged foreign man has a teenage Thai prostitute on his arm), Cuba has emphasized the opposite. President Fidel Castro declared, "Sex tourism will never be permitted, nor drugs nor anything of that sort. This is not gambling tourism; it is healthy tourism, and that is what we want; it is what we promote."

Cuba's healthcare system is now regarded as one of the best in the world, with more than 280 hospitals, 400 polyclinics, 116 dental clinics, and some 1,500 other specialty facilities. Indeed, Cuba's health statistics are almost as good as those of the U.S., and much better than Brazil or Mexico:

	Physicians (per 100,000 pop.)	Life expectancy (years)	Infant mortality (per 1,000 live births)
U.S.	215	76.9	7
Cuba	346	76.3	7
Mexico	160	72.1	29
Brazil	121	67.0	32

Much of this is due to an emphasis on fitness and preventive healthcare. Cuba has invested millions in developing vaccines, a remarkably far-sighted policy in comparison to that of the United States, which buys flu vaccine from British companies instead of producing it domestically. The United States is therefore vulnerable to critical shortages, such as occurred in 2004 when long lines of elderly and disabled people formed outside drug stores waiting for hours for scarce vaccine. Cuba's first breakthrough in medical research was a meningitis-B vaccine, now exported to over 30 countries and widely regarded as more effective than Belgian- and U.S.-produced vaccines.

Elderly Cubans are encouraged to exercise, such as by attending Tai Chi in city parks in Havana. In fact, the law *requires* all people to engage in a sport! (Though not, presumably, aviation or long-distance sailing.) Cuba is still a desperately poor, authoritarian country, and although its citizens may be healthy, a great many of them would like a bit more freedom to enjoy along with their fitness. The need for foreign currency has resulted in a separate economic system for visitors and locals. Medical tourists are catered to with the best of comfort and care, almost entirely out of reach of the Cuban citizenry.

Cuba's pharmaceutical industry manufactures more than 500 different medical products, with cutting-edge products for neck and breast cancer. One of them, the drug TheraCIM h-R3, has caused enormous excitement in the world of biotechnology. If it receives regulatory approval, it could become a standard cancer treatment in Europe in four or five years, with estimated sales of $3 billion a year. Cuba also offers a unique treatment for retinitis pigmentosa, often known as night blindness, which has attracted many patients from Europe and North America. Specialty institutes include the Placental Histotherapy Center, which has provided services for more than 7,000 patients from 100 countries, and the Camilo Cienfuegos International Ophthalmology Center, which combines the comfort of a major hotel with a state-of-the-art medical institution.

Havana

Cira Garcia

Cira Garcia is a clinic adjoining Havana's wealthy Miramar section. In 2004, it hosted 1,300 foreign tourists as inpatients and thousands more as outpatients. Cira Garcia offers everything from herniated disk repair — for $4,750 including anesthesia and a two-week hospital stay — to laser eye surgery and liposuction. Dr. Ramon Prado, the clinic director, said that its prices average about a third lower than those in the United States. For example, according to the American Society of Plastic and Reconstructive Surgeons, a rhinoplasty procedure that costs $3,100 in the United States would cost $1,710 at Cira Garcia, and an abdominoplasty ("tummy tuck") procedure that costs $4,198 in the United States would be $2,340 at the clinic. About 80 percent of the patients come from Latin America and the Caribbean, but the facility has attracted patients from as far away as Japan and Finland.

   ⚕ Cira Garcia
   ✉ Calle 20 No. 4101
       esq. Ave 41 Playa
       Ciudad de La Habana
       Cuba
   ☎ 537-204-2811
   ✆ 537-204-2640
   🌎 www.cirag.cu/ingles/clinica.htm
   @ faculta@cirag.cu

"Want a Radical Face Lift? Try Revolutionary Cuba"

~ Wall Street Journal *headline, January 21, 2000*

Cyprus

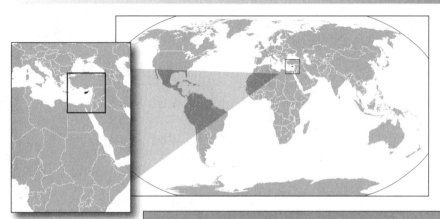

Cyprus is an island in the eastern part of the Mediterranean Sea, 70 miles south of Turkey. English is widely spoken and understood in this island of beautiful beaches, relaxed lifestyle, and excellent cuisine.

Cyprus Politics:

The island is divided into four sectors: the southern Republic of Cyprus, the unrecognized Turkish Republic of Northern Cyprus, the British Sovereign Bases, and the United Nations-controlled Green Line.

Cyprus Travel Requirements:

A valid passport is required. U.S. citizens do not need a visa.

Driving is on the left side of the road, like the United Kingdom, so keep your wits about you if you are not used to this.

Medical tourism in Cyprus has tended to focus on hair transplantation. As the only permanent method of restoring hair, the technique of hair transplants is to take genetically strong hair follicles from the back and sides of the head and place them into the thinning or balding areas. This results in a very natural appearance of growth that is undetectable from the person's existing hair. The process is carried out in a clinic by surgeons who use the latest technology and techniques.

Nicosia

HDC Medical Trichology Center

HDC Medical Trichology Center is located in Nicosia, the capital of Cyprus. The HDC staff pride themselves on patient care and confidentiality. From your initial contact to the aftercare you will be treated with sympathy, professionally and with the utmost understanding.

HDC Medical
Trichology Centre
6 Protagoras Str.
Ayios Antonios
1045 Nicosia
Cyprus
☎ 357-22-34-61-61
✆ 357-22-73-09-20
🌐 www.hdc.com.cy
@ info@hdc.com.cy

Paphos

The capital of Cyprus during the ancient Greek and Roman empires, this city is located on the southeast coast of Cyprus in a beautiful area that is a UNESCO world heritage site with a fast-growing tourism industry. By legend, the harbor of Paphos is where Aphrodite rose from the sea. Archeological research shows that the area has been inhabited since Neolithic times, and visited by the Apostle Paul, who converted the Roman governor to Christianity (it is mentioned in the Acts of the Apostles, XIII 6).

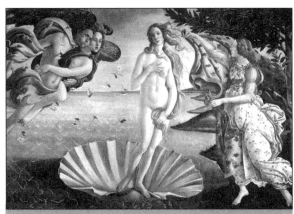

Cyprus is the legendary birthplace of the goddess of beauty, love, sex, and passion, the beautiful goddess Aphrodite, or Kypris, famously depicted by the artist Botticelli in The Birth of Venus.

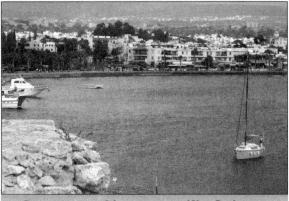

Panoramic view of the ancient port of Kato Paphos — a destination of medical tourists from Biblical times to the present.

The Royal Artemic Medical Center

This very expansive and well-equipped facility specializes in dialysis, using very up-to-date procedures and technology.

Royal Artemic Medical Center
Pavlou Crineou Str.
Cyprus
☎ 357-2696-1600
✆ 357-2696-3670
🌐 www.hemodialysiscenter.com
@ contact@hemodialysiscenter.com

Czech Republic

A top destination choice for: cosmetic surgery, cryotherapy, dental care

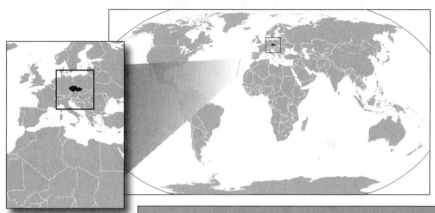

Czech Republic Politics:

After shaking off communist rule, the Czech Republic has once again become a center of art and intellectualism. Oddly, despite the profusion of cathedrals and churches, the majority of Czechs are agnostics or atheists. This is perhaps a consequence of the anti-religious policy during the communist era. The Czech Republic joined the European Union in 2004.

Czech Republic Travel Requirements:

Passport required. Visa not required for a stay of up to 90 days.

In 1993, Czechoslovakia separated into two countries: The Czech Republic and Slovakia. The capital of this small country is the historic city of Prague (*Praha*), a major tourist attraction and also increasingly a major medical tourism destination. As recently as 1997 there was just one clinic in the city treating foreigners; now there are more than 100.

The Czech Republic has a long tradition of plastic surgery. In fact, modern plastic surgery was founded here. Professor František Burian, who established the first Czech chair of plastic surgery at Charles University in 1938, is recognized as one of the pioneers of this specialty. Continuing the tradition of excellence, would-be aesthetic surgeons must undergo five years of special plastic surgery training on top of five years of general surgery after first taking their six-year medical degree.

Prague is a great location for medical tourism because it offers not only high standards and low prices, but also many other things to do. The remarkably well-preserved old town is small enough that inexpensive cafés, restaurants, and places to stay are all within walking distance.

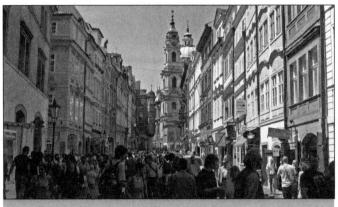

Prague's old city can seem overrun with tourists — and now, medical tourism is yet another attraction.

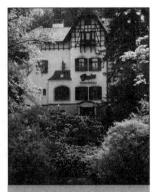

The town of Marienbad is surrounded by 100 healing mineral springs.

The Czech Republic is also promoting assisted fertility care. However, they are facing stiff competition from other countries because of national medical laws. Unlike other countries that offer fertility treatment, Czech law forbids unwed and lesbian couples from receiving sperm donations and bans surrogate motherhood. This might seem surprising in a country in which the majority consider themselves "non-religious" — but evidently the social mores of their Catholic history are as strong as the surviving cathedrals.

Spa Towns

Like other eastern European countries, the Czech Republic also has numerous spas and towns dedicated to health tourism. Services in these towns are typically provided by small operations run by a family, sometimes staying in the same household over hundreds of years. The most prominent are:

- Bílina
- Františkovy Lázně
- Jáchymov
- Hodonín
- Karlova Studánka
- Karlovy Vary (Carlsbad)
- Lázně Běohrad
- Luhačovice
- Mariánské Lázně (Marienbad)
- Poděbrady
- Teplice
- Třeboň

Prague

Beauty in Prague Cosmetic Surgery

With English-speaking staff, Beauty in Prague is a very modern facility that provides a complete service from beginning to end, offering care and support for all its clients while still keeping costs low. The clinic is located near downtown Prague, about five minutes by car, or 15 minutes on foot from apartments supplied by Beauty in Prague. All transportation is provided free.

A sample of prices follows:

Cosmetic Breast Surgery

Breast enlargement / augmentation $2,544
Breast modulation / uplift..$1,764
Breast reduction..$2,148
Correction of inverted nipple...$984
Areola reduction $984

Facial Enhancement Surgery

Nose reshaping $1,932
Ear pinning $1,092
Eyelid reduction, both lids $1,559
Face lift – full $2,604
Lip enlargement...$1,008
Chin and neck $1,643

Body Reshaping for Men and Women

Tummy tuck (abdominoplasty)...$2,328
Arms – inner $2,268
Thighs – inner..$2,508
Cosmetic skin treatments..$138
Scar correction $96

Beauty in Prague also offers body reshaping for women (labial reduction, vaginal tightening, perineorrhaphy), and body reshaping for men (male breast reduction, pectoral implants, testicular implants).

- ⏏ Beauty in Prague
- ✉ Truhlarska 24
  110 00 Prague 1
  Czech Republic
- ☎ 420-222-314-198
- 🌐 www.beautyinprague.com
- @ beauty@beautyinprague.com

Spa towns...

Each of the following towns has several spa resorts, ranging from simple to ornate, from small, family-run bed and breakfasts to large corporate establishments. Most rely on long-term or returning guests, and therefore see little need to advertise themselves.

Františkovy Lázně

Foreigners might find it easier to use the German name of this spa town, Franzensbad. With about 5,200 residents, Františkovy Lázně is world renowned as a spa. The salutary effects of the springs have been known from the 15th century on, and its waters have been sold all over Germany. In 1700, it reportedly sold more water than all other German spas combined! It claims to be the first commercial mud bath in the world, and 12 of its original mineral springs are still in operation.

Karlovy Vary

Also known as Carlsbad, or in German *Karlsbad*, Karlovy Vary is at the confluence of the Ohře and Teplá rivers. It was named after Charles IV, who founded the city in the 1370s, and is famous for its hot springs.

Mariánské Lázně

Better known as Marienbad, this town's top attractions are its 100 or so mineral springs with high carbon dioxide content. Most of the springs are tapped in an orderly fashion and often have pavilions or colonnades built around them.

Dominica

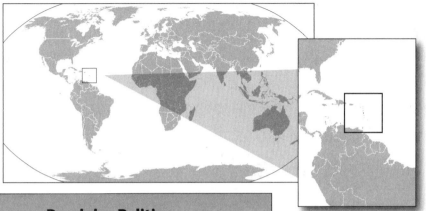

Dominica Politics:

Like most Caribbean micro-states, politics tends to be a local affair focused mainly on sustaining their hallowed tourism industry.

Dominica Travel Requirements:

Passport, onward or return ticket, confirmation of hotel reservation, and another form of picture ID required. U.S. citizens do not need a visa.

The Commonwealth of Dominica (pronounced "do-min-EE-ka") is an island nation in the Caribbean Sea where most people speak Patios, a French creole language. It should not be confused with the Dominican Republic, a larger, Spanish-speaking Caribbean country.

In Latin the name means Sunday, which was the day of its discovery for Europeans by Christopher Columbus. The Carib people living there at the time were less impressed by this discovery and managed to dispatch quite a few of the newcomers. They continued to do so for several centuries, sequentially defeating attempts of colonization by the British and French. This may have had something to do with their penchant for cannibalism and grilling the flesh over open coals. There is not much left of the Caribs now, except their word for grilling — *barbeque*.

Health Tourism

Dominica is a lush island of mountainous rainforests and home of many rare plants, animals, and birds — one of which, the Sisserou parrot, is featured on the Dominica flag. The country is known as "The Nature Island of the Caribbean" due to its extensive natural park system. The most mountainous island of the Lesser Antilles, its

---

volcanic peaks are cones of lava craters and include Boiling Lake, the second-largest, thermally active lake in the world.

Dominica excels in ecotourism and its newer variant of holistic healing resort tourism. There are numerous carefully managed lodges for nature therapy. They say that nothing is more healing to a cancer patient than bathing in the early morning in the mineral-rich La Rivere Blance (White River), viewing the early morning sunrise at Point Mulatre bay amidst the gentle blowing northeast trade winds and sipping from a warm cup of *seimeicountrar* tea.

A Short List of Dominica's Nature Lodges
- Pepper's Cottage
- Roseau Valley Hotel
- Anchorage Hotel & Dive Center
- Crescent Moon Cabins
- Beau Rive
- Zandoli Inn
- Sea Cliff Cottages
- Cocoa Cottages
- Papillote Wilderness Retreat
- Castle Comfort Dive Lodge
- Hibiscus Valley Inn
- Hummingbird Inn
- Snowbirds Bed & Breakfast
- Sutton Place Hotel
- Evergreen Hotel
- Kent Anthony Guest House
- Coconut Beach Hotel
- Oceanview Cottage
- Wind Blow Estate
- Dive Dominica Resort
- Sea World Guest House
- The End Of Eden Guest House
- Stonedge
- Carib Territory Guest House
- Roxy's Mountain Lodge
- Springfield Plantation Guest House
- Ma Bass Guest House
- Nature Island Dive Resort
- Itassi Cottages
- Oceanview Apartments

- Picard Beach Cottages
- Falls View Guest House
- Chez Ophelia Cottage Apartments
- Layou River Hotel
- Casa Ropa
- Cherry Lodge
- Continental Inn
- Floral Garden Hotel
- Gachette's Seaside Lodge

Calibishie Lodges

The following reviews were gleaned from health tourism blogs:

"My wife and I stayed here for 5 amazing days. We booked through Expedia, and it was really easy and user friendly. The staff treat you like family, the food is great and the trips are out of this world. The rooms are perfect, and the pool and grounds are well kept. The trips (We did Batibou Beach, Chaudiere Pool, Victoria Falls, Sari Sari Falls) are world class, and the staff takes care of all the details for you. The other guests at the hotel are really friendly and make for great company at meals. In the end, the only bad part about the Lodges is that you cannot stay forever. Go to Dominica, stay at Calibishie Lodges!!!!!!"

~ *Eli and Yael Weiss, Manhattan, NYC*

"We were in upper lodge number 6. The view was awesome; I must have taken over 50 photos of it in different lights. The views from the other lodges would also be amazing. Other things we remember with joy, watching humming birds while we ate breakfast, the sounds of the crickets and frogs in the evenings, looking down over the village as it came to life in the mornings, hearing and watching the sea."

~ *Barry Pavic, Hasselt, Belgium*

  Calibishie Lodges
  Main Road Calibishie
Dominica
☎ 001-767-445-8537
@ info@calibishie-lodges.com

Dominican Republic

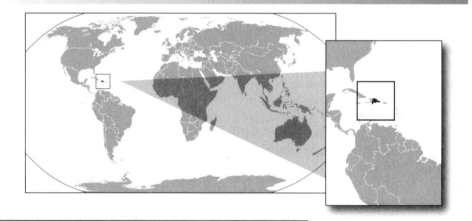

Dominican Republic Politics:

The Dominican Republic is a middle-income developing country primarily dependent on agriculture and, increasingly, tourism. So much of the service trade is dominated by the United States that American money can be readily used, and speaking English is common. The national religion, officially Catholic, is really baseball. Patron saints include Sammy Sosa and many other expats on U.S. ball teams.

Dominican Republic Travel Requirements:

Passport required. U.S. citizens do not need a visa.

Lovingly known simply as DR, the Dominican Republic is the eastern two-thirds of the island of Hispaniola, which it shares with Haiti on the west. This is the second largest of the Caribbean islands, next to Cuba, and has a much bigger economy than the other "micro-states."

The island was the first landfall of Christopher Columbus on his pioneering voyage of 1492. He discovered the peaceful Taíno people and was fascinated by their peculiar custom of inhaling the smoke of a particular plant. The plant was tobacco, and while their smoking habit became popular throughout the world, the Taíno people themselves didn't fare so well and became all but extinct. Today, the majority of the population is mulatto, descended from European and African immigrants.

Plastic Surgery

"Dominican Republic becoming the Mecca of Plastic Surgery" blares the headline from Plasmetic.com — a prominent plastic surgery website. Cosmetic surgery is becoming so popular in DR that one medical tourist, Jo Ann Roselli, even wrote a book about it: *How to Get High-Quality Plastic Surgery...Cheap!*

A group of Hollywood producers is recognizing the value and now offering what is called a "Rejuvenation Vacation", which includes a stay at the Barceló Capella five-star beach resort, entry to numerous restaurants, bars, and water sports at the resort, as well as daily and nightly entertainment.

Barceló Capella Beach Resort

Cosmetic surgery in the Dominican Republic is so new that independent services are only beginning to be established. Instead, they ally themselves with prominent resorts to secure customers and become part of an all-inclusive package. The *Barceló Capella* is the most prominent of these. The 500-room resort is located on the Villas del Mar beach, about 20 minutes from the national airport and 35 minutes from the capital of Santo Domingo. The resort offers complete service to medical tourists.

  📇 *Barceló Capella*
  ✉ Box 4750
     Villas Del Mar
     Santo Domingo
     Dominican Republic
  ☎ 809-526-1080
  📠 809-526-1088
  🌐 www.barcelocapella.com
  @ capella@barcelo.com

Dubai

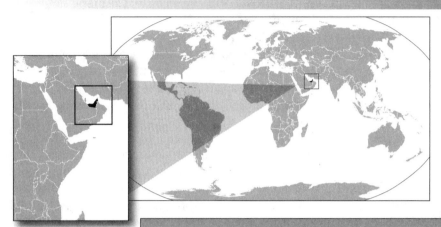

Dubai is not a country in itself, but one of the seven emirates that make up the United Arab Emirates on the Arabian Peninsula. Unlike the other emirates, Dubai gets just 6 percent of its income from oil, and instead it has fo-

Dubai Politics:

Dubai is a middle-Eastern financial hub that has long enjoyed political stability. Investors and entrepreneurs love the fast-track administration, hassle-free visas, streamlined labor process, and simple licensing. There are no taxes on sales, income, or capital gains for individuals.

Dubai Travel Requirements:

Passport required. Visa not required for stay of up to 30 days.

cused on developing the Arabic financial hub known as the Jebel Ali Free Zone (JAFZ) and tourism. Citizens of Dubai account for just 10 percent of the 5 million population; most of the residents are expatriates who run businesses with a local "silent partner." These expatriates may own land, especially on the intricate network of man-made Palm Islands, but they may not be employed in Dubai. The result is a tiny, peculiar country with astonishing wealth and essentially no taxes.

In itself, this is not unusual among oil-producing states that have reaped unimaginable wealth from the resource. What is unique about Dubai is its focus on the future: a heavy investment in new wealth generators — tourism and biomedical technology.

Dubai's Dreams Dwarf Disneyland

Dubai recently opened two of the world's largest indoor shopping arcades: the Mall of Emirates (which includes an indoor ski slope) and the Ibn Battuta Mall. But these pale in comparison to the planned Dubai Mall, which will be the undisputed largest mall in the world. As part of the Burj Dubai complex, it will be home to the tallest building in the world when completed.

Dubailand, an entertainment city clearly inspired by Disneyland, was launched in October 2003. When completed, the master planned development will span over 3 billion square feet with the first phase to be completed in 2008.

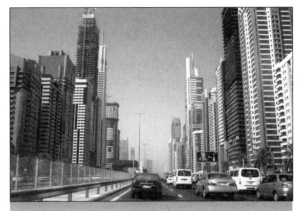

More and more skyscrapers are sprouting up in rapidly developing Dubai, as seen here along Sheikh Zayed Road.

If They Build It, Will Medical Tourists Come?

Dubai is now rapidly developing a high-end medical tourist industry. Its inclusion in this book was questionable — Dubai does not yet have any medical tourism to speak of, and all these plans are still on paper. There are dozens of other countries with similar plans. Dubai, however, does not dabble in projects or approach them lightly. Seemingly within minutes of an announcement of a new venture,

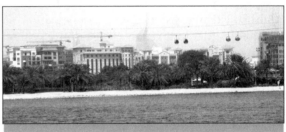

The still-evolving Dubai Healthcare City, allied with Harvard Medical School — is perhaps the only hospital network connected by cable car!

the bulldozers are roaring, and thousands of executives and technicians descend for yet another massive undertaking. That was why the medical tourism world was stunned in November 2003 when His Highness General Sheikh Mohammed bin Rashid Al Maktoum, Crown Prince of Dubai, stated that within seven years Dubai would become a world-class health center. Even the most dynamic cities have spent decades trying to build a state-of-the-art medical complex, and very few succeed. But no one doubts that Dubai will be able to do it. It has already committed $1.8 billion to begin construction of Dubai Healthcare City, a massive 500-acre complex with three major ventures: medical care, medical research, and wellness promotion. Dubai already has a massive hotel and hospitality infrastructure with elaborate shopping arcades, and just about everyone speaks English. These features set the stage for what is expected to become a global center for medical tourism.

At the heart of the project will be the Academic Medical Center, with a 300-bed university hospital. It will be established in partnership with leading global medical institutions and will include a medical college and nursing school to train and develop future doctors and nurses. Its Life Science Research Center is intended to become a major medical research institute.

Sheikh Mohammed is very aware that 1,000 years ago the Arab nations were at the forefront of science. Arab scholars developed mathematics, astronomy, and many other fields. It was only a few centuries ago that Europe took the lead in science, and the Muslim nations fell behind. Now, the Sheikh wants to restore Arab prominence. By 2010, if all goes according to plan, Dubai Healthcare City (DHCC) will become a major medical tourism destination, excelling especially in the fields of cardiology, oncology, diabetes, and health maintenance and rehabilitative services. The Wellness Cluster will include nutrition and safety centers, medical examination centers, spas, health clubs, medical clubs, and even a farm for fresh medicinal herbs.

Characteristic of Dubai, the project was started immediately. DHCC formed an alliance with the Harvard Medical School and held the first scientific symposium in March 2006. DHCC has also invited other internationally respected institutions in healthcare delivery, education, services, and research and development to collocate on the site in order to take advantage of the synergies brought about by physical proximity, interconnectivity, and professional collaboration. Medical centers in Great Britain, Germany, and the United States have expressed interest in participating in DHCC, with particular interest directed to the academic medical center component.

The big question is: If they build the Healthcare City, will medical tourists come? On one hand, Dubai offers a virtually crime-free location with world-class hotels and entertainment facilities. On the other, this is still a desert outpost where Burqa-clad women mingle shyly with less modest Westerners. It is definitely not Las Vegas, Hawaii, or Bangkok. Although it remains to be seen how much market share of medical tourism Dubai will attract, there is no doubt that it will become a major destination.

Derma Health International Group (DHI)

While offering laser treatments for skin conditions, this facility is still largely a work in progress — the website promises many more procedures to be available soon.

🏢 Derma Health International Group
✉ Dhiera
Dubai
UAE
☎ 00-9714-22-43786
🕭 www.dermahealth.org
@ info@dermahealth.org

Egypt

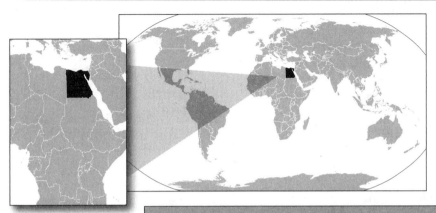

Egypt Politics:

Egypt occasionally has a flare-up of Islamic fundamentalist disturbances, but is generally stable and now has good relations with Israel.

Egypt Travel Requirements:

Passport and visa required. Visas may be obtained upon entry from the Entry Visa Department at the Travel Documents, Immigration and Nationality Administration, or most major ports of entry.

The Arab Republic of Egypt has always fascinated the Western world. A few years ago I was invited to a lavish dinner in Cairo with some of the most economically powerful men in Egypt. It quickly became apparent that I was included as something of a token American to whom they could complain about how the United States ignored Egypt.

"On the contrary," I said. "Egypt has always had a huge significance for Americans — in fact, we put your pyramid on our money." These men, who apparently had never looked closely at a U.S. $1 bill, were astonished and amused to find this to be true.

A visitor to Egypt will quickly realize that the vast majority of the country consists of uninhabited Sahara desert while 77 million people are crammed into a narrow corridor along the Nile River. You can stand on a sand dune on one side of Cairo and look over the city, across the green ribbon of the historic river, past scattered date-palm plantations and all the way to the horizon of sand dunes on the other side. In between are 18 million people, making Cairo one of the most congested, chaotic, and absolutely fascinating places on Earth.

Now tourists come to Egypt not only to visit antiquities but also for inexpensive cosmetic surgery. These services include:

- Botox
- Breast enlargement
- Breast reduction
- Breast uplift
- Calf implants
- Cheek and chin implants
- Collagen replacement therapy
- Ear reshaping
- Eyebag removal
- Facelift
- Hair removal
- Hair restoration
- Labia reduction
- Laser skin resurfacing
- Liposuction
- Mole and cyst removal
- Nose reshaping
- Skin rejuvenation
- Thigh lifts
- Thread vein removal
- Tummy tuck

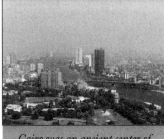

Cairo was an ancient center of medical expertise, and hopes to be again with the growth of medical tourism. The top of the Cairo Tower of the Nile River provides an expansive view of the city.

Typical prices are:

Rhinoplasty (nose reshaping)..$1,440
Breast augmentation..$2,160
Upper and lower eyelids...$1,260
Facelift $2,280

Cairo

Cairo is the Hollywood of the Middle East with an extensive film and entertainment industry. It is also an educational center of the Islamic world, with medical universities producing large numbers of specialists in plastic and reconstructive surgery.

RS Cosmetic Clinic
This is a small group of doctors and nurses who provide cosmetic surgery, along with other health and beauty treatments. "We are completely patient focused and pride ourselves on a service that is led by patient satisfaction, which is continually assessed by patient audit."

The Medical Director, Dr. Mahmoud El Shirbini, is professor of anesthesia and intensive care at Benha University. He suggests that medical tourists plan to stay in Egypt for a few days after surgery to ensure proper care. For small procedures, such as reshaping ears (otoplasty), eyelids (blepharoplasty), or breast augmentation, he advises at least seven to 10 days. For more involved cases, such as breast reduction and abdominoplasty, he suggests staying for 10 to 14 days.

The clinic requires full payment before surgery, with a deposit of $600 eight weeks before travel and the remainder paid after the initial consultation with the surgeon.

- RS Cosmetic Clinic
- 71 Road 9
  Maadi
  Cairo
  Egypt
- 00-20-23-80-67-66
- www.rscosmeticclinic.com
- @ info@RSCosmeticClinic.com

Sharm El Sheikh

Sharm El Sheikh International Hospital

This full-service hospital is a well-equipped, tertiary care facility that can deal with all specialties and emergencies. It is only 15 minutes away from the airport and is within easy reach of all major hotels. More than 60 doctors are available, most of whom speak English.

Since it is considered inappropriate for good Moslem women to be around strange men, especially men who are unclothed and in bed, nurses in Egypt are usually from other countries and speak English as a second (or third, fourth, or fifth) language.

- Sharm El Sheikh International Hospital
- Main Road
  Sharm El Sheikh
  Egypt
- 00-20-696-6089/3
- @ sharm_ih@yahoo.com

Finland

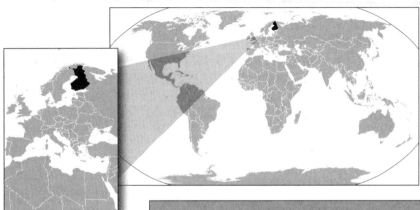

Finland Politics:

Finland has historically played a delicate balance between Scandinavian Europe and the Soviet Union. It now is a prosperous and cosmopolitan country with excellent tourism services.

Finland Travel Requirements:

Passport required. Visa not required for stay of up to 90 days.

The Republic of Finland (*Suomen tasavalta*) is a country with a small population, but it is extraordinarily sophisticated in technology and heath care. Perhaps it needs to be to survive the lengthy winters. Its greatest technological contribution may be the sauna — which also may be the only Finnish word to have entered the English vocabulary. More recently it is the home of Nokia, one of the great driving forces in cell-phone technology.

The Finns are supremely practical people. So it may be no surprise that the government has decided to venture into medical tourism. The Health and Medicine Tourism Project is an internationally competitive program of health tourism services to be built in Kuopio.

Kuopio

Health Kuopio Program

Kuopio has long had been a center of medical expertise, led by innovative programs at the University of Kuopio that focus on health and well-being. A new medical tourism program has been developed that combines the resources of the University,

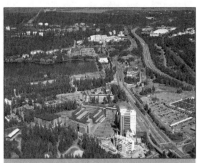

The University of Kuopio is part of a cooperative medical tourism program.

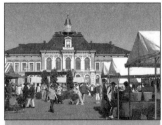

Delightful town center of Kuopio. (courtesy of Riude: Flikr)

the Savonia Polytechnic College, the Teknia Technology Centre, and other businesses and organizations in the region.

Epilepsy surgery is an example of a very specialized medical expertise that will be offered to medical tourists. This will be done at the Kuopio University Hospital.

🚑 Health Kuopio Program

✉ Tulliportinkatu 31
P.O. Box 228
FIN-70110 KUOPIO
Finland

☎ 358-17-182-086

📞 358-17-182-058

🌐 www.kuopio.fi/english.nsf

@ tiedotus.kka@kuopio.fi

Germany

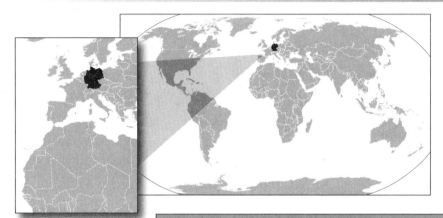

The Federal Republic of Germany (*Bundesrepublik Deutschland*) is one of the world's leading industrialized countries and a crossroads of Europe. It is no surprise to find that German medical staff are fluent in

Germany Politics:

Germany is a founding member of the European Union, and is renowned for efficiency and technological expertise.

Germany Travel Requirements:

Passport required. Visa not required for stay of up to 90 days.

many foreign languages, particularly English, but also Russian, French, and Spanish.

German hospitals are well known for their high standard of medical care and have long attracted international patients. Indeed, scientific medicine had its start in German universities in the 19th century, with discoveries of the germ theory, sterile surgical techniques, and countless other advances that laid the foundation of modern medicine.

The lengthy tradition of treating foreign patients has encouraged many hospitals to have special wards for the treatment of patients from abroad. With about 2,000 hospitals available, a medical tourist can easily be overwhelmed by all the choices.

Amazingly — and perhaps a hint of the future — even the Munich International Airport has become a center for medical tourism. Patients from other countries can fly into Munich, have tests or treatments at the airport, and then fly home, often in a single day! The Munich Airport Clinic has two surgery rooms and 13 beds. Individually designed medical-care packages include diagnosis, inpatient or outpatient surgery, hotel accommodation, transfer to a partner clinic for long-term treatments, and sightseeing programs for patients and their families. The clinic staff will go out of their way to make patients comfortable, even meeting them at the airplane and personally taking them

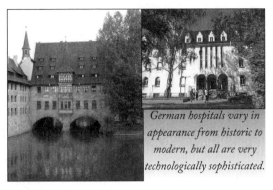
German hospitals vary in appearance from historic to modern, but all are very technologically sophisticated.

through immigration. Specialties include orthopedics, hand surgery, plastic surgery, endocrine surgery, ophthalmology, ear-nose-throat medicine, urology, gynecology, gastroenterology, treatment of cardiovascular conditions, and minimally invasive surgery for various conditions. Remarkably, the clinic has a magnetic resonance imaging (MRI) scanner on the premises.

Characteristic prices:

Rhinoplasty (nose reshaping) $5,780
Breast augmentation..$5,100
Upper and lower eyelids $3,230
Facelift...$5,780

German Hospital Service Ltd.

German Hospital Service is a personal medical tourism facilitation and advisory service. A senior consultant is Johann W. von Krause, who previously served as CEO of a number of hospitals in southern Germany.

🚑 German Hospital Service Ltd.
✉ Traubenweg 1
91623 Sachsen bei Ansbach Germany
☎ 49-9827-927343
📠 49-9827-927344
🌐 www.english.german-hospital-service.com/html/hospitals_12.html
@ info@german-hospital-service.com

German Medicine Net

This service covers a wide range of medical care: cardiac and orthopedic surgery, dentistry, and cosmetic treatments.

🚑 German Medicine Net
✉ GmbH
Yorckstrasse 23
79110 Freiburg
Germany
☎ 49-761-888-730
📠 49-761-888-7316
🌐 www.germanmedicine.net/en/

GMHS Ltd.
GMHS appeals largely to Arabic customers, with a website in English and Arabic.

📇 GMHS Limited

✉ Zweigniederlassung Deutschland
Soonwaldstr. 21
55494 Rheinböllen
Germany

☎ 49-676-496-0681

📠 49-676-496-0682

🌐 www.arabmedicare.com/GMHS/GMHS.html

@ info@gmhs-ltd.com

Surgical Experts International
This service provides a broad range of information on facilities with the following surgical specialties:

- Bone-marrow transplantation
- Brain surgery
- Cardiovascular
- Colon surgery
- Endoprosthetics
- ENT surgery
- Eye surgery
- Gynecologic surgery
- Hair transplantation
- Hand and foot surgery
- Joint replacements
- Neurosurgery
- Obesity surgery
- Oncological surgery
- Orthopedic surgery
- Pediatric surgery

Germans are not as concerned with privacy as are Americans. You probably won't be issued a gown during examinations, and there are usually no curtains around the beds. So bring a nightgown or pajamas and a bathrobe — and, for that matter, your own towels, washcloth, and soap!

On leaving the hospital it is customary to leave a small tip for the nursing staff, such as fruit baskets, candy or baked goods, or a thank-you card and $5-10 for the "coffee fund."

- Reconstructive surgery
- Robotic surgery (DaVinci)
- Spine surgery
- Transplant surgery
- Transsexual surgery
- Thoracic surgery
- Urology surgery
- Vascular surgery

📧 Surgical Experts International
✉ Harderstrasse 11
85049 Ingolstadt
Germany
☎ 49-173-884-6046
📠 49-841-971-2034
🌐 www.surgicalexperts.de
@ patient-service@surgicalexperts.de

Munich

The Munich Airport Clinic
This futuristic clinic, described earlier, has both inpatient and outpatient services.
📧 Munich Airport Clinic
✉ Terminalstrasse West
Terminal 1, Modul E, Ebene 03
München-Flughafen
Germany
☎ 49-89-975-63-328
📠 49-89-439-09-447
🌐 www.airportclinic-m.de
@ info@airportclinic-m.de

A Medical Tourist's Experience in Germany:

Dear Dr. Gahlinger,

In June of last year, my husband Jonathan went to Stenum Hospital in Bremen, Germany, to have two artificial discs put in his neck. My 12-year-old son and I went along. At first the whole prospect of going overseas for surgery sounded very scary, as we had never even been to Europe, but the more we researched it, the more glowing reports we heard from former patients about their excellent results and the wonderful, caring staff at Stenum Hospital.

Overall, we're extremely happy we went to Stenum, because it was the only option for Jonathan, already having had two fusions in his neck. We were willing to take a leap of faith and fly to Germany for the surgery. We felt the hospital was first rate and the staff was warm and compassionate and caring. The setting was beautiful and relaxing, like being at a spa for 2-1/2 weeks. We also felt God leading us to do this and felt him blessing the entire trip as it all flowed so smoothly and everything fell into place.

Sincerely,
Cindy

Greece

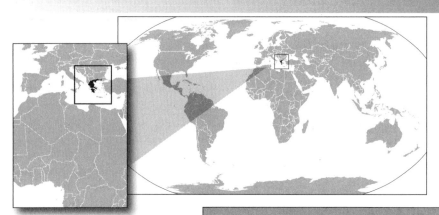

Officially known as the Hellenic Republic (*Hellás*), Greece is generally regarded as the cradle of Western civilization and the birthplace of democracy. Greece has long been a favored tourist destination, and each year, particularly in the summer

Greece Politics:

Greece is a fully integrated member of the European Union.

Greece Travel Requirements:

Passport required. Visa not required for stay of up to 90 days.

months, the country seems to overflow with visitors. In 2004, the country was crammed with people flocking to the Olympics, but the number increased another 14 percent in 2005 and is expected to reach 17 million in 2006. Greece depends on its tourism industry and continues to invest to keep it growing. Last year, the Greek Ministry of Tourism invested another $35 *billion* in infrastructure.

Health tourism is a relatively new concept in Greece, even though our dominant view of medicine got its start here. Even now, American medical students continue to recite the Hippocratic Oath upon graduating, vowing to practice medicine by moral principles, to help the sick regardless of social status and with confidentiality and compassion.

At this time, there are few private cosmetic surgeons who cater to an international clientele, but there are many centers of alternative medicine. Two thalassotherapy

---

Greece was the first country to promote tourism. During the Renaissance, in 17th century England, it became fashionable for young aristocrats to travel to Greece to see the ancient sites and become cultured in the arts. They called their roundtrip a "tour," after the Greece drafting instrument that described a circle, and referred to themselves as "tourists."

---

centers are located in Kriti, with another two under development there. Overall, about 40 medicinal spas are in operation throughout the country.

Athens

Dr. Nodas Kapositas

Nodas Kapositas, MD, PhD, is a certified plastic surgeon, member of the American Society of Plastic Surgeons (ASPS), and member of the International Society of Aesthetic Plastic Surgery (ISAPS). He states: "Our cosmetic surgery clinic in Athens, Greece, offers a complete spectrum of cosmetic surgery procedures for those who wish to regain a youthful appearance in a safe and private environment with affordable excellence in cosmetic surgery."

🕙 Dr Nodas Kapositas MD, PhD
✉ 17 Dim Soutsou Street,
   Mavili Square (USA Embassy)
   Athens 11521
   Greece
☎ 30-21-064-01-004
✆ 30-21-064-00-284
🌏 www.kapositas.gr
@ info@kapositas.gr

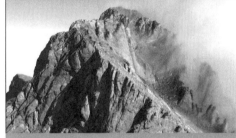

Mt. Olympus is the home of Zeus and 11 other legendary Greek gods. At 9,570 feet, it is about the same height as the Mt. Olympus overlooking Salt Lake City, Utah, which unfortunately has no gods in residence.

Crete

The Fertility Center Chania

A variety of assisted fertility techniques are offered here, with considerable detail in their website (see *Chapter 8* for further explanation).

🕙 Fertility Center Chania
✉ Markou-Botsary 64A
   Chania 73136
   Crete
   Greece
☎ 30-69-722-47-074
✆ 30-28-210-76-106
🌏 www.fertilitycenter-crete.gr
@ info@fertilitycenter-crete.gr

Hong Kong

A top destination choice for:
acupuncture, alternative medicine,
cancer treatment, herbal treatments

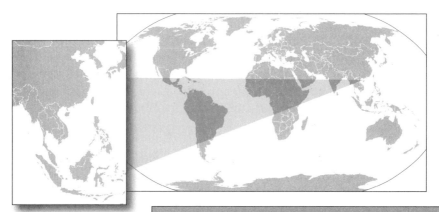

Officially known as "The Hong Kong Special Administrative Region of the People's Republic of China," *Hong Kong* means "fragrant harbor," and while its harbor is no longer quite so fragrant, it is one of the world's great cities and a major international crossroads.

The World Tourism Organization defines medical tourism as any of the

Hong Kong Politics:

Until 1997, Hong Kong was a British colony. Now administered by China under a "one country, two systems" policy, Hong Kong is entitled to a relatively high degree of autonomy; for example, it has its own legal system, currency, customs, air traffic and aircraft landing rights, and immigration laws. Hong Kong even maintains its own road rules, with traffic continuing to drive on the left (as in Britain), while the rest of China and Taiwan drive on the right.

Hong Kong Travel Requirements:

Passport and onward or return transportation by sea or air required. Visa not required for stay of up to 90 days.

following: medical care, sickness and well-being care, rehabilitation, and recuperation. Hong Kong provides all of these — the whole spectrum of services from spas to cosmetic treatments to cardiovascular surgery, and from modern diagnostic services to rehabilitative Chinese herbal treatments. In 2006, Hong Kong hosted both the International Medical and healthcare Fair — a major exposition of medical tourism — and the International Conference & Exhibition of the Modernization of Chinese Medicine & Health Products (ICMCM), which attracted over 300,000 attendees.

However, the country is a little late to the current boom in developing medical tourism, and it stumbles when it refuses to admit anyone who looks ill. It's a paradox: the administration wants to get in on the medical tourism business, but does not want the arrival of sick people. With the rapid development of sophisticated treatment offered in nearby Thailand, Malaysia, and Singapore, it is likely that Hong Kong has missed the boat as a major provider of medical services. But it continues to have a fascinating blend of old and new. For traditional Chinese medicine, this is probably the best place to go.

AmMed International Cancer Center

A U.S. healthcare company, AmMed International has opened Asia's first comprehensive cancer center in Hong Kong, hoping to create an Asian hub for cancer treatment and medical tourism. The center is housed in the Hong Kong Adventist Hospital and is affiliated with the Memorial Sloan-Kettering Cancer Center in New York, which was ranked the number one cancer hospital in the United States.

- AmMed International
  Cancer Center
  Hong Kong Adventist Hospital
- 40 Stubbs Road
  Hong Kong
- 852-2835-3800
- 852-2574-2523
- www.ammed.com
- @ info@ammed.com

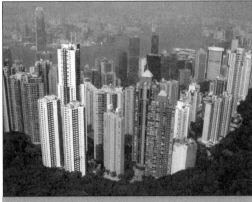

Hong Kong's spectacular skyline, shown here from Victoria Peak, shows its economic power. It is developing world-class facilities for cancer treatment.

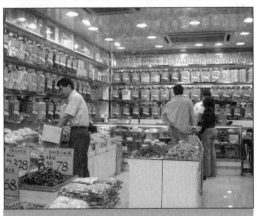

This is a traditional Chinese medicine shop in Tsim Sha Tsui, Hong Kong, where shoppers can find an astonishing variety of health treatments.

Hungary

A top destination choice for:
blepharoplasty, Botox treatment, collagen injection,
reconstructive surgery

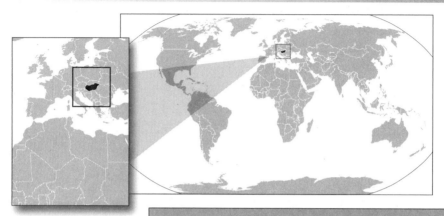

The Republic of Hungary (*Magyar Köztársaság*) is located in the heart of Europe. Its history extends to ancient times, when one of its rulers, Attila the Hun, conquered much of Europe and Asia, rivaling the Roman Empire in power. Hungarians have quite a different view of him as a noble king of whom the barbaric West lived in terror, and Attila is a common name in Hungary.

Hungary Politics:

Hungary entered the European Union in 2004. It is a rapidly developing country with wonderful cultural features and increasing popularity as a tourist destination.

Hungary Travel Requirements:

Passport, onward or return ticket, and proof of sufficient funds required. Visa not required for stay of up to 90 days.

The capital, Budapest, is actually a conglomeration of three cities — Buda, Pest, and Obuda (old Buda) — divided by the River Danube. Budapest is one of the most beautiful European cities. As one tour guide says, "Imagine sipping drinks in one of the many coffee houses which have long time been popular haunts for poets, soldiers, musicians and aristocrats with passionate gypsy music in the background..."

Since Austrian, Swiss, and German patients had already been driving over the Hungarian border for cheaper dental care, it was inevitable that Hungary would develop medical tourism. The key is the lower wages: a Hungarian dental technician earns about $360 per month, while in Germany the same job would pay five times that amount. That allows Hungarian dentists to offer services such as veneers for less than $200, and crowns fashioned by a master ceramicist for $430. Many dentists are jumping into the business and hope their focus on service will overcome the otherwise, let's say, unconventional appearance of a dental clinic. For example, Kreativ, a dental clinic

H **ungry?** When the Muslim Turks invaded Hungary, they left the pigs alone (considering them unclean and not fit to eat). This kept the locals from starving. Now pork is the favorite national food, and found in almost every major dish, especially Goulash.

on the outskirts of Budapest that caters almost exclusively to English-speaking foreigners, has a waiting room over a car repair shop and is filled with fish tanks, flags, and that universal dentist office aroma. This has evidently not deterred foreign patients. A businessman from Dublin, William O'Brien, flew to Budapest for some dental crowns and said he counted 18 people on his flight who had come for dental care.

Many dental clinics are located near the Austrian border to take advantage of easy driving trips. One small city, Mosonmagyarovar, already has over 150 dental practices to cater to foreign patients.

Budapest

Hungarian Health Organization

The Hungarian Health Organization was founded in order to coordinate medical and esthetic services for medical tourists: "We organize their stay, appointments with doctors and other service providers, treatment, leisure programs of their choice. We are committed to help our clients become healthier, smarter, and happier and at the same time have lifelong pleasant memories of their stay in Hungary."

🏬 Hungarian Health Organization
✉ 36 Szemlõhegy str.
  1025 Budapest
  Hungary
☎ 36-20-9934903
☎ 36-70-3896449
📠 36-1-3260705
🌐 www.hungarianhealth.org
@ office@hungarianhealth.org

PerfectProfiles

The Danubius Thermal Hotel on Budapest's Margaret Island recently started offering eye surgery, dental work, and heart evaluations. The medical clinic is managed by PerfectProfiles and provides 24-hour nursing care.

A PerfectProfiles agent meets patients at the Budapest Airport and brings them to the hotel. They are introduced to the clinic and shown the facilities. A daily contact is provided to ensure clinical and hospitality services.

Medical procedures include:
- Abdominoplasty (tummy tuck)
- Blepharoplasty (eyelid surgery)
- Botox
- Breast enlargement
- Breast reduction
- Breast uplift
- Cheek and chin implants
- Collagen replacement therapy
- Facelift
- Liposuction
- Neck lift
- Otoplasty (ear correction)
- Rhinoplasty (nose reshaping)
- Varicose vein removal

One happy client, Ms. A. King, from London, England, wrote: "Perfect Profiles arranged airport transfers and accommodation at the Hotel Thermal, a beautiful spa hotel in Budapest. The surgeon explained everything to me at my consultation, and I forgot any nervousness. The operation was scheduled after the results of my blood tests and the nurse stayed with me until I was feeling well enough to go back to my room. The clinic was located within the hotel so I felt very reassured that there was always someone close by; the hotel staff even brought food up to my room at no extra cost when I didn't feel like braving the restaurant, and I was able to recover by relaxing on my hotel balcony overlooking the River Danube."

Hotel Thermal Medical Centre
Budapest H-1138
Hungary
36-20-919-8695
www.perfectprofiles.eu.com
@ zsuzsa@perfectprofiles.eu.com

Dr. Volom Aesthetic and General Dental Surgery

Dr. Volom is so confident that you will be satisfied, he offers an unprecedented guarantee: if his work is inadequate and you need further treatment, you can go to any dentist and forward the bill to him! Or you can return to him, and he will pay your travel expenses and hotel bill. It certainly would be nice if this practice caught on!

Dr. Volom Aesthetic and General Dental Surgery
Fö utca 37/c
1011 Budapest
Hungary

☎ 36-30-520-2000

📞 36-14-89-3709

🌍 www.dreamsmile.hu

@ info@dreamsmile.hu

BeautyHungary

A brand new service, BeautyHungary offers:
Cosmetic dentistry
- Dental implants
- Crowns
- Veneers
- Teeth whitening
- Bridges
- Orthodontia

Plastic surgery
- Breast enlargement
- Breast reduction and suspension
- Rhinoplasty (nose surgery)
- Face lifting
- Eyelid surgery
- Prominent ear correction
- Calf augmentation
- Buttock contour surgery
- Abdominioplasty
- Facial skin resurfacing
- Liposculpture of the face and body
- Lip enhancement
- Liposuction of the neck
- Forehead lift
- Brow lift
- Hair transplantation
- Gold filaments implantation

Although the website appears to offer these services directly, I suspect this is a referral service since no address or phone numbers are provided.

🌍 www.beautyhungary.com

@ info@beautyhungary.com

India

A top destination choice for:
alternative medicine, assisted reproduction, bone-marrow transplant, cardiac bypass, eye surgery, hip replacement

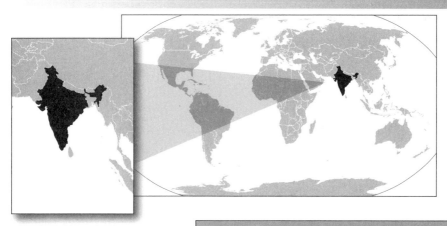

How is it possible to describe India? A country with over a billion people speaking some 300 different languages, a written history going back 5,000 years, and such a diversity of people, culture and religions that it is like trying to describe three Europes in a single paragraph. This is the nation, after all, that gave us the story of the blind men and the elephant: each described what he felt — the leg as a tree trunk, the body as a wall, the tail as a rope, and so on — each completely different from one another, and yet all of them correct. That is India — the greatest profusion of sights, sounds, smells, and sheer kaleidoscope of humanity that you could ever experience. All with a smile and the quirky "no" wag of the head that actually means yes.

The Republic of India has always been a favored destination of tourists.

India Politics:

Formally a post-British colony with a stupendously exasperating bureaucracy, India has reduced trade restrictions and is becoming a global economic power.

India Travel Requirements:

A valid passport and visa are required. It used to be very easy to go to India. Now, with worries about terrorism, etc., getting a visa has become a complicated nuisance, and most people prefer to use one of the many visa agencies — either locally or on the Internet — to handle it for them for a modest fee. If you decide to do it yourself, the instructions are available online at: http://www.indiacgny.org/php/showContent.php?linkid=23.

* Note that you must apply to the specific India office according to where you live they will not accept applications outside of their district! In order to encourage medical tourism, the Indian government has come up with a special visa for this purpose. Unlike the usual tourist visa, which is good for six months, the medical visa is valid for one year and can be extended for another year. However, the paperwork involved in getting this visa appears to be even more complicated than the regular tourist visa, so it hardly seems worth it.

Now it has also become the leading attraction for medical tourists. India has the largest number of hospitals dedicated to international patients and the greatest discounts for services. And it is just beginning. Dozens of new hospitals are being built specifically to accommodate medical tourists. Moreover, India has developed a whole new industry of "medical outsourcing," in which subcontractors provide an unlimited variety of health-related services to wealthier countries: reading x-rays, ultrasound, and MRI scans, transcribing medical notes, and even answering telephone calls made to local hospitals in the United States.

In 2004, about 1.5 million people traveled to India to receive medical treatment — a number expected to increase by about 30 percent per year. Like many developing countries, India has a large body of highly trained doctors who can perform treatments on par with American and European counterparts, but at much lower prices. The India Minister of State for Tourism, Renuka Chowdhury, is encouraging standardization of pricing among Indian hospitals and international accreditation. She said that India receives medical tourists from more than 55 countries, and recommends that tour operators include ayurveda health destinations in their marketing ventures. She is aware of the pitfalls of a loosely regulated medical system: "The marketing of India as a medical tourism destination is done with great care. We cannot have quacks in the gullies."

Quacks, however, are as common in India as sacred cows, and every street seems to have someone peddling a healthful nostrum, offering a healing prayer or *puja*, or pretending to be a *siddhi* yogi with special powers. It is up to you to ensure that you are getting what you want. The tour companies do a great service — sometimes providing a package deal that includes flights, transfers, hotels, treatment, and often a post-operative vacation — but they are businesses, fundamentally, and they will go where the money is, which is not necessarily in the best interest for the patient.

India offers a number of medical procedures that are difficult to obtain in Europe or the United States. Stem-cell treatment, for example, is still essentially unavailable in the U.S., and even research in this field is hobbled by concerns over religious and ethical issues. Indian research institutes and hospitals are far ahead in stem-cell research and development and already have numerous therapeutic offerings.

Hip resurfacing is a new alternative to conventional hip replacement. It speeds healing and

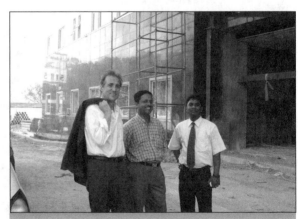

The author (left) inspects Bangalore's newest medical tourism hospital, still under construction.

return to function, and promises much better results overall. In the U.S., this is still an experimental procedure — and costly to those who manage to qualify for a spot in a clinical trial. In India, the procedure is not only commonplace but is also only a fraction of the cost, and entire hospitals are being built just to provide this treatment. As everyone in healthcare knows, quality comes with quantity. Would you prefer to have your hip resurfacing done in Boston, by a surgeon experimenting with the procedure — or in Chennai, by Dr. Bose at the new Apollo orthopedic hospital, who estimates that he does about 200 hip resurfacings a year?

Another treatment that has been questioned in Western countries is lower limb lengthening to achieve a greater

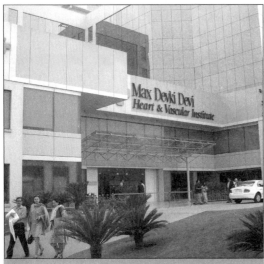

Although Mumbai (Bombay) is the location of world-class hospitals, the ride from the airport is not reassuring.

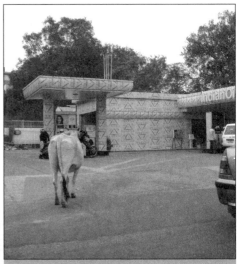

New Delhi's Max Devki Devi Heart & Vascular Institute is as elegant and sophisticated as the world's best ...

... but this is still India — a cow wanders just outside the door!

height. In the science fiction movie *Gattaca*, a man undergoes a painful procedure to become taller — he has his leg bones cut and gradually stretched over a period of about two months in order to gain a few inches. This procedure is available now, in a number of hospitals throughout India. Costing about $60,000, the Ilizarov procedure can add about three inches to your height. It is not for the faint of heart.

Ayurvedic Medicine

India is the birthplace of the ayurvedic system of medicine. The fundamentals of this system include balancing the three main "doshas" — *kapha*, *pita*, and *vata* — which are believed to be imbalanced in illness. This system is thousands of years old and complex enough to demand years of study by those wishing to master it. Some of the therapeutic claims of ayurveda may seem a bit hard to believe, but over a billion people are convinced it works. In any case, many of the therapies are pleasant and relaxing and worth trying on that account alone.

Lakhs and crores

A peculiarity of India is their preference to express large numbers not as thousands or millions but in units of a lakh (100,000) or crore (10,000,000). It can drive you crazy until you get used to it. I find it easiest to think of a lakh as a tenth of a million and a crore as ten million. Since the U.S. dollar has for many years hovered around 50 rupees in exchange, a lakh is about $2,000 and a crore about $200,000. Now, quickly — a hip replacement for 2.5 lakh rupees costs how many U.S. dollars?

India has countless medical tourism opportunities, and more are created almost every day. The only way to keep up is by checking Internet sites. The best are the following:

Medicaltourism.com

This is the one-stop, most comprehensive source of medical tourism for most countries, and especially for India. It is a direct referral site and does not hide information or rely on commissions for favorable placement. Unlike other sites, which actually try to restrict information, this site provides direct links to facilities. It also includes forums for online discussion and other services.

🌐 www.medicaltourism.com

Medical Tourism India

This referral site has a lot of promotional information, but not much else. To learn more, you need to contact them. The website states that the company also is known as Health Tourism India; however, there is no indication of any affiliation with the following referral service.

🌍 www.medical-tourism-india.com

@ gnenterprises@gmail.com

Health Tourism India

This referral service is a branch of Apothecaries' Sundries Mfg. Co., a New Delhi, India, company founded in 1948 to manufacture and export hospital and surgical equipment. With its close relation to the medical industry, the company has entered into medical tourism, acting as a facilitator between patients and hospitals. Services include:

- Suggesting hospitals or clinics for a particular treatment
- Arranging consultations with doctors
- Assisting in planning treatment and scheduling travel
- Airport pick-up
- Arranging accommodation
- Providing translators
- Coordinating all appointments
- Providing additional nurses or guides

The company is also planning to arrange online chats and video conferencing between doctors and international patients so that they can clear doubts before they come to India.

📇 Health Tourism India

✉ Plot No. 46, West Zakir
Nagar, Okhla
New Delhi 110 025
India

☎ 91-931-912-3318

🌍 www.health-tourism-india.com

@ info@tours-travels-india.com

Erco Travels

Despite its website name, "medicaltourismindia," this is just a travel agency. It was formed in New Delhi, India, in 1999, as a branch office of the international travel agency Erco Reizen B.V.

📇 Erco Travels Pvt. Ltd.
Mr. Ravi Gusain

✉ F / 204-206, Ashish Complex, LSC
Mayur Vihar Phase-I
Delhi 110091
India
☎ 91-11-3022-6333
✆ 91-11-2275-5049
🌐 www.medicaltourismindia.com
@ info@medicaltourismindia.com

Med De Tour

Med De Tour is based just outside of London, England. Its major business appears to be sending British patients to Manipal Hospital in Bangalore. This referral service promises to meet and greet patients on arrival and personally arrange doctor's appointments, accommodations, and hospital stay.
🌐 www.meddetour.com
@ usa@meddetour.com

IndUShealth

A referral service that "links uninsured and self-insured Americans to affordable, high-quality medical care in India."
🌐 www.indushealth.com
@ info@indushealth.com

Eye Surgery in India
📠 Health Line India
✉ X-60/61, Okhla Industrial Area, Phase-II
New Delhi 110020
India
☎ 91-11-51611751
✆ 91-11-51612103
🌐 www.eye-surgery-india.com
@ healthlineindia@gmail.com

Ahmedabad

Ahmedabad is the main city in the northeastern state of Gujarat, known for its glorious temples. Excellent opportunities exist for visitors to explore diverse cultures and religions, with almost 3,500 fairs and festivals celebrated each year!

Apollo Hospital (see *Chennai*)

Krishna Heart & Super Specialty Institute
> The Institute is a full-service hospital, located in a park-like campus.
> 🏥 Krishna Heart & Super Specialty Institute
> ✉ Ghuma
> Ahmedabad 380058
> India
> ☎ 91-02717-230877-81
> ☎ 91-98250-22188
> ℘ 91-02717-230876
> 🌐 www.krishnaheart.org/inter.htm
> @ info@krishnaheart.org

Swadesh Healthcare International

Swadesh is a bold new venture in medical tourism that began construction in 2006. Centered in the "town" of Vadodara near Ahmedabad (in India, a town can have 2 million people!), Swadesh will build three major medical centers — the other two will be in Kerala and Goa — and multiple smaller hospitals to capitalize on the expected $3 billion market in medical tourism. The company has allied with some impressive institutes: the Apollo Hospital Group, the Rotunda Human Reproduction Center, the Shroff Eye Center, Wockhardt Hospital & Heart Institute, Escort Heart Institute & Research Center, Kairali Health, Prince Ali Khan Hospital, Ayurveda Gram, and Ananda. These cooperative efforts will give Swadesh a tremendous boost in global competition for medical tourists. Swadesh is specifically planning to target the United States, Canada, and the United Kingdom in its marketing.
> 🌐 www.swadeshinternational.com
> @ info@swadeshinternational.com

Bangalore

The small, southern city of Bangalore has become the "Silicon Valley of India" — a rapidly growing technology center where almost every major electronics firm now has an establishment. Unlike the greater cities of India, Bangalore has little pollution, and the pace of life is much slower. Even more remarkable is the absence of the ubiquitous cows wandering the roads. There is not much for a tourist to do here — Bangalore is not close to beaches, mountains, wildlife parks, ancient monuments, or any of the usual features — except if that tourist is here for medical care. In that case, Bangalore has a huge advantage over its better-known competitors. The high-tech draw has made Bangalore easily reached by direct flights from Singapore and other travel hubs to the brand new international airport, and local travel is also much easier and faster than elsewhere in India. Several new hospitals are springing up to make this city a center for medical technology as well as computer chips and software.

Columbia Asia Medical Center

This is a network of private hospitals offering a variety of services, including rehabilitation.

   Columbia Asia Hospital Pvt. Ltd.
   ✉ Management Office - India
     The Icon, #8, 80 Feet Raod,
     HAL III Stage, Indiranagar
     Bangalore - 560075, India
   ☎ 91-80-4126-9701
   ℘ 91-80-4126-9702
   🌍 www.columbiaasia.com
   @ vinay.khandpur@columbiaasia.com

Manipal Hospital & Heart Foundation

India's first and only multi-specialty, tertiary care hospital to be ISO 9001: 2000 certified for clinical protocols, nursing care, support service (laboratory and pharmacy) and administration. Their slogan is: "Affordable costs in over 39 specialties."

   Manipal Hospital & Heart Foundation
   ✉ 98, Airport Road
     Bangalore 560017
     India
   ☎ 91-80250-23344
   ℘ 91-80412-69702
   🌍 www.manipalhospital.org
   @ info@manipalhospital.org

Golden Palms

This lavish resort and spa is combined with a modern full-fledged surgical center featuring medical and dental procedures. All rooms have a pool-side view, and the entire resort is located in a lush garden setting redolent with scents of hibiscus and jasmine. Lots of marble and elaborate Greco-Roman statues give the place a non-Indian atmosphere, as do the many restaurants that provide sumptuous buffets ranging from Italian to Chinese to Barbeque to suit every taste. Everything is included in the package deal.

Golden Palms was designed and is operated by Dr. Sanjay Pandya, a U.S.-trained cosmetic surgeon and former associate professor of plastic surgery at Northwestern

University in Chicago. The resort is located about 21 miles from the Bangalore airport — which in India means about 45 minutes driving time.

- 🏨 Golden Palms Avenue
- ✉ Hobli, Tumkur Road
  Bangalore 562123
  India
- ☎ 91-80237-12222
- 📠 91-80237-10033
- 🌐 www.goldenpalmsspa.com
- @ info@goldenpalmsspa.com

Hip Resurfacing Center

Dr. G. Balasubramanian is an orthopaedic specialist who has set up this center at Columbia Asia Medical Center, catering to foreigners who want joint reconstructive surgery. A new hospital is also being added, to be completed in 2007. A sister facility is located in Coimbatore.

- 🏨 Colombia Asia Hospital
- ✉ Hebbal Road
  Bangalore 560038
  India
- ☎ 91-80412-69701
- 📠 91-80412-69702
- 🌐 www.hipresurfacingcenter.com
- @ ggbala@hotmail.com

Wockhardt Hospital & Heart Institute (see Mumbai)

Belgaum

This ancient city is located between Mumbai and Goa, without the pollution of the first and the tourist hordes of the second.

Hhope Infertility Clinic

Providing specialty assisted-reproductive procedures (IVF, ICSE, Blastocyst, and TESE) at about one fifth of the cost in North America or Europe.

- 🏨 Keshav Krupa Palace
- ✉ 1st Floor, Plot No.16
  RPD Corner, Tilakwadi
  Belgaum 590 006
  India

☎ 91-83124-22836
📠 91-83130-90273
🌐 www.hhope-infertility-clinic.com
@ dr.varsha@hhope-infertility-clinic.com

Bilaspur

This small city is off the usual tourist trail. It is a pleasant, unhurried, and an inexpensive way to experience traditional India.

Apollo Hospital (see Chennai)

Chennai

Formerly named Madras, Chennai has become a burgeoning technological and medical center.

Apollo Hospitals Enterprise Limited

Apollo is the largest healthcare group in Asia, with over 7,000 beds in 37 hospitals, a string of nursing and hospital management colleges, and dual corporate lifelines of pharmacies and diagnostic clinics. Apollo has long been active in medical tourism, with care given to over 10 million patients from 55 countries. Apollo's business began to grow in the 1990s when the deregulation of the Indian economy drastically cut bureaucratic barriers to expansion and made it easier to import the most modern medical equipment. The first patients were Indian expatriates who returned home for treatment. Soon, patients began to arrive from Europe, the Middle East, and Canada, followed by major investment in new hospitals. Apollo now is expanding even more aggressively to tap into the huge American market, and has also arranged partnerships with hospitals in Kuwait, Sri Lanka, and Nigeria.

Success has brought criticism by Indian politicians that Apollo has focused too much on business and ignored the tremendous health needs of India's poor. Now, Apollo dedicates a portion of earnings to treating the poor, setting aside free beds for those who can't afford care, and pioneering remote, satellite-linked telemedicine across India.

The headquarters for the Apollo Hospitals is located in Chennai, as are several of its flagship facilities: the Institute of Cardiovascular Diseases and the Apollo Cancer Hospital, which was the first hospital in India to be awarded ISO 9002 certification for quality assurance. Additional Apollo hospitals are located in Ahmedabad, Bilaspur, Delhi, Hyderabad, Kolkata, and Madurai.

Apollo is associated with the Mayo Clinic, the Cleveland Heart Institute, and Johns Hopkins University. It is the only international training organization for the Texas

Heart Institute and the Minneapolis Heart Institute for cardiology and cardiothoracic surgery.

Sample treatment costs:

Bone-marrow transplant $25,000
Bypass surgery..$6,000
Breast lump removal..$700
Hemorrhoidectomy $1,000
Knee-joint replacement...$5,000
In-vitro fertilization (IVF) cycle...$1,800
Hernia correction...$1,000
Dental implant $800

In order to facilitate medical tourism, Apollo provides the following services at its International Patient Service Centers:

- Local travel arrangements
- Airport transfers
- Coordination of doctor's appointments
- Accommodation for relatives and attendants
- Locker facilities
- Provision of cuisine options
- Provision of interpreters
- Arrangements with leading resort chains for post-operative recuperation

🏥 Apollo Hospitals Enterprise Limited
✉ 21/22 Greams Lane
   Chennai 600 006
   India
☎ 91-44282-90200
☎ 91-44282-93333
📠 91-44282-94429
🌐 www.apollohospitals.com
@ enquiry@apollohospitals.com

> ## Apollo statistics:
>
> - over 10 million patients treated, as of 2005
> - over 49,000 cardiac surgeries at a 98.5% success rate
> - over 9,400 renal transplants
> - over 130 bone-marrow transplants
> - over 30 liver transplants
> - over 4,000 specialists and super specialists, spanning 53 clinical departments
> - the largest and most sophisticated sleep laboratories in the world
> - pioneered Illizarov and Birmingham hip-resurfacing surgeries

LifeCell

One of the newest types of medical tourism — indeed, a new type of medicine altogether — is stem-cell therapy (see *Chapter 9*). LifeCell is India's first stem-cell transplant hospital, jointly launched by Asia Cryo-Cell Pvt Ltd, and Pioneers and Sri

Ramachandra Medical College and Research Institute (see *Coimbatore*). Dedicated solely to this procedure, it focuses on treating leukemia, spinal cord injuries, and brain injuries.

While the LifeCell head office is in Chennai, it also has facilities in Ahmedabad, Bangalore, Calicut, Coimbatore, Gurgaon, Hyderabad, Jaipur, Kochi, Kolkata, Mumbai, New Delhi, Noida, Panchkula, Pune, and Surat.

📠 Asia CRYO-CELL Private Limited
✉ 26, Vandalur Kelambakkam Main Road
   Keelakottaiyur
   Chennai – 600048
   India
☎ 91-044-27479291-93
☎ (from U.S.) 1-800-425-5323
🌏 www.lifecellindia.com
@ ccche@lifecellindia.com

Madras Institute of Orthopaedics and Traumatology (MIOT)

This modern hospital stands on a sprawling 22-acre site. It was clearly designed for international patients and has drawn a list of celebrities, from presidents of India and chief ministers of several states to popular film stars and diplomats from Germany, United States, United Kingdom, Sri Lanka, Bangladesh, UAE, and the Maldives.

📠 MIOT Hospitals
✉ 4/112 mount Poonamalle Road
   Manapakkam
   Chennai 600 089
   India
☎ 91-44224-92288
📱 91-91442-24911
🌏 www.miothospitals.com
@ miot@vsnl.com

Coimbatore

This small city in southern India has been known as a medical center since the days of Caesar's Rome — and even now, ancient Roman coins and artifacts continue to be discovered in archeological sites in the area. Coimbatore is known for its industrial hub, educational institutions, healthcare facilities, pleasant weather, friendly culture, and hospitality. Often referred to as the "City of Hospitals and Colleges," there are far too many medical facilities to be mentioned here. One of the more prominent is:

Sri Ramakrishna Hospital

This large medical university and hospital complex is named after a 19th Hindu visionary. Known as the "rational mystic," he talked about God like a scientist in discourses later published as The Gospel of Sri Ramakrishna.

The hospital has 400 beds with all major specialties and state-of-the-art diagnostic instruments. The hospital is particularly known as a center for kidney transplants, and the president of India recently opened its new oncology center.

📠 Sri Ramakrishna Hospital
✉ 395 Sarojini Naidu Road
   Coimbatore 44
   India
☎ 91-42221-0075
🌐 www.sriramakrishnahospital.com
@ designer@sriramakrishnahospital.com

Hyderabad

Sometimes jokingly called "Cyberabad," this city rivals Bangalore as a rapidly developing high-tech center.

Apollo Hospital (see Chennai)

L V Prasad Eye Institute

Many medical tourism services in India have been criticized for being too interested in profit and paying little attention to the desperate health needs of the majority of the Indian population. In fact, this argument has been used to criticize the entire medical tourism industry, even going so far as to accuse hospitals built to serve international patients as drawing away physicians who would otherwise be serving poorer people. Regardless of the logic of this argument — which I think is wrong — it certainly cannot be said of the L V Prasad Eye Institute. The Institute's focus, right from the start, has been on providing eye-care services to underprivileged populations in the developing world and to furthering research into eye disease prevention and cure. Set up as a not-for-profit trust, in partnership with the World Health Organization and the International Agency for the Prevention of Blindness, the Institute treats nearly 50 percent of its patients for free. Even with substantial discounts, the income from treating international patients is used to subsidize care for impoverished people with eye diseases.

📠 L V Prasad Eye Institute
✉ L V Prasad Marg, Banjara Hills
   Hyderabad 500 034
   India

" *Looking back, I feel that the tour of L V Prasad was the highlight of my trip to India. The hospital is larger and more modern than I expected, with spacious bright corridors and beautiful artwork. The atmosphere was peaceful and the staff friendly and helpful. The hospital was founded in 1986 and is now a world-class organization with comprehensive patient care, eye research, sight enhancement and rehabilitation, community eye health, education, and product development. L V Prasad Eye Institute serves a wide cross-section of people from India and from countries around the world. It has a community eye health component with outreach to urban slums. I was impressed that all patients are provided the best care possible regardless of the ability to pay. The hospital serves over 500 patients per day and about 50 percent of surgical services are provided free of charge for the underprivileged. People of all ages are treated, and no one is turned away."*

~ Maria Gahlinger, R.N.

☎ 91-40306-12345

✆ 91-40235-48271

🌐 www.lvpei.org

@ communications@lvpei.org

Wockhardt Hospital & Heart Institute (see *Mumbai*)

Kolkata

Formally known as Calcutta, this densely populated city has come a long way from its historical image of extreme poverty and the infamous "black hole." It is now a rapidly developing technology center with medical institutes increasingly specializing in medical tourism.

Apollo Hospital (see *Chennai*)

B. M. Birla Heart Research Centre

The B. M. Birla Heart Research Centre in Kolkata is a super-specialty hospital dedicated exclusively to the diagnosis, treatment, and research of cardiovascular diseases. It deals with the entire spectrum of cardiac ailments, affecting both adults and children, although it is perhaps most renowned for its pediatric reconstructive heart surgery. It recently achieved international recognition with ISO 14001 Certification.

Remarkably for such a large facility, it does not appear to have a direct website. The site www.birlaheart.com just gives some basic health education with no contact information. The email address provided below is for a medical tourism referral agency.

☎ B. M. Birla Heart Research Centre
✉ 1/1, National Library Avenue
Kolkata
India
☎ 91-33245-67777
🌐 www.medical-tourism-india.com/bmbirla.htm
@ gnenterprises@gmail.com

Wockhardt Hospital & Heart Institute (see *Mumbai*)

Madurai

Apollo Hospital (see *Chennai*)

Mumbai

Formerly known as Bombay, this sprawling city served as the gateway to India during the colonial era. It is the nation's largest city and one of the world's great metropolises. Forty percent of international flights to India land here, something to consider if you want to keep your trip as short as possible. It is also one of the most crowded and polluted places on the planet, with infrastructure that has not kept pace with growth for decades. The drive from one side of the city to the other can take two hours, but it doesn't seem so far because the air is too thick to see more than a few blocks anyway. I cannot, for the life of me, see why anyone would want to come here. And yet, it is the most "happening" place in India, home to the gigantic Indian film industry known as Bollywood (which actually produces many more films than Hollywood) and the "City of Dreams" to its devoted residents.

Breach Candy Hospital
Located on the south coast of Mumbai, next to the U.S. Consulate, Breach Candy is a leader in interventional cardiology as well as a wide range of medical care.
☎ Breach Candy Hospital Trust
✉ 60 A Bhulabhai Desai Road
Mumbai 400 026
India

" *W here million-dollar apartments overlook million-population slums."*

~ Time Magazine *description of Mumbai*

☎ 91-22-2367-1888

📠 91-2222367-2666

🌐 www.breachcandyhospital.org

@ info@breachcandyhospital.org

Lilavati Hospital and Research Centre

Lilavati Hospital provides not only medical treatment but also furnishes a very safe and pleasant environment for the patient and family. This world-class medical institution was chosen by the Royal College of Surgeons to conduct its first fellowship examinations outside of Edinburgh, Scotland.

With 300 beds, including 100 intensive-care beds, it has carpeted and unusually spacious patient rooms — each about 1,100 square feet — and a personal nurse devoted to every patient.

🏢 Lilavati Hospital & Research Centre

✉ A - 791, Bandra Reclamation
Bandra (W)
Mumbai 400 0504
India

☎ 91-98-2132-0065

📠 91-22-2640-7655

🌐 www.lilavatihospital.com

@ info@lilavatihospital.com

PD Hinduja National Hospital & Medical Research Centre

An ultramodern hospital on the busiest thoroughfare in central Mumbai, PD Hinduja National Hospital & Medical Research Centre was established by the Hinduja Foundation in collaboration with Massachusetts General Hospital, a teaching facility of Harvard University. The 351-bed hospital offers comprehensive services from diagnosis and investigation to therapy, surgery, and post-operative care. It was the first facility in India to be awarded ISO 9002 Certification.

🏢 PD Hinduja National Hospital & Medical Research Centre

✉ Veer Savarkar Marg, Mahim
Mumbai 400 016
India

☎ 91-22-2445-2222

📠 91-22-2444-9151

🌐 www.hindujahospital.com

@ info@hindujahospital.com

Tata Memorial Hospital

A national center for prevention, treatment, education, and research in cancer, Tata conducts about 8,500 major surgeries each year, and also treats many thousands of others with radiation and chemotherapy. International patients are welcomed with private and deluxe rooms.

- 🏢 Tata Memorial Hospital
- ✉ Dr. E Borges Road
  Parel, Mumbai 400 012
  India
- ☎ 91-22-2417-7000
- 📠 91-22-2414-6937
- 🌐 www.tatamemorialcentre.com
- @ info@tmcmail.org

Wockhardt Hospital & Heart Institute

Wockhardt is among India's leading pharmaceutical and healthcare companies. Owned by a pharmaceutical manufacturer (see Fortis for discussion of a similar arrangement), Wockhardt has become a renowned tertiary-level heart center providing cardiac care to patients of all ages. It has an international alliance with Harvard Medical International. In addition to the Mumbai institute, Wockhardt also operates facilities in Bangalore, Kolkata, Hyderabad, and Nagpur. Vishal Bali, vice president of Wockhardt Hospitals, told me that the large U.S. health insurance company, Blue Cross and Blue Shield, will soon provide coverage for patients who choose to be treated at his hospitals in India. I have not been able to verify this, but if this is the case, it will be a far-reaching shift in American healthcare.

- 🏢 Wockhardt Towers
- ✉ Bandra Kurla Complex
  Bandra East
  Mumbai 400 051
  India
- ☎ 91-22-2659-4444
- 📠 91-22-2414-6937
- 🌐 www.wockhardt.com
  contactus@wockhardt.com
  Wockhardt also has international offices, including one in the United States:
- 🏢 WOCKHARDT USA INC.
- ✉ 75 Ronald Reagan Blvd., Warwick, NY 10990, U.S.A.
- ☎ 908-719-4350
- 📠 908-719-4351
- @ contactusa@wockhardt.com

Wockhardt also has international offices, including one in the U.S.:

🏢 WOCKHARDT USA INC.
✉ 75 Ronald Reagan Blvd., Warwick, NY 10990, U.S.A.
☎ 908-719-4350
📠 908-719-4351

Nagpur

This old, industrial city is almost in the direct center of the country. It is not among the common tourist destinations, perhaps because the summer temperatures regularly hit 114 degrees F. Nonetheless, its highly regarded medical institutions provide superb facilities for inexpensive medical care.

Wockhardt Hospital & Heart Institute (see Mumbai)

New Delhi

New Delhi is undergoing a boom in the number of new world-class hospitals. The buzzword is "First World treatment at Third World prices." Although many of these facilities try to emphasize vacations along with medical care, the reality is that unless you love a chaotic mix of poverty, crowding, pollution, noise, and the delightful insanity known as India — in overdrive — then you may want to get out of Delhi as soon as possible. Luckily, it is not far from Delhi to places with far more tourist appeal, such as the Taj Mahal at Agra or the holy city of Varanasi.

All India Institute of Medical Sciences (AIIMS)

This renowned medical institute has 25 clinical departments and four super specialty centers to manage practically all types of disease. It has 1,766 beds and counts 1,323 doctors among its faculty. As a government institute, profit is not a concern, and therefore costs are low. It is particularly well known for pediatric cardiovascular surgery.

🏢 AIIMS Main Hospital
✉ Aurobindo Marg
Delhi
India
☎ 91-11-2658-8500
📠 91-11-2658-8663
🌐 www.aiims.ac.in
@ webmastr@aiims.ac.in

Escorts Heart Institute and Research Centre (EHIRC)

Currently, Escorts operates three large hospitals in New Delhi, Faridabad, and Amritsar. Together with 11 heart specialty centers and associate hospitals, Escorts manages nearly 900 beds. EHIRC is a leader in the fields of cardiac surgery, interventional cardiology and cardiac diagnostics, and has been ranked as the best cardiac hospital in India. The Institute has introduced innovative techniques of minimally invasive and robotic surgery. The Institute's latest addition of the state-of-the-art Cardiac Scan Centre provides the combined power of CV-MRI and Smart Score CT Scanner to diagnose coronary artery disease at a very early stage. This facility is the first of its kind outside of the United States. The Institute has nine operating rooms and carries out nearly 15,000 procedures every year.

Escorts was founded by Naresh Trehan, a former assistant professor at New York University Medical School, who said he earned nearly $2 million a year from his Manhattan practice before returning to India to found Escorts in 1988. Dr. Trehan, who still has a youthful exuberance at age 58, claims "our surgeons are much better" than those in the U.S.

    🏥 Escorts Heart Institute and Research Centre

    ✉ Okhla Road
       New Delhi 110 025
       India

    ☎ 91-11268-25000

    📠 91-11268-25013

    🌐 www.ehirc.com

    @ contact@ehirc.com

Fortis Healthcare

In the United States, a lot of negative publicity attends the increasing relationship between pharmaceutical companies and major medical centers. It is considered an unseemly conflict of interest, or even illegal, since the practice of medicine should be independent of the production and sale of drugs and supplies. In India, however, there is no such restraint — and Fortis exemplifies this. Fortis Healthcare is owned and operated by Ranbaxy, India's largest pharmaceutical company with manufacturing in seven countries and products marketed in more than 100 countries. Fortis is also closely affiliated with Partners HealthCare System, Inc., which includes Massachusetts General Hospital and Brigham & Women's Hospital, both of which are teaching hospitals of the Harvard Medical School.

Ranbaxy — and therefore Fortis — is owned by brothers Malvinder and Shivinder Singh. They view the combination of pharmaceutical giant and major hospital complex as a synergistic and beneficial operation which ultimately results in lowered costs. Their goal is to become a "Top-five" global player in generic pharmaceuticals. Fortis Healthcare also has ambitious growth plans in the hospitals segment. The brothers intend to build a number of multi-specialty Fortis Healthcare hospitals over the next three to five years through an investment of close to U.S. $217 million. This will increase capacity to 4,000 beds in 10 hospitals, up from the existing 600 beds in four hospitals. As part of this initiative, Fortis will be setting up a "medical city" at Gurgaon in Haryana based on the Johns Hopkins Medical Center in the United States. The medical city will be called Fortis International Institute of Medical and Biosciences (FIIMBS). It will house a medical college, an attached hospital, and an allied sciences institute, among other facilities.

Fortis's flagship hospital, at Mohali (Chandigarh), is claimed to be India's most advanced cardiac hospital. Additional hospitals are located throughout India, and two new major hospitals specifically for medical tourists are planned on the outskirts of New Delhi. The new construction will be overseen by Harpal Singh, who also happens to be Malvinder Singh's father-in-law.

🏥 Fortis Jessa Ram Hospital, New Delhi

✉ WEA, Karol Bagh
New Delhi 110 005
India

☎ 91 11257 45265

🌐 www.fortishealthcare.com

@ fipsc@fortishealthcare.com

Indraprastha Medical Corporation

This huge medical complex is part of Apollo Hospital Enterprises (see *Chennai*), and is the third-largest corporate hospital outside the United States.

Max Devki Devi Heart & Vascular Institute

This astonishing new hospital epitomizes India's development of medical tourism. Although the hospital serves the general population, it clearly focuses on international patients — and it does so with care that is among the best in the world. The brand new facility has not spared expenses on luxury and state-of-the-art cardiovascular research and treatment.

🏥 Max Devki Devi Heart & Vascular Institute

✉ 2, Press Enclave Road, Saket
New Delhi
India

☎ 91-11265-15050

📠 91-11265-10050

🌐 http://maxhealthcare.in/mddhvi/index.html

Pune

If Mumbai, Delhi, and Bangalore are the preferred destinations for medical tourism, Pune's popularity is more for its niche offering — specifically, knee and hip replacements, obesity surgery, dental surgery, heart surgery, and in-vitro fertilization (IVF). The costs here are also less than in the more renowned cities.

Sancheti Institute for Orthopaedics and Rehabilitation
The Sancheti Institute offers an amazingly wide range of orthopedic services, and its capability in hip replacements is renowned.

🚑 Sancheti Institute for Orthopaedics and Rehabilitation
✉ 16, Shiavji Nagar
   Pune 411005
   India
☎ 91-20-2553-3333
📠 91-20-2553-3233
🌐 www.sanchetihospital.org
@ sanchetihospital@eth.net

Vellore

You probably won't find Vellore mentioned in most tourism literature or guidebooks. The fame of this far-southern city is from two of India's most prestigious educational facilities that are located here: the Christian Medical College & Hospital and the Vellore Institute of Technology.

Christian Medical College & Hospital (CMCH)
A 1,700-bed multi-campus complex, CMCH Vellore is committed to healing the total person. Tertiary-level care includes organ transplants and advanced cardiothoracic and neurological care. Despite its name, this is a nondenominational institute and welcomes people of all faiths.

🚑 Christian Medical College & Hospital
✉ Vellore 632 004
   India
☎ 91-41-6222-2102
📠 91-41-6223-2035
🌐 http://cmch-vellore.edu

Iran

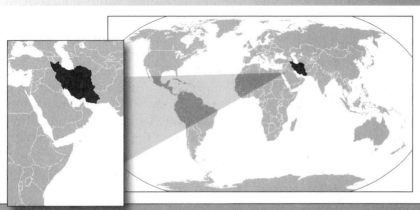

Iran Politics:

It is hard to imagine a country less promising to the development of a tourism industry than present-day Iran. The president is an unrelenting critic of western countries, publicly denies the Jewish holocaust, funds the terrorist group Hizballah, repeatedly calls for the destruction of major economic powers — especially the United States — and it is actively trying to build an atomic bomb. As if this was not enough, the official state religion, Shia Islam, is perhaps the most repressive outside of the Afghan Taliban, hated not only by its persecuted religious minorities but also by 90 percent of other Muslims, who are Sunni and at loggerheads with Shi'ites since the death of Mohammed in 632. And yet, the Iranian government somehow believes that it can compete with countries such as India and Thailand to attract medical tourists. This belief may be as delusional as their notions of world history.

Iran Travel Requirements:

Passport and visa required. The United States does not maintain diplomatic or consular relations with Iran. For visa information, contact the Embassy of Pakistan, Iranian Interests Section, 2209 Wisconsin Avenue, NW, Washington, DC 20007 (202-965-4990). Internet: www.daftar.org. Attention: U.S. citizens may need a U.S. Treasury Department license in order to engage in any transactions related to travel to and within Iran. Before planning any travel to Iran, U.S. citizens should contact the Licensing Division, Office of Foreign Assets Control, U.S. Department of Treasury, (202-622-2480) or www.treas.gov/ofac. Authorities may confiscate U.S. passports of U.S.-Iranian dual nationals upon arrival. Therefore, the Department of State suggests leaving U.S. passports at the nearest U.S. Embassy or Consulate overseas prior to entering Iran and using an Iranian passport to enter.

The Islamic Republic of Iran was formerly known as Persia. Shi'a Islam is the official state religion.

Iranians consider themselves the proud inheritors and guardians of an ancient and sophisticated culture. This includes historical prominence in medicine — and now,

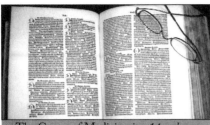

The Canon of Medicine *is a 14–volume medical encyclopedia by Persian physician Abu Ali ibn Sina — better known as Avicenna. Written in 1020, it became the authoritative medical text in Europe and made Iran the center of scientific medicine for the next 700 years. But can Iran compete in the modern era of medicine?*

following an official proclamation in February 2005, Iran intends to again become a global center for healthcare and medical tourism.

The problem is that Iran is not currently a popular destination for any sort of tourism whatsoever. Governmental restrictions on travel make it difficult to get there, let alone move around freely inside the country. In terms of tourist-hosting capacity, Iran ranks 70th worldwide and 13th among Muslim countries. This is a pity, because the country does have many attractions.

Esrafil Shafi Zadeh, director of Iran's medical tourism group, also promotes the traditional medicinal spas that dot the country. He acknowledges that Iran does have an infrastructure and image problem: "Iran's water therapy centers are trying to better their qualities; the more international relations, the better the quality of the services aimed at attracting more tourists." In other words, the spas need to be spiffed up and international relations improved in order to attract more tourists. True enough. But this is going to require quite a change from the current regime.

Iran's numerous medicinal hot springs are used mainly by locals and appear somewhat neglected in comparison to spas in other countries.

City	Name of Spa	Water Temp	Curative for conditions
Takab	Takhteh Solyman	118 F	Neurology
Bandar-e-Abbas (Geno)	Geno	113 F	Rheumatism, gynecology
Bandar-e-Abbas (Khorgoo)	Khorgoo	118 F	Rheumatism, gynecology

While traveling in Iran, I was careful not to disobey the many restrictions on public dress and behavior. However, Iran apparently does have some liberties not allowed in the U.S. As I stood at a bus stop in downtown Teheran, I was joined by a man pulling a large black goat with a rope. I was wondering how he was going to take the goat on the bus, when he casually pulled out of his pocket two heavy duty plastic bags and a long curved knife. To my astonishment he then slit the animal's throat. The blood ran into the gutter as he dismembered the goat and put the meat into one of the bags and the offal, skin, hoofs, and horns into the other. Then the bus arrived and we both got on, with him carrying two manageable bags.

City	Name of Spa	Water Temp	Curative for conditions
Bandar-e-Abbas (Khamir)	Leshtan	115 F	Rheumatism, gynecology
Khalkhal (Senjid)	Givi Souei	138 F	Neurology
Khalkhal (Khoresh ostam)	Miansaran	79 F	Neurology
Ardebil (Sare Eiyn)	Ab Chashm	64 F	Neurology
Ardebil (Sare Eiyn)	Pehen Souei	86 F	Neurology
Ardebil (Sare Eiyn)	Jeneral	108 F	Joint pains
Ardebil (Sare Eiyn)	Sari Sou	106 F	Neurology
Ardebil (Sare Eiyn)	Ghara Sou	117 F	Neurology
Ardebil (Sare Eiyn)	Ghahveh Souei	111 F	Joint pains
Ardebil (Sare Eiyn)	Gavmishgoli	109 F	Neurology, Rheumatism
Ardebil (Sare Eiyn)	Besh Bajilar	104 F	Neurology
Ardebil (Sare Eiyn)	Viladarag	66 F	Gastro-intestinal, Kidney
Ardebil (Sare Eiyn)	Savalan Water Therapy	115 F	Neurology
Ardebil (Markazi)	Sardabe	68 F	Hepatic
Meshkin	Shahr Eilando	93 F	Neurology
Meshkin	Shahr Torsh Sou	54 F	Neurology
Meshkin	Shahr Dobdo	109 F	Neurology
Meshkin	Shahr Shabil	118 F	Joint pains
Meshkin	Shahr Ghotour Souei	102 F	Skin diseases
Meshkin	Shahr Ghinarje	183 F	Joint pains
Meshkin	Shahr Malek Souei	100 F	Neurology
Meshkin	Shahr Mo Eil	106 F	Neurology

Iran Paradise

This service provides information on medicinal springs.

☎ 98-21-2206-7254
℡ 98-21-2206-7256
🌍 www.iranparadise.com
@ Contact@IranParadise.com

Israel

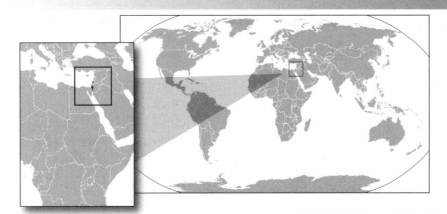

The State of Israel is a tiny country with a huge history. It seems remarkable that Israel, with roughly the same population as neighbor Jordan, should have such a tremendous influence on global politics. This is

Israel Politics:

Israel is a parliamentary democracy and the world's only Jewish state. Since its inception in 1948, it has suffered chronic political turbulence.

Israel Travel Requirements:

Passport, onward or return ticket, and proof of sufficient funds required. Visa not required for stay of up to 90 days.

largely due to the influence of the world's two dominant religions — Christianity and Islam, each with over a billion believers — whose sacred sites lie on the same patch of ground. Every step seems rich with history. Walking along a construction site, I found shards of pottery embedded in the road. I plucked out a big piece and later had it analyzed by a friend who is an archeologist. It dated from approximately 200 A.D. This country has so much history that artifacts of antiquity are used as road fill!

The founding of the State of Israel, in 1948, was followed by the immigration of thousands of scientists and physicians from Germany, Russia, and numerous other countries. They produced many advances in technology and medicine, and Israel now has first-rate medical facilities. Medical tourism would therefore appear to be a logical industry. Indeed, a substantial number of foreigners, particularly Jewish tourists, travel there for healthcare. Assisted reproduction is one such treatment: an IVF procedure can be had for about $2,560 — one fourth of what it would cost in the U.S. However, the major hindrance to tourism is the on-going political tension. Few tourists want to be in a war zone.

W ith regard to the Israeli tourism industry, ironically, the Dead Sea has the most life.

The great exception is the Dead Sea, which draws ever more tourists each year, most of them coming for healthcare or wellness. The sea is called "dead" because its high salinity prevents fish and other creatures from living in it, although it is not sterile and some types of bacteria and fungi can thrive. The Dead Sea is the lowest surface area on Earth and has the most mineral-laden water, with an astonishing salt content of over 30 percent. The water is so dense that "swimming" is a bit of a misnomer — you can simply sit on the water with most your body floating above it.

Shraga Kelson, public relations director of the Radisson Moriah Gardens Dead Sea Hotel at Ein Bokek, explains that Dead Sea tourists feel safe and far removed from terrorist bombings and other troubles. Many are regulars, coming every year for the rejuvenating influence of sun and the water. It is perhaps the only place where a fair-skinned person can sunbathe freely in intense sun without fear of sunburn, since the heavy atmospheric density screens out ultraviolet radiation. Most health tourists come for a month or longer, quickly filling up the 4,000 hotel rooms. The result is a boom in construction to accommodate ever more visitors. Many European countries even pay for patients with skin diseases to spend time at Dead Sea resorts.

The salutary properties of the Dead Sea have been known for thousands of years. Roman soldiers would transport samples of water to Italy for home use. During British rule in the last century, military officers from all over the Empire were brought to the Dead Sea for rest and recuperation, some of them flown right onto the water by seaplane.

Once difficult to get to, the popularity and access to the Dead Sea have steadily grown. Further growth will be even more dramatic with the construction of thousands of new hotel rooms and major medical facilities to accompany existing health spas.

Einbokek
The following Internet address does not include phone numbers or a mailing address, but it will give you just about everything you would want to know. This is typical Israeli efficiency!

 www.einbokek.com

> " *These tourists don't care about [reports of violence].* As far as they're concerned, the Dead Sea is 400 meters below the news; it's another reality."
> ~ Shraga Kelson

Tel Aviv

Rabin Medical Center
Located just outside Tel Aviv, this is the largest medical center in Israel and welcomes medical tourists. Virtually all types of medical care are offered, including very advanced organ transplants. With 1,300 beds and 37 operating rooms, it performs more than 34,000 operations per year.

The Rabin Medical Center, locally just called RMC, has two campuses — Beilinson and Golda-Hasharon — together comprising the largest medical center in Israel. RMC is affiliated with the Tel-Aviv University Sackler School of Medicine and serves as a referral center for patients throughout the country and the region.

- 🏥 Rabin Medical Center
- ✉ Jabutinski St.
  Petah-Tikva 49100
  Israel
- ☎ 972-3-9377-377
- 📠 972-3-9376-364
- 🌐 www.clalit.org.il/rabin/DefaultEng.asp

Ramat Hasharon (Dead Sea)

Health Vacation Center Ltd
More than 60,000 patients have been treated here for psoriasis and arthritis.

- 🏥 Health Vacation Center Ltd
- ✉ 53A Hagefen Street
  Ramat Hasharon
  Israel
- ☎ 972-3-5400-135
- 📠 972-3-5401-069
- @ hvc1@netvision.net.il

Italy

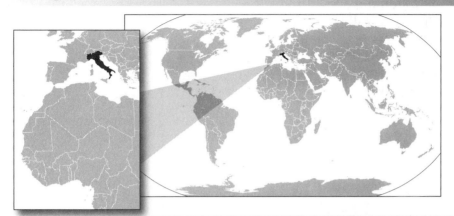

Italy Politics

It is highly ironic that this core of the Roman Empire, the foundation of all Western political structure, should have the most unstable government in Europe.

Italy Travel Requirements:

Passport required. Visa not required for stay of up to 90 days.

The Italian Republic (*Repubblica Italiana*) is always described as a boot-shaped peninsula on the Mediterranean Sea, and it includes the islands of Sicily and Sardinia. Within Italy are the tiny independent countries of San Marino and the Vatican City, not much larger than the postage stamps from which they derive a big part of their income.

Medical tourism in Italy cannot compete with state-of-the-art facilities in Europe or cost-discounts in Asia. At this time, it is mostly concentrated on small, independent clinics that do minor cosmetic surgery and hair transplants. Although the costs are higher than in some other countries, this is a nice adjunct to an Italian vacation and a good excuse to visit this beautiful part of the world.

Scerne di Pineto

This pleasant seaside town is located on the Adriatic Coast in central Italy.

Laser CosMedics
Dr. Donato Zizi specializes in hair restoration, at an approximate cost of $5,400 to $7,200.

Dr. Donato Zizi

✆ Laser CosMedics

✉ via Volturno
64020 Scerne di Pineto (TE)
Italy

☎ 0039-085-9461049

🜨 http://xoomer.virgilio.it/lasercosmedics/

@ donatozizi@virgilio.it

Jordan

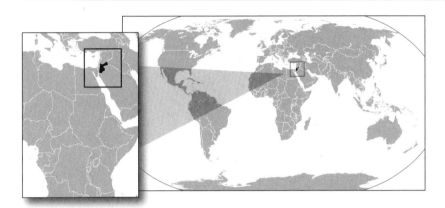

The Hashemite Kingdom of Jordan lies between Israel and Saudi Arabia, which helps explain its peculiar blend of Islamic rigidity and Western modernity.

Jordan's 56 private hospitals are massively promoting medical tourism. According to the Jordan Private Hospital Association

Jordan Politics:

Jordan continually finds itself embroiled in Middle East politics, particularly between its Israel and its Arabic neighbors, although it tries to steer a course of moderation and appeasement to all sides.

Jordan Travel Requirements:

Passport and visa required. Visitors may obtain a visa for Jordan, for a fee, at most international ports of entry upon arrival except at the King Hussein/Allenby Bridge.

(PHA), about 100,000 patients have been arriving each year from other Arabic countries, attracted by the low cost and high quality of the hospitals. Major draws are sophisticated treatment in coronary care, kidney and corneal transplants, and spinal cord injuries. Now these hospitals also want to attract patients from non-Arab countries. To help facilitate this industry, the Ministry of Health has set up promotional bureaus in the north and south terminals of the Queen Alia International Airport for arriving patients. Jordanian officials in foreign embassies guide prospective patients to the Kingdom's most specialized hospitals, including the Royal Medical Services Hospital, the Arab Surgical Hospital, Khalidi Hospital, the Islamic Hospital, the Specialized Hospital, Ibn Haitham Hospital, and the expansive new Estishari Hospital, all of which are located in the capital, Amman.

A problem is that many of these arriving medical tourists have been defrauded, abused, and otherwise taken advantage of — even by the physicians and treating hospitals. This has given Jordan a terrible reputation in medical tourism. To prevent further abuse, the Health Ministry recently standardized medical fees of private hospitals so that patients would not be overcharged. However, it will be difficult to overcome this reputation in the face of rapidly increasing medical tourism offerings in other countries.

Because individual hospitals do not make arrangements for medical tourists, it is best to contact the Jordan embassy for current information and recommendations at www.jordanembassyus.org

Latvia

A top destination choice for:
dental care

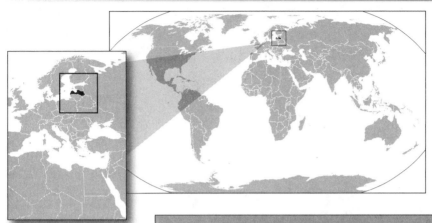

The Republic of Latvia (*Latvijas Republika*) is a small country across the Baltic Sea from Sweden. Travel from Europe is easy, and savvy tourists are discovering that Latvia provides European-quality healthcare at much lower prices. The country's medical tourism at this point is largely dental work, but additional services are underway.

Latvia Politics:

Latvia is one of three small Baltic countries (the others are Estonia and Lithuania) that have won independence from Russia and are now turning culturally and economically to Europe.

Latvia Travel Requirements:

Passport with minimum validity of three months required. Visa not required for a stay of up to 90 days.

Riga

Villadent

Villadent is an affiliation of several dental clinics in Latvia. Services include standard and cosmetic dentistry.

- 🚑 Villadent
- ✉ Riga, Dzelzavas 38
  LV-1035
  Latvia
- ☎ 371 757 9809
- 🌍 www.villadent.com
- @ villa@villadent.com

Malaysia

A top destination choice for:
cancer treatment, cardiac bypass, hip replacement

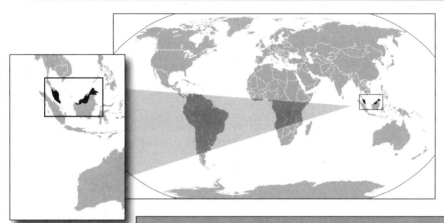

Malaysia Politics:

Although the national religion is Islam, the government downplays any form of extremism in order to appeal to non-Islamic people and industries.

Malaysia Travel Requirements:

A valid passport is required. U.S. citizens do not need a visa.

The Federation of Malaysia was formed in 1963 out of several Malayan-speaking regions that had suffered colonization and occupation by various powers until after the Second World War. Singapore, at the tip of the Malayan peninsula, was initially part of Malaysia, but the pronounced ethnic and cultural differences between the predominantly Muslim Malays and the predominantly Chinese in Singapore led to a split. Malaysia consists of two geographical regions divided by the South China Sea: West Malaysia, or Peninsular Malaysia, between Thailand to the north and Singapore on the south; and East Malaysia, on the island of Borneo.

A spectacular country of tropical rainforests, sandy white beaches, and countless islands, Malaysia has long been a favored tourist destination. More recently, the government has aggressively encouraged the technology industry, with plans to become a developed nation by 2020. Examples of this abound: in Kuala Lumpur, the capital, the recent economic boom has created a jungle of high-tech buildings — including the Petronas Towers, the tallest twin towers in the world. Close on the heels of the technology industry is a new emphasis on medical tourism, headed by a wide network of high-quality hospitals.

The Malaysian healthcare system requires doctors to perform a compulsory service of three years in public hospitals, providing universal healthcare for its population.

Foreign doctors are also encouraged to work in Malaysia, and many have been attracted by the low cost of living and the tropical environment.

Private hospitals, formerly considered a poor investment, are now rapidly expanding to accommodate medical tourists. Most of these hospitals do not have a budget or program in place for the active promotion of medical tourism, but they encourage foreign patients and treat them with the utmost hospitality. Many cater to long-term care residents, which is especially advantageous for medical tourists who need lengthy nursing or hospice care.

In this large and varied country, the best strategy for someone seeking inexpensive medical care is to choose the location first and then inquire directly with the local hospital.

The following hospitals specifically welcome medical tourists:

Johor
Century Medical Centre Sdn Bhd
Hospital Pakar Larkin
Hospital Penawar Sdn Bhd
Johor Specialist Hospital
Klinik C S Koh & Rumah Bersalin
Klinik Rakyat & Hospital Bersalin
Pelangi Medical Centre
Pusat Pakar Kluang Utama
Pusat Pakar Perbidanan & Sakitpuan Raja
Puteri Specialist Hospital
Siow Specialist Hospital
Southern Hospital
Tan Clinic & Maternity Home
Tey Specialist Maternity & Gynae Centre
Wisma Maria Medical Specialist Centre

Kedah
Kedah Medical Centre
Metro Specialist Hospital
Putra Medical Centre
Strand Hospital & Retirement Home

Kelantan
Kota Bahru Medical Centre
Perdana Specialist Hospital
Pusat Rawatan Islam An-Nisa

Kuala Lumpur
  Apollo TTDI Medical Centre
  Damai Service Hospital
  Dato' Dr Harnam ENT Clinic
  Cheras Geriatric Centre
  Chinese Maternity Hospital
  Gleneagles Intan Medical Centre
  Hospital Danau Kota
  Hospital Pantai Indah
  Imran Ear, Nose & Throat Specialist Hospital
  Institut Jantung Negara
  Klinik Alam Medic Sentul
  Lourdes Medical Centre
  Pantai Cheras Medical Centre
  Pantai Medical Centre
  Poliklinik Kotaraya
  Pudu Specialist Centre
  Pusat Pakar Tawakal
  Pusat Rawatan Islam
  Roopi Medical Centre
  Sambhi Clinic & Nursing Home
  Samuel Clinic & Specialist Maternity & Clinic for Women
  Sentosa Medical Centre
  Sentul Hospital
  Taman Desa Medical Centre
  Tung Shin Hospital

Melaka
  Hospital Pantai Ayer Keroh
  Mahkota Medical Centre
  The Southern Hospital

Negeri Sembilan
  Columbia Medical Centre, Seremban
  Hospital Pakar Seremban
  N.S. Chinese Maternity Hospital
  Nilai Cancer Institute
  Pusat Pakar Seremban

Pahang

Kuantan Medical Centre
Kuantan Specialist Hospital
Pusat Perubatan Fadzilah
S T Chong Maternity & Surgery

Penang

Bagan Specialist Centre
Bukit Mertajam Specialist Hospital
Gleneagles Medical Centre
Hope Children Hospital
Hospital Pantai Mutiara
Hospital Peninsula
Island Hospital
KS Wan & Liow Specialist Maternity Centre
Lam Wah Ee Hospital
Loh Guan Lye Specialist Centre
Mount Miriam Hospital
Peace Medical Centre
Penang Adventist Hospital
Srigim Medical Centre
Tan & Tan Specialist Maternity Centre
Tanjung Medical Centre

Perak

Apollo Medical Centre
Hospital Fatimah
Hospital Pantai-Putri
Ipoh Specialist Hospital
Kinta Medical Centre
Maxwell Maternity & Surgical Centre
Perak Chinese Maternity Hospital
Pusat Pakar Rajindar Singh
Taiping Medical Centre

Sabah

Damai Specialist Centre
Sabah Medical Centre

Sarawak

Columbia Asia Medical Centre
Lions Nursing Homes
Kuching Medical Centre
Miri City Medical Centre
Normah Medical Centre
Rejang Medical Centre
Timberland Medical Centre

Selangor

Ampang Puteri Specialist Hospital
Andalas Medical Centre
Arunamari Specialist Medical Centre
Assunta Hospital
Az-Zahrah Islamic Medical Centre
Damai Service Hospital (Melawati)
Damansara Fertility Centre
Damansara Specialist Hospital
Darul Ehsan Medical Centre
Kajang Specialist Maternity & Surgery
Kelana Jaya Medical Centre
Klinik Damo & Pusat Bersalin
Klinik Kartini Medan
Klinik Pakar Razif & Norana
Klinik Pakar Wanita Sheela & Rumah Bersalin
Klinik Puravi & Maternity Home
Lam Surgery & Maternity Home
Mawar Medical Centre
Pantai Klang Specialist Centre
PJ Nursing Home
PMMC Shah Alam
Pusat Rawatan Islam (MAIS)
QHC Medical Centre
Salam Medical Centre
Selangor Medical Centre
Shah Alam Medical Centre

Sri Kota Medical Centre
Subang Jaya Medical Centre
Sunway Medical Centre
Tee Maternity & Gynae Specialist Centre
Tun Hussein Onn National Eye Hospital

George Town

In 1786, Captain Francis Light of the British East India Company obtained the island of Penang from the Sultan of Kedah, and named his settlement on the island after King George III. Penang has since become one of Malaysia's premier tourist destinations, while George Town has retained a pre-colonial charm. A new monorail system will soon ease travel within the region.

Penang Adventist Hospital

A private medical institution that is part of an international network of more than 500 hospitals and healthcare facilities operated by Adventist Health System, Penang Adventist Hospital is associated with The Loma Linda University & Medical Centre in California, and The Florida Hospital in Orlando. The hospital has specialists in microvascular surgery, coronary bypass, laser heart surgery, and open-heart surgery.

Penang Adventist's mission statement reads:

"Our hospital gives medical care to the community regardless of race, colour, or creed, and promotes the prevention of disease through health education. Our mission: 'To make man whole' is to follow the ideals of God, the Master Physician, and to provide for your well-being by ministering to your spiritual and emotional needs, in modern and pleasant facilities."

🏥 Penang Adventist Hospital
✉ 465 Burma Road
   10350 George Town
   Malaysia
☎ 604-226-1133
✆ 604-226-3366
🌐 www.pah.com.my
@ AdventistHealth@pah.com.my

Ipoh

Ipoh is a town in the highlands of Malaysia, near the central mountain range. It is renowned for its pure waters, numerous waterfalls, and limestone caverns.

Fatimah Hospital

Nestled in lush greenery in the business center of Ipoh Garden, Fatimah hospital has easy access to transport, shops and popular eateries. It was founded by a religious congregation, The Congregation of the Brothers of Mercy, with the goal of delivering high-quality and compassionate healthcare to patients from all levels of society, irrespective of race, religion, or creed.

Its mission statement: "In Hospital Fatimah, we aim to give what is often described as 'holistic' care. We endeavour to minister to the many dimensions of a person's needs by providing physical, spiritual, emotional, and psychological care."

- 🏥 Fatimah Hospital
- ✉ Jalan Dato Lau Pak Khuan
  Ipoh Garden
  31400 Ipoh
  Perak
  Malaysia
- ☎ 605-545-5777
- ℡ 605-547-7050
- 🌐 www.fatimah.com.my
- @ enquiry@fatimah.com.my

Ipoh Specialist Hospital

This is a 210-bed full-service hospital that delivers emergency, acute, inpatient, and outpatient care all in one central location.

- 🏥 Ipoh Specialist Hospital
- ✉ 26 Jalan Raja Dihilir
  30350 Ipoh
  Perak
  Malaysia
- ☎ 604-227-6111
- ℡ 604-226-2994
- 🌐 www.ish.kpjhealth.com.my
- @ ish@ish.kpjhealth.com.my

Johor

Johor Specialist Hospital

Johor Specialist Hospital (JSH) opened its doors to the public in 1981 as the first private hospital in Johor. Located on a five-acre site off Jalan Abdul Samad Johor Bahru, JSH has a commanding view of the lush sculptured surroundings of Royal Johor Country Club, Johor Bahru. JSH is associated with 11 other private specialist hospitals in Malaysia — the KPJ Healthcare Group of hospitals in the Healthcare Division of Johor Corporation.

🚑 Johor Specialist Hospital
✉ 39-B, Jalan Abdul Samad
   80100 Johor Bahru
   Malaysia
☎ 607-225-3000
📠 607-224-8213
🌐 www.jsh.kpj.com.my
@ jsh@jsh.kpj.com.my

Kuala Lumpur

The capital and by far the largest city of Malaysia, Kuala Lumpur means "muddy river confluence." The city, which is experiencing a technology boom, is colloquially called KL.

Gleneagles Intan Medical Centre

Gleneagles has 110 specialist consulting suites, a 180-seat auditorium on the top floor, and a retail pharmacy, a bank, and a car park on the ground floor. Specialist physicians are independent practitioners.

🚑 Gleneagles Intan Medical Centre
✉ Wilayah Persekutuan
   282-286 Jalan Ampang
   50450 Kuala Lumpur
   Malaysia
☎ 603-4257-1300
📠 603-4257-9233
🌐 www.gimc.com.my
@ jessmooi@gleneaglesintan.com.my

Pantai Medical Centre

The Pantai Group's flagship hospital operates 264 beds and has a medical staff of more than 130 specialists. It is located in the cozy, residential neighborhood of Bangsar, yet is close to the city center. The hospital houses the WorldCare Health Telemedicine hub linked to the major U.S. institutions, including the Johns Hopkins Medical Center, Duke University Hospital, Cleveland Clinic, and the Massachusetts General Hospital.

🚑 Pantai Medical Centre
✉ 8 Jalan Bukit Pantai
   59100 Kuala Lumpur
   Malaysia

☎ 603-2296-0888
📠 603-2282-1557
🌐 www.pantai.com
@ pmc@pantai.com.my

Penang

Gleneagles Medical Centre, Penang

This was the first private hospital in the island of Penang. Along with other Gleneagles hospitals, it is owned by Parkway Holdings Limited of Singapore.

📇 Gleneagles Medical Centre
✉ 1 Jalan Pangkor
10050 Pulau Pinang
Malaysia
☎ 604-227-6111
📠 604-226-2994
🌐 www.gleneagles-penang.com
@ admin@gmc.po.my

Island Hospital

This is a 240-bed private medical center known for its warmth, friendliness, and compassion. For about $75, you can get a complete "Executive Screening Programme" done, which includes a full medical exam and a dozen lab tests.

The Island Heart Centre is a prominent, highly regarded facility that provides comprehensive cardiac care, surgery, and rehabilitation.

📇 Island Hospital
✉ 308 MacAlister Road
10450 Pulau Pinang
Malaysia
☎ 604-228-8222
📠 604-226-7989
🌐 www.islandhospital.com
@ info@islandhospital.com

Mount Miriam Hospital Cancer Centre

This hospital specializes in cancer treatment, providing radiotherapy, brachytherapy, interventional radiology, and oncology palliative care.

📇 Mount Miriam Hospital
✉ 23, Jalan Bulan Fettes Park
Tanjong Bunga

11200 Pulau Pinang
Malaysia
☎ 604-890-7044
📠 604-890-1583
🌐 www.mountmiriam.com
@ mmiriam@tm.net.my

Selangor

Ampang Puteri Specialist Hospital
This six-story hospital is designed and furnished to resemble the highest-quality hospitals internationally. It is located near the Ampang Point Shopping Complex.

🏥 Ampang Puteri Specialist Hospital
✉ No. 1, Jalan Mamanda 9
68000 Ampang
Selangor
Malaysia
☎ 603-4270-2500
📠 603-4270-2443
🌐 www.apsh.kpj.com.my
@ apsh@apsh.kpj.com.my

Assunta Hospital
Founded by the Franciscan Missionaries of Mary in 1957, this hospital started the first private nursing school in the country. The Assunta College of Nursing is now highly regarded for its professional nursing standards and caring service.

The Assunta philosophy
Every person is created by God and is equal in the sight of God.

The object of the hospital is to serve all in need of treatment with the respect, care and devotion owed to a creature of God.

Since all are equal in the sight of God, all persons, whatever their nationality, race, belief or social status are deserving of equal respect.

Patients must be treated as whole persons with particular care for their feelings as well as their physical needs.

Cheerfulness, courtesy and warmth of service constitute an important part of every patient's treatment.

🏥 Assunta Hospital
✉ Lot 68 Jalan Templer
46990 Petaling Jaya

Selangor
Malaysia
☎ 603-7782-3433
℡ 603-7784-1749
🌐 www.assunta.com.my

Columbia Asia Medical Center
This is a network of private hospitals offering a variety of services, including rehabilitation.

🏢 Columbia Pacific Healthcare Management Sdn. Bhd.
✉ Suite W701, West Tower, 7th Floor
Wisma Consplant 11
No. 2. Jalan SS 16/4
47500 Subang Jaya
Selangor
Malaysia
☎ 603-5632-3800
℡ 603-5632-4800
🌐 www.columbiaasia.com
@ info@columbiaasia.com

Damansara Fertility Centre (DFC)
Established in January 1994, DFC has grown and developed into a one-stop center providing the entire spectrum of the most technologically advanced treatment options for couples with fertility problems. They perform laparoscopic (keyhole) surgery, intra-uterine insemination (IUI), in-vitro fertilization (IVF), gamete intra-fallopian transfer (GIFT), intra-cytoplasmic sperm injection (ICSI), blastocyst transfer, pre-implantation genetic diagnosis (PGD) and freezing of embryos and sperm. The center also provides other ancillary services in the management of infertility, including an embryo and a sperm bank.

Secondary facilities are the Damansara Fertility and Women's Specialist Center in Johor Bahru, just five minutes' drive from the Singapore Causeway, and in Kepong, Kuala Lumpur.

🏢 Damansara Fertility Centre
✉ 55, Jalan SS21/56B
Damansara Utama
Selangor
Malaysia
☎ 603-7729-3199

☏ 603-7727-8066
🌐 www.damansarafertility.com

Sunway Medical Centre (SUNMED)

SUNMED is a private hospital offering specialized tertiary healthcare services. The medical complex is an eight-story building with 240 beds and 45 specialist consultation suites.

🏥 Sunway Medical Centre Berhad
✉ 5, Jalan Lagoon Selatan, Bandar Sunway
46150 Petaling Jaya
Selangor
Malaysia
☎ 603-74919191
☏ 603-74918181
🌐 www.sunway.com.my/sunmed
@ smc@sunway.com.my

Sungai Petani

Metro Specialist Hospital

This modern hospital is equipped with MRI, mammogram, lithotripter, and other state-of-the-art technology, especially for the treatment of kidney stones. They are particularly proud of their Swiss "Lithoclast Master," a sort of high-tech vacuum cleaner for kidney stones that allows minimally invasive removal.

🏥 Metro Specialist Hospital
✉ No. 1, Lorong Metro 08000
Sungai Petani Kedah
Malaysia
☎ 604-423-8888
☏ 604-423-4848
🌐 www.hospitalmetro.com
@ metro@hospitalmetro.com

Malta

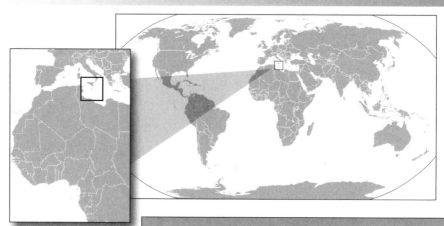

Malta Politics:

These strategically located islands have been fought over for thousands of years. Malta now is the smallest European Union country in both population and area.

Malta Travel Requirements:

Passport required. Visa not required for stay of up to 90 days.

The Republic of Malta is a small and densely populated group of islands in the middle of the Mediterranean Sea. The Maltese language is closely related to Arabic.

Malta has many museums, shops, beaches, and leisure activities in a densely packed area. It is a well-known popular vacation destination among Europeans.

Saint James Hospital

This is a network of hospitals and clinics in the communities of Zabbar, Sliema, Gozo, Mosta, and Transforma.

- 🏨 Saint James Hospital
- ✉ St James Square
  Zabbar ZBR 05
  Malta
- ☎ 356-21692055
- 📠 356-21692030
- 🌐 www.stjameshospital.com
- @ info@stjameshospital.com

Mexico

A top destination choice for:
alternative medicine, Botox treatment,
cosmetic surgery

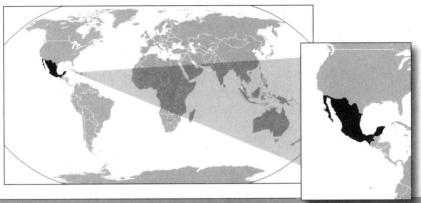

Mexico Politics:

The histories and economies of the United States and Mexico have been closely intertwined for over a century. This relationship is likely to intensify as trade barriers decrease.

Mexico Travel Requirements:

Passport is required. You must also have a tourist card, valid for three months for single entry up to 180 days. The card, which has a $20 fee, can be obtained in advance from a Consulate or Tourism Office, but most airlines serving Mexico provide them upon arrival. For additional information, check with the Embassy of Mexico, 1911 Pennsylvania Ave., NW, Washington, DC 20006 (202-736-1000) or nearest Consulate General:

 Arizona (602-242-7398)
 California (213-351-6800, 415-392-5554, 619-231-8414)
 Colorado (303-331-1110)
 Florida (305-716-4977)
 Georgia (404-266-1913)
 Illinois (312-855-1380)
 Louisiana (504-522-3596)
 New York (212-689-0460)
 Puerto Rico (809-764-0258)
 Texas (210-227-1085, 214-630-7341, 713-542-2300, 512-478-9031, 915-533-4082)
 Internet: www.embassyofmexico.org

Mexico serves as an important lesson in the pros and cons of medical tourism. It is one of the first countries to engage in modern medical tourism. Its location — directly south of, and sharing a long border with, a country with a high standard of living but a costly and inadequate healthcare delivery system — should clearly place Mexico among the top medical tourist destinations.

But it is not. In fact, Mexico is not even in the top 20 or 30 countries that cater to international patients. What went wrong?

For over a century, cost-conscious Americans have crossed the border for cheaper services or procedures unavailable in the United States To capitalize on the healthcare industry, clinics have sprung up from Tijuana on the Pacific coast to Mata Moros on the Gulf Coast, and every border town in between. Some are legitimate medical and dental clinics. However, the biggest moneymakers — and greatest attraction for Americans — are the countless clinics and pharmacies offering miraculous new treatments for fatal illnesses such as cancer. It doesn't matter that investigators consider them bogus or outright frauds. Americans go to them anyway, often reasoning that a person dying of cancer has nothing to lose, so every chance of a cure, no matter how unlikely, is better than no chance at all. And this desperation is precisely what the clinics prey on. They dangle the hope of an exotic (but costly) treatment to people with terminal illness, reminding them that they have nothing to lose. Any ethical concerns about fleecing the dying are swept aside by the general attitude that *Norteamericanos* are rich and stupid, and this is merely a way of redressing the economic imbalances. No doubt, a few patients do improve or even recover. This is normal in terminal illness — there are always a few people who spontaneously recover. However, these clinics shamelessly exploit such recoveries (or any real or imagined improvement) and claim it was due to their treatment.

A famous example was Steve McQueen. The great film actor suffered from mesothelioma, a rare and fatal type of lung cancer probably caused by his exposure to asbestos when he was a young Navy serviceman. Although his doctors strongly advised Mr. McQueen against it, he felt desperate and spent millions of dollars on worthless treatments in Mexico. By the time he died, he was already being followed by thousands of Americans seeking similarly hopeful cures. Yet his death did nothing to discourage the phenomenon — the news only served to alert people about the clinics' existence, and, ironically, resulted in an even much greater flow of healthcare-seeking Americans to Mexico.

Steve McQueen was treated by laetrile, a cyanide-containing extract from apricot pits. Mexican clinics are still promoting this useless substance. Ever more fanciful remedies are invented every day, often mimicking the medical news or popular science discoveries. For example, the ethical concerns around using human stem cells in research have become a major political issue. Although few medical tourists have any understanding of stem cells, this does not prevent numerous clinics from offering an outlandish variety of "stem-cell treatments" — usually from sheep! — which are taken as a drinkable potion or injected. Any reputable scientist or physician would laugh at this, but the practice is popular and is viewed as an alternative to the domineering American medical establishment.

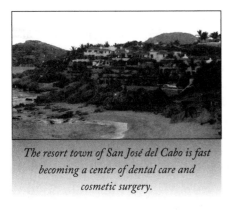

The resort town of San José del Cabo is fast becoming a center of dental care and cosmetic surgery.

A more notable and sad example of a duped medical tourist is Coretta Scott King, the wife of assassinated civil rights leader Martin Luther King, Jr. Since his death, Mrs. King continued his work to promote a non-violent solution to discrimination, and she was a tireless and respected leader in her own right. At age 78, suffering from a debilitating stroke and terminal ovarian cancer, she died on January 30, 2006, at Rosarito Beach, Mexico, while undergoing treatment at a "holistic" clinic. Her very expensive treatment with sham remedies did nothing to help her, but it did contribute to the wellbeing of her so-called doctors.

Entire busloads of elderly and infirm Americans and Canadians go on chartered tours of border towns where they are taken from one "clinic" to another — most of which do not have medical accreditation even in the lax Mexican regulatory environment. The same is true of drugs, since many Mexican pharmacies are unscrupulous in selling to Americans whatever they want. Because of this, Mexico has come to be known as the destination of last resort, scamming terminally ill patients with bogus treatments.

This is the only form of medical tourism that most Americans have heard of, and it has given the practice a bad reputation. More specifically, it has given Mexico a bad reputation. The once-favored country for discount treatment has become known as the place to avoid if you want quality care.

Now Mexico is trying to divest itself of this image and capitalize on the surge of modern medical tourism. In this regard, it is lagging behind other faster-moving countries in the region such as Costa Rica and Panama. All of these countries feature mostly dental and cosmetic work at much lower prices than in the U.S. The most successful Mexican clinics seem to be located in resort communities with high populations of Americans, such as Cabo San Lucas. But Cabo is a small niche market, appealing mainly to wealthy tourists who can afford resort vacations. The more accessible border towns, meanwhile, continue to suffer from a profusion of quack clinics.

Beginning in 2006, a new trend is appearing. American healthcare has become so expensive that even the major medical insurance companies are looking for an escape. Blue Shield is exploring ways to have its patients treated in Mexico, and many counties in the U.S. are planning to refer uninsured patients to the nearest hospital south of the border. In response, the large Mexican hospital chain, Grupo Empresarial Angeles, is building half a dozen hospitals in the border cities.

Clearly, Mexico is trying to leave the past behind and develop medical tourism in a big way. Ultimately, this trend may bring as much change to the U.S. as it does to Mexico.

CosmeticSurgery.com

This cosmetic surgery referral site is primarily for the U.S.-based clinics, but also refers to some other countries, including Mexico. Click on "Find a Doctor," then "Select a Location," then "Mexico," and then "Search." You will be shown a list of supposedly reputable cosmetic surgeons in Mexico.

Dr. Miguelangelo Gonzalez is one of them. He has personal offices on the grounds of Cabo San Lucas's venerable palm-shaded waterfront Hotel Hacienda Beach Resort. A private recovery room and 24-hour nursing care help reassure patients who have any concern about being in Mexico. Patients often elect to stay at the hotel to recuperate and relax by the pool overlooking the bay and the famous Land's End rock formations that mark the tip of the thousand-mile-long Baja California peninsula.

- 🌐 www.cosmeticsurgery.com

Miguelangelo Plastic Surgery Clinic

- 🏢 Miguelangelo Plastic Surgery Clinic
- ✉ Hotel Hacienda Beach Resort, Int. #6
  Cabo San Lucas
  Baja California Sur
  México
- ☎ 52-624-143-4303
- 📠 52-624-143-4391
- 🌐 www.miguelangeloclinic.com
- @ info@miguelangeloclinic.com

Angels Touch Dental Clinic

Not far from Cabo San Lucas lies the lesser-known tourist town of San José del Cabo. The formerly secret hideaway of John Wayne, Bing Crosby, Desi Arnaz and other Hollywood stars is now a popular medical tourist destination. Dr. Rosa Pena runs three dental clinics catering to entire families of Americans.

- 🏢 Angels Touch Dental Clinic
- ✉ Plazas Doradas Building local #7
  San José del Cabo
  México
- ☎ 52-624-142-6192
- 🌐 www.angelsdental.com
- @ info@angelsdental.com

Tijuana

Tijuana, a city of 1.5 million on the California border, is the first to build a hospital designed specifically to accommodate American medical tourists.

Hospital Angeles Tijuana

This new $70 million facility is specifically designed to provide discounted health-care for nearby Californians. Located in the upscale Rio Zone, it is the first hospital in Tijuana to have its own pharmacy, blood bank, x-ray equipment, neonatal intensive care unit, nuclear medicine lab, monitoring equipment, emergency department, and operating rooms all in the same nine-story building. On opening day, Mexico's health minister Julio Frenk declared: "Today, Mexico offers options that rival those of any institution in any part of the world." Hospital Angeles is now negotiating with Medicare to be allowed to provide treatment for Medicare patients — the first time Medicare will pay for standard treatment in a foreign country.

   📇 Hospital Angeles Tijuana
   ✉ Ave. Paseo de los Héroes 10999
      Zona Río Tijuana
      22010 Tijuana, B.C.
      México
   ☎ 011-664-634-7806
   📠 011-664-634-2251
   🌐 www.hospitalangelestijuana.com.mx

Los Algodones

Just across the border from Yuma, Arizona, is the small town of Los Algodones ("The Cottons"). Today, most of the cotton there is turned into dressings used in dental work. Amazingly, more than 350 dentists now practice there, providing everything from basic dentistry to the most advanced treatment. The vast majority of the patients are, of course, Americans. They come not only from nearby Phoenix and San Diego but also from much farther away for an all-inclusive dental vacation. The cost is about 75 percent less than the equivalent dental work in the United States.

MexAdvantage

MexAdvantage helps people choose among the many dentists in Los Algodones for a $5 fee. It is located in Yuma and provides transportation across the border. You can make an appointment online.

   📇 MexAdvantage
   ✉ Advantage Complex
      1292 Fifth Avenue
      Yuma, AZ 85364
   🌐 www.dentistsofalgodones.com

New Zealand

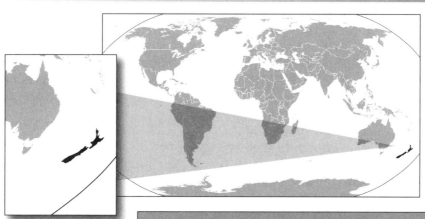

New Zealand is a country of two large islands (North and South Islands), and many much smaller islands in the southwestern Pacific Ocean. The country is notable for its geographic isolation; although it is always considered close to Australia, the distance to its larger neighbor is 1,250 miles.

Most of New Zealand's people are of European descent, having supplanted the indigenous Maoris, who are now the largest minority. Many other Polynesian and Asian peoples are also significant minorities, especially in the larger cities.

New Zealand Politics:

New Zealand has always been something of a pacifist nation, occasionally a nuisance to Western powers because of its opposition to nuclear testing and other military operations. In general, it is a very peaceful, friendly nation with a population that treasures its geographic remoteness from the rest of the world.

New Zealand Travel Requirements:

Passport and arrival card (to be completed upon arrival) are required. A visa is not required for a stay of up to three months, but you must have an onward or return ticket, a visa for the next destination, and proof of sufficient funds. Oddly, New Zealand regulations also state that "All visitors who travel to New Zealand for healthcare and who are not New Zealand citizens or New Zealand residents require a Visitors Visa. There are no exceptions. It is also necessary to have proof that funding is available for medical care prior to arrival in New Zealand." This implies that you normally do not need a visa, but you do if your purpose is healthcare. It may be worth sending an e-mail to the New Zealand embassy (nz@nzemb.org) to clarify this if you have any questions.

Although New Zealand derives a large part of its foreign income from tourism, relatively few people come specifically for medical treatment. The costs are low — about

40 to 50 percent of the cost in the United States — but this is not quite enough to compete with other major medical tourism destinations. However, the combination of medical treatment and a vacation in the land where *The Lord of the Rings* was filmed is a great attraction.

Auckland

About one third of the New Zealand population lives in Greater Auckland, a very pleasant city of 1.2 million.

New Zealand Health Tourism Company

The New Zealand Health Tourism Company (NUAZ) acts as a facilitator to coordinate travel, accommodation, specialist consultation, private hospital, public hospital, and recovery arrangements for medical tourism. A NUAZ representative will meet you on arrival at the airport and escort you to your accommodation. This is a commercial referral service to New Zealand healthcare providers, such as the privately owned Ascot Integrated Hospital.

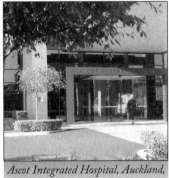

Ascot Integrated Hospital, Auckland, New Zealand, is a favored destination for medical tourists.

- 📠 NUAZ Ltd
- ✉ PO Box 24 498
  Royal Oak, Auckland
  New Zealand
- ☎ 64-9-636-0388
- ☎ 64-27-477-5390
- ☎ 64-9-636-5039
- 📠 64-8-326-1577
- 🌐 www.nuaz.co.nz
- @ janet@nuaz.co.nz

Panama

A top destination choice for:
cosmetic surgery, dental care, eye surgery,
hip replacement

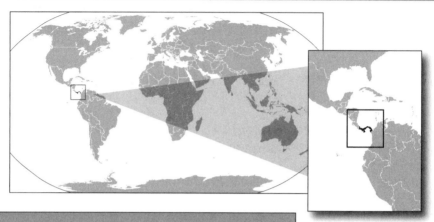

Panama Politics:

Since the building of the Panama Canal, the Canal Zone was owned by the United States and effectively split the country in two. In the 1970s, the Canal Zone was returned to Panama, helping to integrate the country and sustain its economy, which is largely based on shipping fees. However, Panama continues to have a strong American presence and a very cosmopolitan culture as an international crossroads.

Panama Travel Requirements:

Passport or proof of U.S. citizenship and photo ID, tourist card or visa, proof of sufficient funds, and an onward or return ticket is required. A visa and tourist card is valid for 30 days. Visas are issued at the Embassy of Panama or one of the Consulates. Tourist cards are available from airlines serving Panama for a $5 fee.

Panama (*Panamá*) is a narrow country forming the bridge between North and South America and separating the two greatest oceans of the world — the Atlantic and Pacific. As such, it has a very cosmopolitan atmosphere, especially in Panama City where voices can be heard in languages from around the world. Many goals and interests bring people to Panama, and now there is a new one: health tourism.

Most of Panama's doctors speak excellent English, are board certified in their specialties, and many have trained in the United States. Panama offers savings of about 50 percent in comparison with the U.S., and the American dollar is widely used. Furthermore, getting there is easy; it is just two and a half hours by air from Miami. Panama has become a favorite retirement area for Americans, and each increase in the number of expats makes Americans feel more at home.

Approximate prices of some common treatments:

Cardiology
Echocardiogram...$300
Stress echocardiogram $500
Echocardiogram with dobutamine $450
Holter monitor $200
Exercise stress test...$200

Laparoscopic Surgery
Gall bladder removal..$3,500
Hernia...$4,000
Nissen fundoplication $5,000
Gastric bypass...$15,000

Plastic Surgery
Neck or face lift $6,800
Blepharoplasty..$2,300
Cervicoplasty..$2,150
Rhinoplasty $3,100
Breast augmentation $3,900
Breast reconstruction..$3,000
Breast reduction...$5,600
Breast lift...$3,800
Liposuction...$2,900
Thigh lift..$4,000
Dermabrasion $1,500
Chemical peel...$600
Fat injections $400
Buttock augmentation...$3,900

Gastroenterology
Esophagogastroduodenoscopy (EGD) $325
Colonoscopy..$550
Colonoscopy and polypectomy $750
ERCP and stone extraction..$1,000
Bravo capsule imaging..$300
Capsule endoscopy...$400

Assisted reproduction

Intrauterine insemination $850
In-vitro fertilization...$5,000
In-vitro fertilization with donated egg $7,500

Dental implants and periodontics

Dental implant $1,000
Periodontal surgery $450
Periodontal plastic surgery $500
Periodontal regenerative procedure $600
Free gingival graft $450

Clinical laboratory

Kidney function $66
Liver function...$63
Bone metabolism (osteoporosis) $94
Heart function and coronary risk..$61
Choosing the sex of your baby $960

Pulmonology

Bronchoscopy..$350
Pleurodesis...$300
Thoracentesis...$150
Percutaneous lung biopsy $1,000

Orthopedic surgery

Hip or knee replacement...$12,000
Arthroscopy $5,000
Herniated disc repair $6,500
Carpal tunnel release..$3,000

Ophthalmology

Cataract surgery...$2,500
Glaucoma surgery..$2,000
Eyelid surgery $2,500

Panama City

Pana-Health

Pana-Health is a referral service to "Panama's top health professionals."

www.pana-health.com
info@pana-health.com

Nacional Hospital

Nacional is a private, full-service hospital located in the heart of Panama City. The hospital is run by Family Hospital Corporation (FHC), a U.S. hospital administration firm that works throughout Latin America and insures quality. It is affiliated with Harvard Medical Faculty Physicians at Beth Israel Deaconess Medical Center.

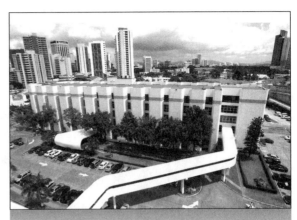

The Centro Médico Patilla is one of Panama Health's superb medical centers oriented to international patients.

🚑 Nacional Hospital
✉ Cuba St.
Panama City
Panama
☎ 507-207-8100
📞 507-207-8337
🌎 www.hospitalnacional.com
@ mercadeo@hospitalnacional.com

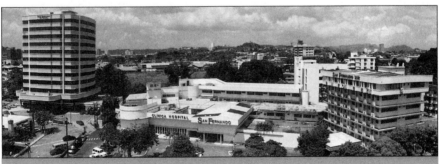

The Hospital San Fernando Fachada is one of Pana-Health's network of facilities welcoming international patients.

Philippines

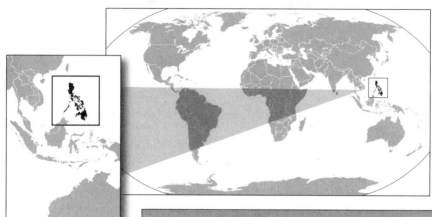

The Republic of the Philippines (*Republika ng Pilipinas*) consists of 7,107 islands, approximately 700 of which are inhabited. The great majority of the people live in densely crowded cities — especially in Quezon City and the capital of Manila. Fil-

Philippines Politics:

The Philippines was a colony of Spain (named in 1543 after King Philip II of Spain), and then of the United States. The former shows its influence in the national language, Tagalog, and the national religion, Catholicism, while the latter is evident by continued strong cultural ties.

Philippines Travel Requirements:

Passport and onward or return ticket required. A visa is not required for stay of up to 21 days.

ipinos work in service industries around the world, and a significant part of the Philippine economy consists of remittances sent home from these overseas workers.

The Philippines is among the poorer countries of Asia, and it has viewed with envy the development of medical tourism in Thailand, Malaysia, and Singapore. Aiming to catch up, officials unveiled an ambitious plan on January 23, 2006 to make the Philippines the "new hub of wellness and medical care in Asia." The newly designated Philippine Health Tourism Program is expected to bring into the country about $2 billion annually within five years, based on an estimate of 700,000 medical tourists per year. The government predicts that the Philippines will catch up to its more developed neighbors within three years. According to Health Secretary Francisco Duque, "It will catapult us to the world stage of medical tourism."

If only it were so easy! Clearly, such government promises will be very hard to keep. The Philippines already has tremendous difficulty in taking care of its own people — 50 percent of deaths occur in people who have received no medical treatment at all — and the country overall has an enormous "brain drain" of unemployed doctors who are forced to emigrate in order to find work. The situation is so bad that Philippine doctors often take foreign jobs far beneath their skill level. When I visited the Cebu Institute of Medicine, a prominent medical university, I was astonished that the most popular course was in retraining doctors to become nurses. The reason, as it was explained to me, is that doctors can find overseas work much more easily as nurses.

This situation, along with generally unimpressive medical facilities, makes it difficult to believe that the Philippines can compete with Thailand or Singapore for medical tourists, and certainly not within three years. Evidently, there are a few more levelheaded people in the government who have started the process with more modest goals: 10 hospitals (five government and five private) will be marketed as centers for medical tourism:

- Capitol Medical Center
- St. Luke's Medical Center
- Asian Hospital
- Medical City
- Makati Medical Center
- Lung Center
- Philippine Heart Center
- National Kidney Institute
- Philippine Children's Medical Center
- East Avenue Medical Center

They will try to emphasize the country's hospitable, English-speaking medical professionals and facilities, and the very competitive costs for treatment. However, the government continues to make odd statements that do not resonate well with prospective medical tourists. For example, the new director of the program announced that kidney transplants would be available for about $60,000 — about half the cost in the U.S. Then, perhaps realizing that extra kidneys are as scarce in the Philippines as they are anywhere, he added, "We don't want Filipinos to be sacrificed in favor of medical tourism," so medical tourists seeking transplants should "bring your own kidney donor."

Cebu

Cebu has five-star hotels, casinos, white sand beaches, world-class golf courses, convention centers, and shopping malls. *Condenast Travellers Magazine* named Cebu the seventh best Asian-Pacific island destination in 2004.

Cosmetic Surgery Center of Asia

This is a one-stop plastic surgery clinic, conveniently located in Mactan Island, Cebu, just minutes from the international airport. It is a private clinic owned by Dr. Alfonso Amores, FACS, and Luz Amores, RN, BSN. All surgeries are performed by Dr. Amores.

   ✉ Cosmetic Surgery Center of Asia
   ✉ E Vano Bldg, ML Quezon Highway
     Pusok, Lapu-Lapu City
     Metro Cebu 6015
     Philippines
   ☎ 632-536-2398
   🌐 www.cosmeticsurgeryasia.com

Costs for common cosmetic procedures:

Blepharoplasty	$400
Botox injection	$200
Breast augmentation	$2,100
Breast lift (mastopexy)	$1,700
Breast reduction	$2,500
Buttock lift	$2,500
Cheek implant	$900
Chemical peel	$250
Chin augmentation	$560
Dermabrasion	$1,000
Ear surgery	$1,500
Face and neck lift	$2,500
Forehead lift	$1,350

Manila

With over 10 million people, metro Manila is considered one of the world's great cities. Unfortunately, it also suffers from overpopulation, traffic congestion, pollution, and crime.

World Citi Med

World Citi Med is a 15-story tower located at the very heart of Metropolitan Manila. This is a full-service hospital with a mission statement that reads: "Because Filipinos are considered the best health givers of the world for their compassionate heart, advanced medical know-how and flexibility in any culture, here at World Citi Med we show the world these very abilities from our treasured staff."

☎ World Citi Med
✉ 960 Aurora Boulevard
Quezon City 1109
Philippines
☎ 632-913-8380
🌐 http://worldcitimed.rxpinoy.com/
@ info@worldcitimed.com

Eye Republic Ophthalmology Clinic
☎ Eye Republic Ophthalmology Clinic
✉ 3/F Don Santiago Building Unit 310
1344 Taft Avenue, Ermita
Manila 1000
Philippine
☎ 632-536-2398
🌐 www.medicaltourism.ph
@ help@EyeRepublic.com.ph

Poland

A top destination choice for:
alternative medicine, aromatherapy,
balneotherapy, cosmetic surgery

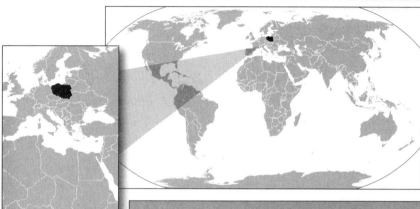

The Republic of Poland (*Rzeczpospolita Polska*) has a 200-year history of health tourism, with spas dating back even further to the 13th century.

Poland Politics:

Poland at one time was one of the largest, wealthiest, and most powerful countries in Europe. The past couple of centuries have seen tremendous turmoil as it fell into the political spheres of its neighbors, especially the Soviet Union. It is now a prosperous and rapidly developing nation, having joined the European Union in 2004.

Poland Travel Requirements:

Passport required. Visa not required for stay of up to 90 days.

In 75 locations around the country there are more than 321 health spas offering unique health facilities and treatments. There is even an underground spa in a former salt mine.

Poland is ranked seventh in Europe in terms of numbers of health spas. The largest are found at:
- Nałęczów
- Krynica-Zdrój
- Augustów
- Kołobrzeg
- Ciechocinek
- Rabka
- Duszniki-Zdrój
- Wieliczka

These health spas are usually located in regions bordering national parks and reserves. They offer the opportunity to spend time outdoors and take advantage of the virtues of eco-tourism by the sea, in the mountains, or lakes. Tourists can choose between brine pools, thermal baths, the natural mineral water springs, or cryotherapy (cold water) chambers. The cost of such treatment is $30 to $50 per day, including room and board, and two or three treatments.

A popular destination is one of the underground salt chambers for asthma treatment. Because the treatment is rendered over time, the managers have a number of social and tour programs available for their patients.

Cosmetic surgery has recently joined spa tourism. The cost of liposuction of the inner thighs is about $3,300, breast enlargement about $3,200, and nose reconstruction about $2,500.

Warsaw

Warsaw has many historical sites to offer the traveler. One needs only to stroll along the Royal route — a thoroughfare lined by beautiful palaces, churches, houses, statues and parks — to appreciate the legacy of Polish civilization. Warsaw

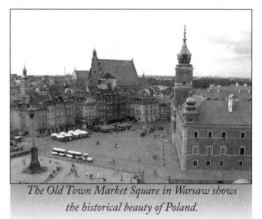

The Old Town Market Square in Warsaw shows the historical beauty of Poland.

also has an impressive cultural scene with its many museums, galleries, theatres, concert halls, and nightclubs. However, the most enchanting part is "old town," a UNESCO World Heritage site, with its cobblestone streets, hidden nooks, and charming gothic and baroque architecture. Closed off to traffic, it is ideal for walks and horse-drawn carriage rides. The heart of this area is the Old Town Market Square, with its traditional Polish restaurants, quaint cafes, enticing shops, street vendors, and street artists.

History buffs will want to visit the Jewish Ghetto, the Jewish Historic Museum, Jewish Cemetery and Path of Remembrance. Also worth visiting is the birthplace of Chopin in Zelazowa Wola — a tiny village about 35 miles west of Warsaw.

Jolly Med Clinic
This plastic surgery clinic opened in 1999 in the center of Warsaw, in the district of Stara Ochota.

☎ Jolly Med
✉ Lelechowska 5
   Warsaw
   Poland
☎ 22 659 7889
🌐 www.jollymed.pl
@ jollymed@pro.onet.pl

Damian Medical Center

This multi-specialty outpatient clinic is the first private hospital in Warsaw. It has 40 beds in single and double rooms, three operating rooms, an obstetric clinic, general and surgical departments. Over 2,000 operations are done per year, mostly in cosmetic surgery. The hospital has recently expanded to two additional locations in Warsaw. All medical staff are fluent in English.

☎ Damian Medical Center
✉ "Medoc" 03-152
   310/312 Modli ska Str.
   Warsaw
   Poland
@ turystyka@damian.com.pl

Wieliczka Salt Mine

Six miles from Krakow, this former salt mine features bacteria-free salty air, which reputedly helps heal asthma and other respiratory diseases, allergies, and skin diseases. Comprehensive packages include transportation, hotel and full accommodations, and 14 daily sessions in the mine's 440-foot-deep Lake Wessel Chamber.

☎ Wieliczka Salt Mine
✉ Ul Danilowicza 10 32-020
   Wieleczka
   Poland
@ urystyka@kapalnia.pl

Saudi Arabia

A top destination choice for:
cosmetic surgery, dental care

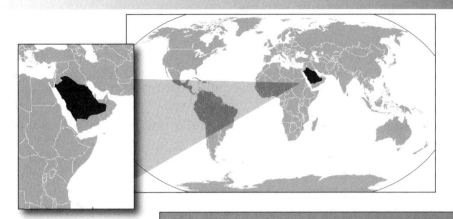

The Kingdom of Saudi Arabia is a vast country — one third larger than Alaska — known to Americans mostly for its enormous oil wealth. This desert land, of which just two percent is inhabitable, is equally significant as the "the land of the 2 holy mosques" — Mecca and Medina — which are Islam's two holiest places.

Saudi Arabia might seem to be an unlikely candidate for medical tourism. The Kingdom has never particularly welcomed foreigners and has essentially no tourism industry. The single exception is the hajj — the obligation of every able-bodied Muslim to make a pilgrimage to Mecca at least once in his or her lifetime. This might be considered a form of religious tourism, and it has now led to a convenience-based medical tourism. When people travel to Mecca, they increasingly stop in Jeddah, Riyadh, and other cities to take advantage of the opportunity for high-quality and low-cost medical care.

Saudi Arabia Politics:

The Basic Law adopted in 1992 declared that Saudi Arabia is a monarchy ruled by the sons and grandsons of the first king, Abd Al Aziz Al Saud, and that the Qur'an is the constitution of the country, which is governed on the basis of Islamic law (Shari'a). This is not a good country in which to run afoul of the local laws.

Saudi Arabia Travel Requirements:

A passport valid for at least six months and visa are required for entry. Visas are issued for business and work, to visit close relatives, and for transit and religious visits. Visas for tourism are issued only for approved tour groups following organized itineraries. Airport and seaport visas are not available. All visas require a sponsor, can take several months to process, and must be obtained prior to arrival. American citizens may be refused a Saudi visa if their passports show travel to Israel.

Medical and cosmetic surgery centers have sprung up around the country to handle the demand from the world's one billion Muslims.

Young women, in particular, seek out visits to dental clinics. Dr. Zaina Zogby, a Saudi female dentist, said most of her patients are women seeking orthodontics treatment. "We're booking appointments for visitors six months before summer," which is the peak time for the hajj. Nabeel Khouri, manager of a Jeddah cosmetic surgery center, also has noted the strong influx associated with the pilgrimage. Dr. Waheed Mustafa said his eye clinic receives more than 70 visitors per day, and he conducts more than 15 operations per day.

Recent statistics indicate these medical centers take in about $ 350 million annually.

Jeddah

Because of its location on the Red Sea, Jeddah is the most popular tourist destination in Saudi Arabia. There are more than 40 large hospitals in Jeddah, not counting private medical clinics. Many medical tourists say that the wide variety of choices is one reason they choose Jeddah.

Saudi German Hospitals Group
The Saudi German Hospitals Group is considered the largest private healthcare company in the Middle East and North Africa. The Jeddah facility offers a full range of medical care.
- ☎ 966-2-682-9000
- ℘ 966-2-683-5874
- 🌏 www.sghgroup.com
- @ webmaster@sghgroup.com

Riyadh

Riyadh is the capital of Saudi Arabia. This fast-growing city has about five million residents, a fifth of the country's population.

GAMA Dental Center
This extensive dental clinic is operated by mostly expatriate dentists from the United States and Canada.

GAMA Dental Center
FAL Shopping Center
King Abdul Aziz Road
P.O. Box 41726
Riyadh 11531
Saudi Arabia
☎ 966-1-454-2929
✆ 966-1-456-9563
🌍 www.gama-dental.com
@ gama_dental@yahoo.com

Singapore

A top destination choice for:
bone-marrow transplant, cosmetic surgery,
heart surgery, hip replacement

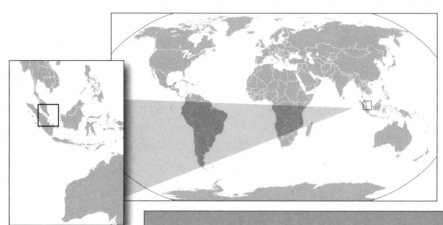

The Republic of Singapore is an island city-state and the smallest country in Southeast Asia, located just 85 miles from the Equator.

The name Singapore was derived from the Malay word *singa*, "lion," and *pura*, "city," because its founder in the 3rd century thought he saw a lion. Over 2,000 years, the fishing village and trading port has grown to a population of 4.5 million and become one of the greatest global centers of transportation, finance, and technology. It is astonishing how a country less than one fifth the size of Rhode Island can support not only an enormous urban and industrial complex but also find room for wildlife parks, a military range, and a major airport.

Singapore Politics:

In 1819, Sir Thomas Stamford Raffles, an official with the British East India Company, made a treaty with the Sultan of Johore and turned a sleepy fishing village into an international port. Its strategic location attracted the attention of many other countries, of which the United Kingdom was the most powerful. In 1867, Singapore was made a British crown colony. Japan occupied it during the Second World War, after which it briefly joined the formation of Malaysia before becoming entirely independent in 1965. Lew Kuan Yew took control of the government from the start, and even now continues to run the country like a family corporation: clean, safe, and ruthlessly efficient. This makes it a favorite for foreign companies and expatriates.

Singapore Travel Requirements:

Passport with a minimum validity of six months, proof of sufficient funds for stay, and onward or return ticket required. Visa not required for stays of up to 30 days, normally, but the length is determined by the discretion of the immigration officer.

Tourism is one of the largest industries in Singapore. Visitors are attracted by the colonial history, duty-free shopping, and cultural diversity, with enclaves of Chinese,

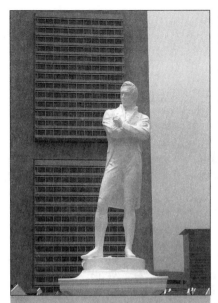

Statue of Thomas Stamford Raffles, at the spot where he first landed at Singapore. He is recognized as the founder of modern Singapore.

Malay, Indian, Eurasian, and Arab living in perfect harmony. Perfection, in many foreigners' impressions, is what Singapore is all about. When I first went there, I was bored by the ultra-clean environment. Singapore is notorious for punishments by fines for everything from spitting on the street to not flushing a toilet. The common joke holds Singapore as the "world's finest city," with a new meaning of "have a fine day." Long-haired backpackers were required to have a haircut at the airport in order to be allowed entry. As for drug smugglers, justice was quick and fatal.

By about my third visit, this efficient, clean, and crime-free city began to grow on me. Once you've dealt with the confusion of India, the incompetence of Indonesia, the incoherence of Malaysia, and the scams of Thailand, Singapore is like a breath of fresh air — quite literally, since you are also relieved from the lung-muddying air pollution of almost all other Asian cities.

Of course, Singapore is not 100 percent wholesome. You can gamble if you want, or drink yourself into a stupor at countless bars, including the famous Long Bar at the Raffles Hotel. As for all those pretty girls of every ethnicity who are so friendly — they're hookers.

A notable characteristic of Singapore is its energetic drive to be the best. People here feel that if they stop running they will fall behind, and their island nation will have no resources to support them. The Chinese word for this is *kiasu* — "afraid to lose." One in four people here is a foreigner, attracted by the high-tech industries and by the ability to do business in a place that *works*. Singapore Airlines is the choice of the sophisticated

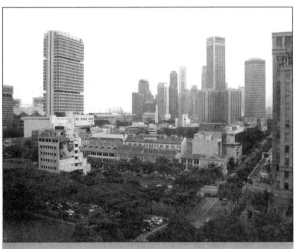

This is a view of the "city-state" Singapore and its astonishing diversity — from a hospital room.

traveler, and Chiangi Airport's network of 77 airlines will take you to 178 cities in 56 countries; it is consistently rated as one of the best international airports in the world. The cuisine is also superb and caters to every taste — and perhaps a few distastes. As the saying goes, "If a Chinese sees a snake in the grass, he'll think of a way to eat it."

Now Singapore is planning to develop a whole new industry: medical tourism. They know they are not alone in this, so their approach is the same one that they use for other industries: they simply intend to be the best. This means that Singapore will not be your first choice for discount dentistry or cosmetic surgery. But if you are concerned about quality, you cannot go wrong by choosing one of Singapore's world-class medical facilities. Indeed, the World Health Organization ranks Singapore as having the best health system in Asia, well ahead of Japan.

Alan Tan, director of the Singapore Tourism Board, explains that even without the great cost discounts, patients will "still come to Singapore in record numbers for more advanced medical care, such as organ transplants, heart surgery, and cancer treatment." For example, Parkway Group Healthcare's Asian Centre for Liver Disease and Transplantation performs at least one live-donor liver transplant every week. Almost all of the patients come from overseas. Neuroscience is another area in which Singapore is a world leader. The critical care unit at the National Neuroscience Institute (NNI) is the only unit of its kind in the Asia Pacific region to provide integrated, state-of-the-art monitoring facilities for brain tissue oxygenation, brain temperatures, blood flow, and microdialysis.

Singapore is encouraging medical tourism by providing dedicated international patient service centers to assist medical tourists with travel, admission, appointments, transport, and interpreters. "Ultimately," adds Alan Tan, "we are looking at providing a person who is sick, anxious, and in an unfamiliar country with a seamless package that goes far beyond basic healthcare."

Sample treatment costs:

Breast lump removal...$1,000
Haemorrhoidectomy $1,500
Knee-joint replacement $7,000
Hernia correction..$2,500
Dental implant $1,600

To make the most of your medical treatment, you may want to add a side trip to Kusu Island (also called Turtle Island), one of the tiny islands just a 30-minute ferry ride from Sentosa. There, you can buy baby turtles to release into the Tortoise Sanctuary — it is supposed to bring good health.

There is a 5 percent goods and services tax (GST). If you leave by air, you can get a refund on this, so be sure to ask. The refund is by cash, check, or added directly to your credit card.

Parkway Group Healthcare Medical Referral Centre

The international Medical Referral Centre (MRC) is a service provided by Parkway Group Healthcare for its international patients. It is a call center that operates a 24-hour hotline and one-stop service center that helps patients access specialist expertise, personalized patient care, and cutting-edge technology at its hospitals in Singapore. Parkway Group Healthcare, one of Asia's leading healthcare providers, is committed to bringing customers quality service and state-of-the-art facilities. The Group's three hospitals — Mount Elizabeth, Gleneagles and East Shore — are the first private hospitals in Asia Pacific to achieve the ISO 9002 international quality certification. They have collectively performed the largest number of cardiac surgeries and neurosurgeries in the private healthcare sector in the region. The Gleneagles facility is the location of The Asian Centre for Liver Disease & Transplantation (ACLDT).

Parkway is particularly known for its stem cell transplant center, providing highly advanced treatment (unavailable in the U.S.) for cancers of the pancreas, kidney, colon, and ovaries, and for blood disorders such as Thalassemia Major and Sickle Cell anemia. The Haematology and Stem Cell Transplant Centre (HSCT), headed by world-renowned specialist Dr. Patrick Tan, reports up to 80 percent cure for many leukemias.

🖳 Parkway Group Healthcare
   Medical Referral Centre (MRC)
✉ 302 Orchard Road
   Tong Building #16-01/02/03
   Singapore 238862
☎ 65-6735-5000 (24-hour hotline)
📠 65-6732-6733
🌐 www.imrc.com.sg
@ mrc@parkway.com.sg

Raffles International Patients Centre

Providing a full range of personalized services to international patients and their accompanying family members, this one-stop service center has a dedicated team of professional patient relations officers to ensure that every international patient's visit is comfortable, pleasant, and hassle-free. Raffles Hospital offers a full complement of specialist services combined with some of the most advanced medical technology. The hospital also has a host of multi-disciplinary outpatient specialty clinics which include:

- Raffles Specialist Centre
- Raffles Aesthetics Centre
- Raffles Cancer Centre
- Raffles Children's Centre
- Raffles Counselling Centre
- Raffles DentiCare

- Raffles Eye & ENT Centre
- Raffles Heart Centre
- Raffles Health Screeners
- Raffles Internal Medicine Centre
- Raffles Japanese Clinic
- Raffles Surgery Centre
- Raffles Women's Centre

🚑 Raffles International Patients Centre

✉ Raffles Hospital
585 North Bridge Road
Singapore 188770

☎ 65-6311-1666

📠 65-6311-2333

🌐 www.raffleshospital.com

@ enquiries@raffleshospital.com

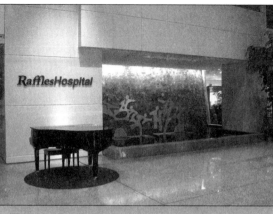

The foyer of the Raffles Hospital, Singapore, greets patients with luxury.

National Healthcare Group International Patient Liaison Centre (IPLC)

The IPLC is located at the National University Hospital (NUH), a 943-bed tertiary care hospital and the only university hospital in Singapore. Founded on corporate objectives that focus on patient care, research, and education, it strives to provide accessible and cost-effective care within an environment of intensive research and medical education.

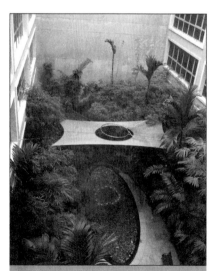

Raffles Hospital patient rooms open to an indoor garden with center waterfalls.

🚑 National Healthcare Group International Patient Liaison Centre

✉ National University Hospital
5 Lower Kent Ridge Road
Singapore 119074

☎ 65-6779-2777 (24-hour hotline)

📠 65-6777-8065

🌐 www.nuh.com.sg

@ iplc@nuh.com.sg

Singapore Health Services (SingHealth)

The International Medical Service (IMS), situated at Singapore General Hospital (SGH), offers international patients a one-stop service that is totally committed to meeting patients' needs. It is the country's largest tertiary care hospital and national referral center, with more than 1,500 beds and a pool of about 400 specialists. A multi-disciplinary approach to medical care provides patients with ready access to a wide range of specialties and support services. SGH has a comprehensive range of clinical specialties in 25 specialty departments and is the national referral center for plastic surgery and burns, renal medicine, nuclear medicine, pathology and hematology.

📇 Singapore Health Services (SingHealth) International Medical Service

✉ Singapore General Hospital
   Block 6 Level 1
   Outram Road
   Singapore 169608

☎ 65-6326-5656

📠 65-6326-5900

🌏 www.singhealth.com.sg

@ ims@sgh.com.sg

South Africa

A top destination choice for:
assisted reproduction, cosmetic surgery,
gastric bypass surgery, heart surgery

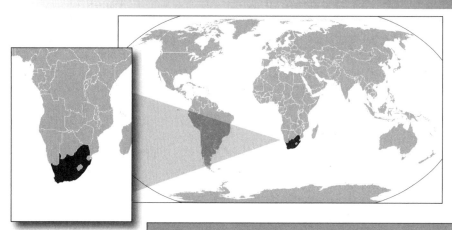

Located on the southern tip of the African continent, South Africa is a subtropical country filled with rugged mountains, lush river valleys, and endless beaches. It is here that some of the first humans walked the earth 300,000 years ago. They could hardly have picked a more beautiful place. South Africa has amazing diversity and a perfect climate. Because of the lingering problems of previous racist regimes, and now crime and AIDS, South Africa has

South Africa Politics:

South Africa is a classic example of colonial politics of the entire world. Beginning in the 16th century, European colonists began to populate the southern tip of Africa. At the same time, equatorial Bantu-speaking Africans were migrating south. The indigenous, diminutive, coppery-skinned Koisan people were squeezed out, and now they represent only a small part of the population, largely in the Kalahari Desert. The inevitable conflict between various nations ultimately resorted in a crude attempt to keep ethnic Europeans in power, called apartheid. True democracy was instituted in the early 1990s, but there continue to be large economic disparities. Despite widespread crime and AIDS, South Africa is nonetheless the most successful country in Africa.

South Africa Travel Requirements:

Passport required. Visa not required for stay of up to 90 days.

only a fraction of the tourism industry it would otherwise enjoy. Where else can you take a safari to see giraffes, lions, elephants, whales, and sea lions — all in their natural habitat — and then go surfing or visit a world-class vineyard, all in the same day?

South African universities have long had world-class medical treatment and research hospitals. It was here, after all, that the world's first heart transplant was performed and many other medical discoveries made. Now these same facilities are encouraging medical tourism.

Typical costs in South Africa:
Rhinoplasty (nose reshaping)..$3,570
Breast augmentation...$3,740
Upper and lower eyelid shaping $2,975
Facelift $5,610

Since medical tourism is relatively new in South Africa, as it is in most of the world, the traveler must be careful to choose a reputable surgeon. This is not so easily done when your only source of information is a website that promises the very best. One way to help ensure quality in South Africa is by checking the following:

Make sure the surgeon belongs to the South African Medical Association (SAMA). You can check this on www.sama.co.za

Make sure the surgeon is qualified and listed in the Association of Plastic and Reconstructive Surgeons of South Africa (APRSSA). You can find this at: www.aprssa.co.za and also at www.plasticsurgeons.co.za

Cape Town

Cape Town is one of the most scenic cities on earth, and is where the majority of South Africa's medical tourism industry is focused.

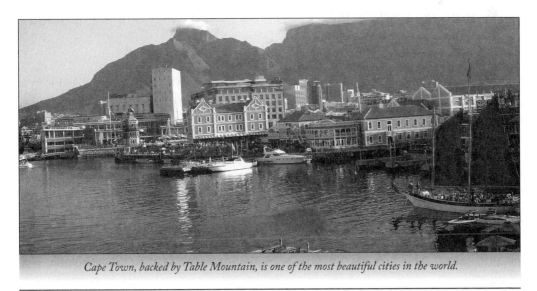

Cape Town, backed by Table Mountain, is one of the most beautiful cities in the world.

Cape Doctor Health Tours

Ruby Khan, the owner of this referral service, says fertility treatment has the highest popularity among medical tourists. The typical cost is $2,560 to $3,520 per treatment cycle. Many other types of surgery are also offered.

- 📠 Cape Doctor Health and Tours
- ✉ P. O. Box 19161, Tygerberg 7505
  Cape Town
  South Africa
- ☎ 27-21-447-6699
- 📠 27-21-447-6433
- @ info@capedoctor.net

Mediscapes

A very comprehensive referral service that offers full packages to accommodate almost every request. Although the website emphasizes cosmetic surgery, it does offer most forms of medical services.

- ☎ 27-21-434-0821
- 📠 27-21-434-5680
- 🌐 www.mediscapes.com
- @ info@mediscapes.com

Nu Look Surgery

This is a referral service for cosmetic surgery in Cape Town and Natal.

- ☎ 27-21-791-4111
- 🌐 www.nulooksurgery.com
- @ info@nulooksurgery.com

Panorama Medi-Clinic

A 424-bed multidisciplinary private hospital located in Cape Town, this belongs to the Medi-Clinic chain of private hospitals in Africa. There is a total of 43 throughout South Africa and two in Namibia. Panorama Medi-Clinic offers magnificent views of Cape Town's Table Mountain, the Cape Peninsula, and the beautiful Cape coastline. It also has excellent accommodations surrounding it, ranging from hotels to bed-and-breakfast establishments.

- 📠 Panorama Medi-Clinic
- ✉ Rothschild Boulevard
  Panorama, Parow 7500
  PO Box 15041, Panorama 7506
  Cape Town
  South Africa

☎ 27-21-938-2111

🌐 www.panoramamc.co.za

@ hospmngrpanor@mediclinic.co.za

Johannesburg

Fondly nicknamed Jo'burg or Jozi, this is South Africa's largest city, and indeed, the dominant city for all of Africa.

Evolution Cosmetic

Launched in January 2001, Victoria Wagner organizes trips to South Africa for medical tourists seeking cosmetic, dental, or ophthalmic surgery.

🏢 Evolution Cosmetic

✉ 23 Winslow Road
Parkwood
Johannesburg 2193
South Africa

☎ 27-11-804-7117

📠 27-11-656-9378

🌐 www.evolutioncosmetic.com

@ victoria@evo.co.za

Serokolo Health Tourism

Dr. Tshepo P. Maaka is the founder and Managing Director of this woman-owned health and medical tourism company. Serokolo's goal is to provide holistic, comprehensive, and quality health services to the international community. Dr. Maaka's formal training includes anesthesiology, the provision of health services, public health management and health management strategy consulting. She refers patients to private and public medical centers, clinics, and specialists at affordable and competitive prices.

☎ 27-11-442-5682

📠 27-11-447-4364

🌐 www.serokolo.co.za

@ info@serokolo.co.za

Surgical Attractions

This referral service assists patients in arranging a wide range of cosmetic, bariatric, and dental procedures.

🏢 Surgical Attractions

✉ 45 Bristol Road

Parkwood
Johannesburg 2193
South Africa
☎ 27-11-880-5122
📠 27-11-788-9043
🌐 www.surgicalattractions.com
@ info@surgicalattractions.com

Surgeon & Safari

Located in a suburb of Johannesburg, this referral service organizes cosmetic and other surgery, followed by a recuperative stay at The Westcliff Hotel in Johannesburg or the Cellars-Hohenort in Cape Town — both of them sumptuous resorts — and a variety of safari wildlife tours.

🚙 Surgeon & Safari
✉ PO Box 97646
Petervale 2151
South Africa
☎ 27-11-463-3154
📠 27-11-706-5582
🌐 www.surgeon-and-safari.co.za
@ info@surgeon-and-safari.co.za

South Korea

A top destination choice for:
acupuncture, cosmetic surgery,
hip replacement

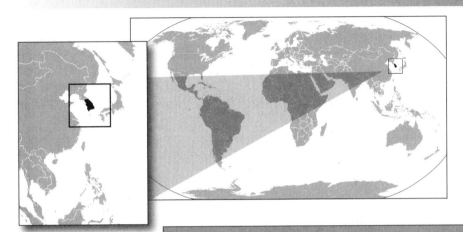

South Korea Politics:

The Republic of Korea is the southern half of the Korean Peninsula, and more usually known as South Korea. Just a few miles north of Seoul is the border of North Korea, which separated from the South in 1945 in a lengthy and brutal civil war that still smolders. Now, South Korea is one of the most economically and industrially advanced countries in Asia while North Korea languishes in extreme political oppression, poverty, and outright starvation.

South Korea Travel Requirements:

Passport and onward or return ticket required. Visa not required for stay of up to 30 days.

South Korea once was one of Asia's poorest countries but is now the 11th largest economy in the world and one of the most technologically advanced. If you want to see what cell phones and other high-tech gadgets will be like in two years, go to South Korea now. Koreans are considered the most "wired" in the world. Although South Korea has several major cities, by far the largest is Seoul, with about one-third of the entire population of the country. As far as cities go, I find it rather bleak and depressing. But the sightseeing here is indoors. The national religion seems to be consumption and technology. This is a place that hums with commerce and deserves its name as an "Asian tiger."

As it has with technology, South Korea is taking the same bold approach to medical tourism by offering procedures that are very advanced and difficult to obtain elsewhere, even in the United States. This is particularly true of stem-cell therapy. The first hospital in the world exclusively focused on stem-cell therapy, Histostem, was completed in 2007. Patients are already being treated on an experimental basis, using

---

umbilical cord blood stem cells to treat liver cirrhosis, Buerger's disease, diabetes, chronic renal failure, and a dozen other diseases. It is especially promising for spinal cord injuries and Alzheimer's Disease.

Seoul

Anacli

Anacli is a Seoul-based clinic for skincare and plastic surgery. The ability to read Korean is helpful in reviewing their website. The hospital treats about 1,000 medical tourists annually, apparently most of them Japanese and Chinese who are eager to resemble Korean movie stars.

"For us, the market for foreign patients is inexhaustible," said Lee Sang-jun, chairman of the private hospital which operates five branches in Seoul.

🌐 www.anacli.com
@ info@anacli.co.kr

Wooridul Spine Hospital

Wooridul Spine hospital is one of the few Korean hospitals that provide a one-stop service to overseas patients. Well-known for its innovative spinal care treatment, the hospital helps its overseas customers obtain a visa, picks them up at the airport, and even introduces them to a travel agent for a downtown tour. This hospital has a large international patient service, often with direct referrals from physicians in other countries. It specializes in minimally invasive spinal surgery (MISS) for spine problems, including:

- Percutaneous endoscopic lumbar discectomy (PELD)
- Percutaneous endoscopic cervical discectomy (PECD)
- Percutaneous endoscopic thoracic discectomy (PETD)
- Percutaneous endoscopic laser-assisted annulopalsty (PELA)
- Microscopic laser discectomy
- Laparoscopic spinal discectomy and fusion
- Video-assisted thoracoscopic discectomy and fusion

☎ 82-2-513-8385
📠 82-2-513-8386
🌐 http://en.wooridul.com
@ wipc@wooridul.co.kr

Spain

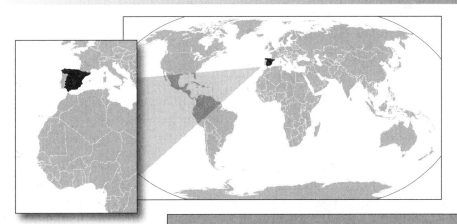

The Kingdom of Spain (*España*) includes the Balearic Islands in the Mediterranean Sea, the Canary Islands in the Atlantic Ocean, and a number of uninhabited islands on the Mediterranean. Spain has long been a favored destination for tourists from northern Europe, especially from the United Kingdom. With

Spain Politics:

Spain is a member of the European Union. Several minority groups around the country are agitating for greater autonomy and survival of their language — for example, Catalan in the northeast and the Basque in the northwest — but the trend seems to be an increasing absorption into a "United States of Europe."

Spain Travel Requirements:

Passport required. Visa not required for stay of up to 90 days.

the development of the European Union, it has also become much easier for other Europeans to live and work in Spain. The result is a large expatriate community, with the common language of English.

Due to familiarity with Spain and the many English speakers, medical tourism has largely been targeted toward the British. Most cosmetic surgery referral agencies or clinics have offices in England, and some even have physicians in the United Kingdom to do pre-screening.

Spain has somewhat less attraction for Americans: costs are higher than in Asia, and Spain is much further to travel than Central America.

Typical prices for some common cosmetic surgeries:
Rhinoplasty (nose reshaping) $4,000
Breast augmentation $4,900
Upper and lower eyelid shaping $3,600
Facelift $5,400

Barcelona

According to legend, this beautiful city was founded by Hercules 400 years before the building of Rome. It is one of the most intriguing and historic cities in the world.

Belliance
Belliance is a referral service, and like most such services it has a flashy website but very little information on the actual surgeons or clinics. Their "associate" clinics — in other words, the clinics they refer patients to — are in Barcelona, Málaga, Córdoba, and in the popular tourist region of the Costa del Sol ("Sun Coast"): Marbella, Fuengirola, and Torremolinos.
☎ 34-902-235-542
🌎 www.belliance.com

Cosmetic Surgery Abroad
A referral service. Largely targeted to residents of the United Kingdom, it has follow-up services in London.
🏥 Cosmetic Surgery Abroad
✉ c/ Escuelas Pias 103
08017 Barcelona
Spain
☎ 34-932-54-5411
@ drbenito@cirugia-estetica.com

Clínica Fundació Fiatc
This is a private clinic in an exclusive part of town. It has 43 nicely appointed patient rooms, three operating rooms, and an intensive care unit.
🏥 Clínica Fundació Fiatc
✉ Av. Diagonal, 648
08017 Barcelona
Spain

☎ 93-2053213

✆ 93-2806280

🌐 www.cosmeticsurgeryabroad.org

@ info@cosmeticsurgeryabroad.org

Institut Dexeus

Dexeus is a 110 all–private-bed facility that has very strong OB/GYN and reproductive medicine service.

🏥 Institut Dexeus

✉ C/ Calatrava 83
08017 Barcelona
Spain

☎ 93-227-4747

🌐 www.cosmeticsurgeryabroad.org

@ info@cosmeticsurgeryabroad.org

Marbella

Marbella is a beach resort on the famed Costa del Sol. Archeological evidence shows that it has been a favorite tourist destination since the European Paleolithic, some 50,000 years ago. It continues to attract legions of tourists, especially from northern Europe.

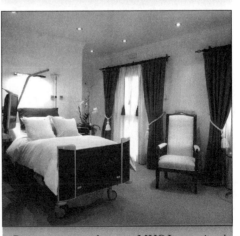

The pretty harbor of the Marbella beach resort on the Costa del Sol, Spain, has long attracted people — who now provide the market for a growing medical tourism industry.

MHC International Private Hospital

Bookings for British patients are made through the Mills & Mills Medical Group, owned by David and Debra Mills. They offer packages that include:

- Free consultation in the United Kingdom with a qualified surgeon.
- Return flights and travel arrangements to Marbella.
- Chauffeur service from Malaga airport to the hospital and your hotel.
- Free hospital room, if arriving the night before (subject to availability).
- Your procedure performed at a five-star hospital in Marbella, Spain.

Patient rooms are elegant at MHC International Private Hospital in Marbella.

- A beautiful private room in the hospital, with qualified doctors on hand 24 hours a day.
- Recover in style and comfort in your luxury four-star holiday hotel.
- Chauffeur service back to Malaga airport for your flight home.
- Free aftercare with your surgeon in the United Kingdom.
- A comprehensive finance and insurance option, making the dream of cosmetic surgery even more affordable, and with added peace of mind.

Apparently, this enterprising couple contracts with surgeons at the hospital to provide the actual services.

🖴 Mills & Mills Medical Group S.L.
✉ MHC International Private Hospital
Casa Sta. Isabel
Urb. Las Mimosas
29660 Nueva Andalucia
Marbella
Spain
☎ 34-952-908-538
📠 34-952-908-628
🌍 www.millsmedical.com
@ info@millsmedical.com

Syria

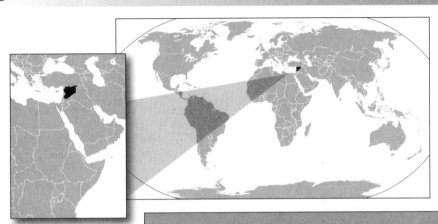

The Syrian Arab Republic is located east of Lebanon and northeast of Israel, which stills occupies Syria's Golan Heights border area. The government of Syria claims to have 460 public and private hospitals, 1,560 health centers, and 90,000 healthcare employees. The Ministry of Health has decided to promote medical tourism in Syria as a major feature of the new economy in its 10th five-year plan (2006–2010).

Syria Politics:

Syria is in the center of the Middle East conflicts and has veered between supporting and antagonizing the Western powers. This sort of political instability does not help tourism or other economic development.

Syria Travel Requirements:

Passport and visa required. Obtain your visa in advance. A single- or double-entry visa, valid for three months, requires two application forms, two photos, and a $100 fee (money order only). Enclose SASE with $6 postage (not metered stamps for certified mail) for return of passport by mail, $14 for express mail. For additional information, contact the Embassy of the Syrian Arab Republic, 2215 Wyoming Ave., NW, Washington, DC 20008 (202-232-6313). Internet: www.syrianembassy.us

At the time this book is being written, there has once again been political instability in the region. Currently, no facilities are advertising medical tourism in Syria. However, they apparently have big plans! With the simultaneous competition for medical tourists in nearby Jordan, Turkey, and Iran — not to mention Dubai — Syria may have a difficult time attracting a part of the market.

Taiwan

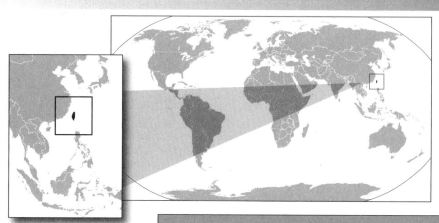

Taiwan Politics:

The political status of Taiwan remains a contentious issue. In 1971, Taiwan was dismissed from the United Nations and was replaced by the People's Republic of China, which continues to claim that Taiwan is merely a renegade province and occasionally threatens to bring it back by force. Taiwan therefore is careful not to claim independence, even as it functions as a separate country.

Taiwan Travel Requirements:

Passport, onward or return ticket, and valid visa for next destination, if applicable, are required. A visa is not required for stays of up to 30 days.

Taiwan is an island nation off the coast of mainland China, north of the Philippines. Officially known as the Taiwan Province of the Republic of China (ROC), this status is contested by the People's Republic of China (PRC), which claims it as one of its provinces. Lost in this dispute is the fact that the greater Republic of China no longer exists, and the government of the country now known as China — the PRC — does not, and has never, exercised control over Taiwan. Confusing? Yes, but this mutual pretense seems to have worked satisfactorily for the last half-century to prevent an all-out war.

In the last few years, the government, universities, and hospitals of Taiwan have looked enviously at the growth of medical tourism in Singapore and Thailand. There was no reason, they figured, why they could not also develop this industry. The result was a Health Tourism Guidance Task Force, convened in 2004, to rapidly explore and promote medical tourism. The first such step has been at the National Taiwan University Hospital, but much more is to expected follow.

Taipei

It is somewhat amusing to watch the competition between the PRC, whose 1.2 billion population and massive size dwarf the relatively tiny island of Taiwan, yet Taiwan's "Asian Tiger" economy is up for the challenge. The result is often a competition of symbols, especially in the prominence of tall buildings. Currently, Taipei 101 is the tallest in the world, with Shanghai trying to catch up.

National Taiwan University Hospital

The National Taiwan University Hospital has begun a new international service aimed at medical tourists. In the initial stages, this service will mainly focus on foreign businessmen who happen to be in Taiwan for other professional reasons. In the future, the hospital will launch an international publicity campaign to promote medical tourism.

📠 National Taiwan University Hospital
✉ No.7, Chung San South Road
Taipei
Taiwan (Republic of China)
☎ 02-2312-3456, ext. 5992
🕏 http://ntuh.mc.ntu.edu.tw/english
@ service@mailer.mc.ntu.edu.tw

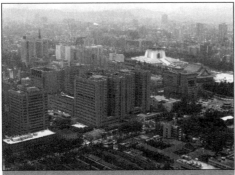

National Taiwan University Hospital, Taipei, Taiwan, is central to a massive government plan to develop medical tourism.

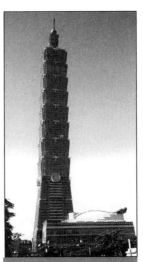

Taipei 101, currently the world's tallest building, is a sign of Taiwan's tremendous growth.

Thailand

A top destination choice for:
alternative medicine, cosmetic surgery, dental care, gastric bypass surgery, heart surgery, hip replacement

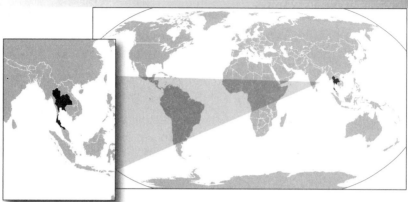

Thailand is one of the renowned tourism destinations of the world. Throughout history, travelers have been fascinated by the ancient Buddhist kingdom with its unique combination of cultural purity and open-minded tolerance. What can you say about a country that expects young men to spend an obligatory period as monks, instead of soldiers, yet respects every religion in the world? Where any public touch between men and women is highly frowned upon, yet sexual tourism flourishes? Where hedonism seems to reign supreme in the midst of the most calculating market economy? This is Thailand — a pleasure ground for Westerners that is rapidly becoming a technological powerhouse.

I first visited Thailand in 1976. The Vietnam War had just ended, and the country was gripped in political instability. Bangkok was so crowded with smoke-spewing,

Thailand Politics:

Thailand has a unique government run by an impenetrable coalition of religious, bureaucratic, and capitalist forces. The degree of respect awarded to the King borders on worship — a point to be well taken by tourists whose lack of respect can seem very offensive. Officially, government is chosen by democratic elections. In practice, it is largely composed of a number of dominant ruling families who control the economy. When this arrangement goes well, the country prospers, and it is the envy of its neighbors. When it goes badly, it can result in violent demonstrations to the point where the king has to step in to maintain order. In other words: rule is autocratic, for good or bad.

Thailand Travel Requirements:

Passport, onward or return ticket, and valid visa for next destination, if applicable, are required. A visa not required for a stay of up to 30 days.

three-wheel *tuk-tuks* that you could barely see across the street through the blue clouds of exhaust. The best way to travel at that time was on the skein of canals that gave the city the smells and appearance of a fetid swamp festooned with temples. At midnight the military curfew kicked in, and the only vehicles left prowling the streets were machine-gun turreted jeeps and the only sound a distant staccato burst of gunfire.

On my return in early 2006, I couldn't recognize the city. All but the largest canals have been paved over. The traffic is still thick but the *tuk-tuks* are gone, replaced by clean new motorbikes, propane-burning taxis, and the elevated Skytrain. Now you can actually see across the city, although most of the temple spires have become hidden by the glass towers of high-tech industry. Remarkably, this formerly squalid city has become a rival to Singapore.

The rest of the country has experienced the same growth. Koh Samui has been transformed from a hippie hangout to a modern constellation of resorts, as has Phuket, Chiang Mai, and many other former backpacker destinations. The new Thailand is well on its way to becoming a technologically advanced Asian nation like Japan,

---

A **Affordable Sex-Change Operations.** In the 1975 film, *Dog Day Afternoon*, starring a young Al Pacino and based on a true story, a man could not afford a sex-change operation for his male lover, so he tries to rob a bank. Today, he would not have to go to such extreme measures. His lover could fly to Bangkok and for about $5,000 have his surgery performed at any of several high-quality hospitals. Remarkably, sex-reassignment surgery has become one of the top 10 procedures for medical tourists in Thailand.

South Korea, and Taiwan. And a major backbone of this new economy is not just tourism — with some 13 million visitors per year — but specifically medical tourism. Over a million people a year travel to Thailand for everything from cosmetic surgery to the most advanced stem cell heart treatment.

The modern Thai medical system began when Prince Mahidol of Songla, the King's father, earned his M.D. degree at Harvard Medical School. He started a trend of Thai physicians becoming trained in the United States and then returning home to build an affiliation between Thai and American hospitals. According to the U.S. Consular information sheets, the crime rate in Bangkok is lower than that in many U.S. cities.

Thailand has become the poster-child for medical tourism, mentioned by almost every article and news program on this trend. Why has Thailand been so successful when there are over 50 other countries trying to capture the medical tourism market? The U.S.-trained doctors are a factor, along with the many JCI-accredited hospitals.

Another reason is the country itself; it is already a popular destination with a low crime rate. Finally, there is just something about the sensitive (and sensuous) Thai hospitality that has attracted health-seeking visitors for a thousand years.

Thailand's medical tourism industry provides the entire spectrum of services from traditional Thai massage and ayurvedic treatments to the most sophisticated surgical centers, and even such avante-garde procedures as stem-cell therapy. Thailand's hospitals have now also become the favored facilities for sex-change operations.

Because of the open attitudes of Thai people to foreigners — welcoming *farangi* has been a tradition for centuries — and because of the single-minded pursuits of young soldiers during the many nearby wars, Thailand has developed an unfortunate reputation for sex tourism. Hundreds of rural villages depend on income earned by sending young girls to Bangkok, Pattaya, and other major tourist regions to satisfy foreign men. Public health campaigns have done much to reduce sexually transmitted diseases — especially AIDS — that are spread by prostitution. However, this is simply a feature of the urban landscape, and tourists who are offended by prostitution should avoid those areas in which it flourishes.

Despite the apparent easy-going nature of Thais, and the flaunting of sex services, it may come as a surprise to many visitors that Thais are actually very puritanical. A few things to remember in Thailand:

- Bowing slightly with hands folded in prayer, a gesture called *wai*, is the traditional Thai greeting from inferior to superior. Since moneyed tourists are considered socially superior to the lower-income service and sales people, you will be *wai*'d hundreds of times a day. It is tempting to return the *wai*. Don't do this, or you will be denigrating the welcome by implying social equality — and certainly don't exaggerate the *wai*, which is not only impolite but shows ridicule of what is a gracious gesture. Instead, acknowledge a *wai* with a smile and a nod of the head.
- Thailand is officially a Buddhist country, where young men typically undergo a period of material renunciation. They become monks in the same way that young men in other countries have mandatory military service. Monks beg, but are not to be pitied or treated as objects of curiosity. They are regular young men and (less often) women, from all ranges of society, including the wealthy, and are doing their religious service.
- Thais feel the head is sacred and touching it is offensive. In fact, any sort of physical contact between genders in public is frowned upon. If you see a man with a Thai woman holding hands or kissing in public, she is a prostitute.
- Thais feel that the feet are dirty. It is disrespectful to even expose the soles of your feet to others. Care should be taken in restaurants or when seated outside to avoid showing the soles of the feet.
- "Saving face" is very important, so Thais will try to avoid saying anything negative

as much as possible. If you ask a question, a respectful Thai may give you a lengthy answer even though he doesn't have a clue about what you want to know. He is answering just to make you happy.

Thailand is not Disneyland. The legions of tourists who forget to respect the local culture are an embarrassment to everyone.

Advanced Medi-Travel

Formerly called All About Beauty Cosmetic & Plastic Surgery Consultant Pty Ltd (and still often referred to by that name), this service is directed by Crista Bradley, better known down under as "Australia's Queen Of Plastic Surgery." Crista (www.christabradley.com) has had 29 surgeries and 62 cosmetic procedures and knows what she's talking about. She often makes arrangements with the surgeons at the Bumrungrad International, the Bangkok Phuket hospital, and the Body Line Retreat to provide comprehensive medical tourism services. Even if you decide not to use her services, I suggest that anyone considering cosmetic surgery look at Advanced Medi-Travel's website (www.allaboutbeauty.com.au). It provides a tremendous amount of information on everything from what sort of clothing to bring to downloadable travel forms.

- 📖 All About Beauty Pty Ltd
- ✉ 19 Pearce Road
  Kanwal 2259
  N.S.W Australia
- ☎ 612-4392-9436
- 📠 612-4392-9436
- 🌐 www.allaboutbeauty.com.au
- @ allaboutbeauty@optusnet.com.au

Bangkok

Although an increasing number of flights go directly to Phuket and other popular resort areas, for the vast majority of visitors Bangkok will be the first experience of Thailand. This sprawling city is quite complex. Most tourists congregate in Sukumvit, a central neighborhood with countless hotels and good access to the major medical tourist hospitals. With sidewalks blocked every few feet by venders selling everything from pirated DVDs to fresh pineapple, it is much easier to travel by taxi, or even hop on the back of a motorbike for a small fee. You will be whisked through a maze of small streets, called *soi*, and taken over the sidewalk and right to the doorstep of your destination. If walking is your preference, try the paths along the canals, called *khlong*. The grand canal, Saen Saep, meanders more than 10 miles. The walkway along this canal is just 200 yards from Bumrungrad Hospital.

Bangkok Hospital

This is a very large network of state-of-the-art hospitals with advanced procedures that are sometimes not yet available in the United States. Its flagship hospitals in Bangkok — also known as Bangkok General Hospital and Bangkok International Hospital — feature instrumentation such as Novalis shaped-beam surgery and non-invasive stereotactic radiosurgery. Bangkok Hospital already has 22 major medical centers, and construction is underway for many more. Only those that serve primarily medical tourists are included here.

   📠 Bangkok Hospital
   ✉ 2 Soi Soonvijai 7
      New Petchburi Road
      Bangkok 10310
      Thailand
   ☎ 662-310-3000
   📠 662-755-1310
   🌐 www.bangkokhospital.com
   @ contactcenter@bangkokhospital.com

Bangkok Heart Hospital

Bangkok Heart Hospital brings together the best internationally experienced doctors, consultants, and skilled clinical specialists. Advanced diagnostic technologies include a 64-slice Multidetector CT Scanner, 3-Tesla Cardiovascular MRI, a cardiac catheterization Lab., electro-physiologic and radio-frequency catheter ablation

---

Time Magazine (Asia) *reports: "When Bob Grinstead landed in Bangkok, he might have been mistaken for a typical tourist … but he wasn't in any shape for sightseeing."* The 70-year-old from Atlanta had suffered a heart attack, followed by two bypass surgeries and numerous angioplasties. Walking a few steps left him exhausted, but his doctors told him there was nothing more they could do. At his age, he was not eligible for a heart transplant. So, Bob opted for stem-cell treatment offered by TheraVitae in Thailand The trip to Bangkok was more of a vacation than a treatment: his room at Bangkok Heart Hospital was like a luxury hotel suite, even including adjacent rooms for his wife and daughter. The procedure was a simple matter of blood drawn after his arrival, and re-injected a few days later. That was all. Then it was just a matter of reconditioning physical therapy as the heart began to grow healthy new tissue. Eight months later, to the amazement of his Atlanta doctors, Bob was taking half-hour walks and enjoying life.

---

equipment, and ability to implant AICD, CRT, and pacemakers. These are all examples of state-of-the-art equipment that U.S.-based hospitals would be proud to have. In addition, the Bangkok Heart Hospital features the Da Vinci Robotic Cardiac Surgery System for high-precision, minimally invasive surgery.

🏥 Bangkok Heart Hospital
✉ 2 Soi Soonvijai 7
   New Petchburi Road
   Bangkok 10310
   Thailand
☎ 662-310-3323
📠 662-310-3088
🌐 www.bangkokhearthospital.com
@ heart@bangkokhospital.com

Bangkok Hospital Pattaya *(see Chonburi)*

Bangkok Hospital Phuket *(see Phuket)*

Bangkok Hospital Samui *(see Koh Samui)*

Bangkok Christian Hospital (BCH)
A private hospital since 1949, BCH emphasizes medical tourism, and just about the entire staff speaks excellent English. This is a smaller hospital than some others, but the fees are also lower.

🏥 Bangkok Christian Hospital
✉ 124 Silom Road
   Silom, Bangrak
   Bangkok
   Thailand
☎ 662-264-0560
📠 662-236-2911
🌐 www.bkkchristianhosp.th.com/NEWBCH/English/AboutBCH/Information.html
@ Info@Bkkchristianhosp.th.com

Bangkok Christian Guest House (BCGH)
The BCGH is famous for its expansive green lawn and garden space providing an oasis in the center of Bangkok. It was recently rebuilt, but its goal is to offer the same relaxed, Christian, homey atmosphere at reasonable rates for which the Guest House has long been known. The capacity has grown to include 50 guest rooms, expanded meeting rooms, dining facilities, lounge space, chapel, children's activity room, exercise room,

gift and handicraft shop, and more. Larger rooms and connecting rooms are available for families and their children.

First established by Presbyterian missionaries, the BCGH was built to serve as a temporary base in Bangkok for international Christian mission and development workers. It has been providing temporary housing and shelter in downtown Bangkok at very economical rates for missionaries, social workers, aid providers, medical personnel, families, and others traveling in Asia for nearly 75 years. The Guest House has helped many expectant mothers and families celebrate the arrival of new babies both through natural means and by adoption.

The BCGH is centrally located just off the business and tourist area of Silom Road. The Saladaeng stop on the Skytain is just a three-minute walk. The Guest House also helps arrange tours in the city or to outlying attractions. BCGH has dining facilities, but there is also an endless variety of restaurants within a short walk. U.S. fast-food chains are close by, as are restaurants featuring food from all around the world at all price levels.

   🏨 Bangkok Christian Guest House
   ✉ 123 Saladaeng Soi 2
       Bangkok 10500
   ☎ 662-233-6303
   📠 662-237-1742
   🌐 www.bcgh.org
   @ reservations@bcgh.org

BNH Hospital

This superb facility grew from humble origins as the Bangkok Nursing Home. Its patient rooms are nicer than many luxury hotels. Among its patients are many international diplomats, and it seems to be the preferred hospital for expatriates living in Bangkok.

   🏨 BNH Hospital
   ✉ 9/1 Convent Road
       Silom, Bangrak
       Bangkok 10500
       Thailand
   ☎ 662-632-0550
   📠 662-632-0577
   🌐 www.bnhhospital.com
   @ info@bnhhospital.com

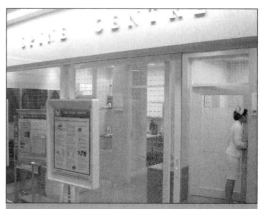

The BNH Spine Centre, Bangkok, Thailand has long been a favorite for resident foreigners, and now attracts patients from dozens of countries.

Bumrungrad Hospital

Virtually every article on medical tourism mentions Bumrungrad — it is the global standard to which all other high-end medical tourism facilities are compared. Bumrungrad International is one of the largest hospitals in Bangkok and the first to achieve the coveted Joint Commission International (JCI) accreditation, the highest mark of quality assurance.

Bumrungrad was designed specifically to accommodate medical tourists. At this time, the majority of patients come from the oil-rich states of the

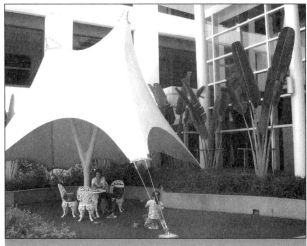

An interior oasis in the Bumrungrad hospital, Bangkok, Thailand, provides a peaceful place to relax.

Persian Gulf, especially UAE, Oman, and Saudi Arabia. Standing at the entrance, you will see an almost constant stream of luxury taxis and limousines bringing well-dressed men and women — many of whom are entirely covered in *burqa*, a black robe with just a narrow, veiled slit for the eyes. The grand hospital front has flags of two dozen countries. You might notice that the flag of the United States is conspicuously absent. This is probably done to cater to an Islamic clientele who would prefer to avoid association with the U.S. Little do they know that the hospital is managed by Americans.

At 12 stories, this is the largest private hospital in Southeast Asia. Since it opened in 1997, it has treated over a million patients per year. One third of these are medical tourists from over 150 different countries. Just a list of the beds is impressive: 554 inpatient beds, 26 adult intensive-care beds, 14 cardiac-care (CCU) beds, 57 deluxe rooms, 21 VIP Suites, and two Royal Suites. Taking care of these patients are 700 doctors and dentists, and 2,600 nurses.

A patient here enjoys a luxurious experience. On the lower floors, shops and personal services cater to every whim, from hairdressers and massage parlors to more complex treatments at the Vitalife Wellness Center. Patients are provided with an international concierge service, embassy assistance, VIP airport transfers, Internet services, international insurance facilitators, and international medical coordinators. Family members accompanying the patient may stay at 74 fully serviced two-room and studio apartments connected to the hospital. Further accommodation is available at the Bumrungrad Hospitality Suites, including 51 fully serviced apartments with swimming pool and fitness facilities.

Bumrungrad is not the cheapest of facilities, but it still costs much less than one would pay in the U.S. For example, a U.S. surgeon's fee for a full face-lift averaged $4,822 in 2004, not including hospital costs, according to the American Society of Plastic Surgeons. The total cost could approach $10,000 for all-inclusive services. At Bumrungrad, the surgeon's fee for a full facelift is about $1,200, and includes a neck lift and upper and lower eyelid lifts. With hospital and other fees, the total bill is about $4,000. This discount — about 40 percent of the U.S. cost — is typical of Bumrungrad; it is higher than many other facilities in Thailand, which run about 20 percent of U.S. costs, but it is still quite a bargain.

Ruben Toral, the media liaison for the hospital, told me that Americans still account for a very small proportion of overseas patients — just 58,000 in 2005, 83 percent of whom came for non-cosmetic treatments — but he expects that to change with Bumrungrad's new promotional campaigns. The hospital currently has International Representative Offices located in Eschende, Netherlands, and Sydney, Australia, and intends to open similar offices in the United States.

Part of the revenue from medical tourism goes to the Bumrungrad Hospital Foundation, which has provided over 100,000 Thais with free medical services, including heart valve replacements for children.

   ☏ Bumrungrad International Hospital
   ✉ 33 Sukumvit 3 (Soi Nana Nua)
      Wattana
      Bangkok 10110
      Thailand
   ☎ 662-253-0250
   ✆ 662-667-2525
   🌐 www.bumrungrad.com
   @ info@bumrungrad.com

Chao Phya Hospital

Chao Phya Hospital is a beautiful full-service hospital in a park-like setting. Although it is largely dedicated to medical tourists, the website's information is posted only in Thai!

   ☏ Chao Phya Hospital
   ✉ 113/44 Soi Rungphracha
      Boromrachachonnnee Road
      Bangkok Noi Bangkok 10700
      Thailand
   ☎ 662-434-1111
   🌐 www.chaophya.com
   @ webmaster@chaophya.com

Dental Hospital

Opened since 1990, Dental Hospital offers comprehensive dental services — in fact, it is the only hospital I know of that is solely devoted to dental treatment. The four-story building has 24 dental treatment rooms. It is open from 9 a.m. to 8 p.m., Monday to Saturday, and 9 a.m. to 4:30 p.m. on Sunday, and also has 24-hour emergency service.

Dental Hospital is located nearby the well-known Samitivej Hospital (see below) in Sukhumvit.

🚑 Dental Hospital
✉ 88/88 Sukhumvit 49
   Sukhumvit Road
   Bangkok 10110
   Thailand
☎ 662-260-5000
℻ 662-260-5026
🌏 www.dentalhospitalbangkok.com
@ dental@loxinfo.co.th

Phyathai Hospitals

This is a network of three new full-service hospitals with luxurious services for medical tourists.

🚑 Phyathai 1 Hospital
✉ 364 Sri Ayuthaya Road
   Ratchathevee, Bangkok 10400
   Thailand
☎ 662-640-1111
℻ 662-640-1100
🌏 www.phyathai.com
@ onestop@phyathai.com

Piyavate Hospital

A beautiful full-service hospital with specialty institutes including oncology, cardiology, esthetic surgery, orthopedics, and Chinese medicine.

🚑 Piyavate Hospital
✉ 998 Rama 9 Road
   Bangkapi, Huay Kwang
   Bangkok 10320
   Thailand
☎ 662-625-6500
℻ 662-246-9253

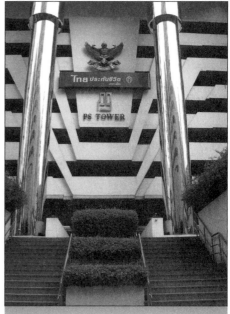

www.piyavate.com
@ info@piyavate.com

Rutnin Eye Hospital

Founded in 1964 by Harvard-trained Professor Dr. Uthai Rutnin, the Rutnin Eye Hospital was Thailand's first private hospital exclusively devoted to ophthalmology. The hospital has 29 board-certified surgeons in every subspecialty of the eye, including the cornea, glaucoma, neuro-ophthalmology, vitreo-retina, oculoplastics, pediatric ophthalmology, and excimer laser refractive surgery. The hospital is affiliated with the world-renowned Gimbel Eye Centre, in Calgary, Canada.

Rutnin Eye Hospital
80/1 Sukhumvit 21 Road (Soi Asoke)
Bangkok 10110
Thailand
☎ 662-639-3399
📠 662-639-3311
www.rutnin.com
@ contact@rutnin.com

Samitivej Hospitals

Located in the popular district of Sukumvit, this is a beautiful full-service complex that is especially well-regarded for its dental and esthetic clinics.

Samitivej Hospitals
133 Sukumvit 49
Klong Tan Nua, Vadhana
Bangkok 10110
Thailand
☎ 662-381-6807
📠 662-391-1290
www.samitivej.co.th
@ info@samitivej.co.th

Theravitae's imposing entrance is a symbol of the future power of stem–cell therapy.

TheraVitae

TheraVitae may become the harbinger of 21st century medicine. This remarkable new U.S. and Israeli venture is located in Bangkok. The increasing concentration of medical expertise in this city, combined with Thailand's liberal regulatory apparatus in medical innovation, make it an ideal place to develop new therapies. TheraVitae's product is peripheral blood stem-cell treatment. Stem cells harvested from a patient's own blood sidestep thorny ethical issues and may also prove safer than cells taken from embryos. Like all stem cells, this tissue can theoretically be used to regrow any part of the body. TheraVitae has developed proprietary methods to extract stem cells from the patient's blood (taking about one cupful), then reproducing them in their laboratory to create millions of stem cells, and then injecting these cells straight into the heart. The result has astonished heart specialists around the world; patients who were given "no option" and doomed to an early death have experienced a remarkable recovery.

> For decades, Don Ho has entertained countless visitors to Hawaii with his gentle island melodies. By 2005, his heart was failing to the point where he could no longer climb a single flight of stairs. It looked like the show was over for the 75-year-old crooner of standards such as "Tiny Bubbles" and "I'll Remember You." The best cardiologists of Hawaii said nothing more could be done — but then recommended that he consider a new procedure offered at the Bangkok Heart Hospital. There, heart surgeon Kitipan Visudharom injected stem cells developed by Theravitae. Two months later, Mr. Ho was back to doing five shows a week!

As Robert Clark, president and chairman of TheraVitae, explained to me, their procedures are still considered experimental. So far, they have had excellent results in heart disease patients, and they are planning to build on this foundation to treat a wide variety of degenerative and neurological conditions. Dr. Thein Htut, the marketing director of TheraVitae, emphasized to me that they will only accept, at this time, patients who have been diagnosed as "no option" with current available care in their home countries. The cost for the treatment is about $30,000.

TheraVitae is primarily a research facility. The actual clinical treatment — which consists of drawing blood and then injecting the stem cells — is done at the nearby Bangkok Heart Hospital.

📞 TheraVitae Co.,Ltd.
✉ 36/72 PS Tower, 21st Floor
Sukhumvit 21 Rd.
Klongtoey-Nua, Wattana
Bangkok 10110
Thailand

☎ 662-664-4290
📠 662-664-4289
🌐 www.theravitae.com
@ enquiries@theravitae.com

Vejthani Hospital

Vejthani has very modern facilities and attracts medical tourists for computer-assisted knee surgery, in vitro fertility, and its dental center.

🏥 Vejthani Hospital
✉ 1 Ladprao Road 111
   Klong-Chun, Bangkapi
   Bangkok 10240
   Thailand
☎ 662-734-0000
📠 662-734-0044
🌐 www.vejthani.com
@ webmaster@vejthani.com

Vibhavadi Hospital

This full-service, 350-bed hospital is in joint venture with Chao Phyra Hospital, Vibharam Hospital, Synphaet General Hospital, and Ramkhamhaeng Hospital. Its Advanced Lasik Center (www.wavefronthai.com) is among the best in the world. This highly ranked facility offers Thai massage and has a training school for a variety of massage therapies.

🏥 Vibhavadi Hospital
✉ 51/3 Ngamwongwam Road
   Kwaeng Lat Yao
   Khet Chatuchak
   Bangkok 10900
   Thailand
☎ 662-941-2800
📠 662-561-1466
🌐 www.vibhavadi.com
@ info@vibhavadi.com

Yanhee International Hospital

Yanhee offers comprehensive services for medical tourists. Ayurvedic medicine is also available. One of the more unusual procedures popular at Yanhee is hymenoplasty, also known as the "revirgination" procedure, at a cost of about $200.

☎ Yanhee International Hospital
✉ 454 Charansanitwong Road
Bang-O, Bangplad
Bangkok 10700
Thailand
☎ 662-879-0300
🌐 www.yanhee.net
@ info@yanhee.net

Chiang Mai

The small city of Chiang Mai is in northern Thailand, near the mountains and therefore higher and cooler than the rest of the low-lying country. For decades, it has been a favorite side trip for tourists wanting to go on treks to see the hill tribes, enjoy elephant rides, and view elephant logging operations. Now the city has added medical tourism and features several high-quality hospitals.

Chiangmai Ram Hospital
This facility, adjacent to the School of Medicine at the university, was built in 1994 specifically for medical tourism. In 1998, it began collaborating with the Japanese Labor Welfare Organization to provide discounted healthcare.
☎ Chiangmai Ram Hospital
✉ 8 Boonruangrit Road
Sripoom Distric
Chiang Mai 50300
Thailand
☎ 665-322-4821
📞 665-322-4880
🌐 www.chiangmairam.com
@ chiangmairam@chiangmairam.com

Lanna Hospital
All doctors speak English in this small hospital, with consultants in over 50 specialties from Chiang Mai University. Specialty clinics exist in IVF, obesity, and other fields.
☎ Lanna Hospital
✉ 1 Sukkasem Road
Kwang Nakornping Amphur Muang
Chiang Mai 50300
Thailand

☎ 665-335-7234
📞 665-340-8432
🌐 www.lanna-hospital.com
@ lanna@lanna-hospital.com

Chonburi

Chonburi is on the coast of Thailand, not far from the hugely popular tourist region of Pattaya. This area was perhaps responsible for the reputation of Thailand as a hotbed of sex tourism and general debauchery. During the Vietnam War, American soldiers began to frequent Pattaya for its beautiful sandy beaches, about a two-and-a-half hour bus ride from Bangkok. It has grown enormously since then and still attracts the majority of tourists visiting Thailand.

Bangkok Pattaya Hospital

This is part of the Bangkok Hospital Group, a growing conglomerate of medical centers. Bangkok Pattaya is a world-renowned medical center with excellent state-of-the-art services in virtually every medical specialty — and then some. It also has become perhaps the most popular place for persons seeking sex reassignment surgery (sex change operations).

🏥 Bangkok Pattaya Hospital
✉ 301 Moo 6, Sukumvit Road, K.M. 143
   Banglamung, Chonburi 20150
   Thailand
☎ 663-825-9999
📞 663-842-7770
🌐 www.bangkokpattayahospital.com
@ inquiry@bph.co.th

Pattaya International Hospital

Known as the "hospital in the park" for its natural surroundings, this is a full-service hospital specially directed to medical tourists.

🏥 Pattaya International Hospital
✉ Sol 4 Pattaya 2 nd Road
   Pattaya City, Chonburi 20260
   Thailand
☎ 663-842-8674
📞 663-842-2773
🌐 www.pih-inter.com
@ picpih@loxinfo.co.th

Koh Samui

During the great backpacker tourism explosion of the 1970s, when hordes of young people traveled on the cheap between Europe and Australia, Koh Samui became known as an idyllic island of laid-back Thai hospitality and beautiful beaches. In fact, it appears to have been the inspiration for the 2000 movie, *The Beach* (the movie was actually filmed near Phuket). Now the tourism industry of this small island of 45,000 inhabitants has become highly developed with a modern jetport, numerous resorts, and several sophisticated hospitals catering to medical tourism.

Bangkok Hospital Samui
A member of the Bangkok Hospital Group, this is a modern 50-bed facility with a broad range of services for medical tourists.
- Bangkok Hospital Samui
- 57 Moo 3, Thaweerat Phakdee Road
  Bophut, Koh Samui, Surattani 84320
  Thailand
- ☎ 667-742-9500
- 667-742-9505
- www.samuihospital.com
- @ info@samuihospital.com

Samui International Hospital (SIH)
Established in 1997, this modern hospital was built specifically to serve the international community. It accepts insurance from over 150 providers, mostly European, and financial arrangements for others who prefer a "cashless" transaction. A full range of medical and dental services is provided.
- Samui International Hospital
- Northern Chaweng Beach Road, 90/2 Moo 2
  Bophut, Koh Samui, Surattani 84320
  Thailand
- ☎ 667-742-2272
- 667-723-0049
- www.sih.co.th
- @ info@sih.co.th

Thai International Hospital
Located near the airport, this hospital is specifically directed to medical tourists.
- Thai International Hospital
- 25/25 Opposite Tesco Lotus Moo 6

Bophut, Koh Samui, Surattani 84320
Thailand
☎ 667-741-4400
📠 667-724-5690
🌐 www.thaiinterhospital.com
@ thaiinterhospital@yahoo.com

Phuket

Outside of Bangkok, Phuket is the best-known city in Thailand and now has direct flights from many other countries. The name — pronounced "boo-get" — is sometimes misspoken in a derogatory way to emphasize its reputation for sexual tourism. However, visitors who are seeking this form of entertainment would be better off going elsewhere. Phuket is a small city surrounded by superb recreational areas including expansive beaches, elephant jungle trips, rock climbing at nearby Railei Beach, and all manner of ocean sports on the Andaman Sea. This region suffered terribly from the great tsunami of December 26, 2004. However, it has almost entirely recovered — thanks in large part to the many excellent hospitals engaged in medical tourism.

Bangkok Phuket Hospital

Part of the Bangkok Hospital Group, this very modern facility is largely designed to serve the increasing numbers of medical tourists. The major focus is cosmetic surgery, sex-change surgery, and dentistry.

🏥 Bangkok Phuket Hospital
✉ 2/1 Hongyok utis Road
   Muang District, Phuket 83000
   Thailand
☎ 667-625-4421
📠 667-625-4430
🌐 www.phukethospital.com
@ info@phukethospital.com

Phuket International Hospital

Peter Davison, a tall elderly gentleman from Sweden, is the manager of the international services. He is optimistic about the growing numbers of medical tourists from Europe and Australia, and is particularly interested in reaching out to Americans. An expansive new wing of the hospital is specifically designed for medical tourists, with beautifully appointed rooms and gardens.

🖩 Phuket International Hospital
✉ 44 Chalermprakiat Ror 9 Road
Phuket 83000
Thailand
☎ 667-624-9400
✉ 667-621-0936
🕹 www.phuket-inter-hospital.co.th
@ info@phuket-inter-hospital.co.th

The Bodyline Retreat

This superb facility is the harbinger of a whole new dimension of medical tourism: the post-surgical recovery resort. Located right on the beach just minutes from the major hospitals, the resort consists of a large open-air restaurant and communal building near a central pool and garden, around which is a collection of beautifully designed individual cabins. The ambience provides both privacy and social mingling, depending on the desires of the guest, and everything is set up to enhance recovery after surgery. Patients are taken to the hospital for treatment and follow-up care, doctors and nurses are available around the clock, and the entire staff is trained in post-op care. The attraction to many patients is the comfort of sharing the medical tourist experience with others — there is no need to feel awkward when coming to the restaurant with a face swathed in bandages. Some people come with the intent of just staying a few days after their procedure, but they end up liking it so much that they stay for weeks — and return year after year even if they are not having surgery.

The Bodyline Retreat was built from the former Aochalong Village Resort (and locals still know it by that name) by Australian twin sisters Janese and Judith, and Janese's husband Mike. The sisters have decades of experience in international tourism and global entrepreneurial ventures. They designed Bodyline as a model of the interface between medical treatment and the tourism/hospitality components of medical tourism. Their success is obvious — hospitals in the region compete with each other to send their patients to the retreat for post-surgical recovery.

🖩 The Bodyline Retreat
✉ 5/26 Moo 9, Soi Porn Chalong
East Chaofa Road, Muang
Phuket 83000
Thailand
☎ 667-638-1691
✉ 667-638-1692
🕹 www.thebodylineretreat.com
@ info@thebodylineretreat.com
Skype lytwayt/bodyline935

Tunisia

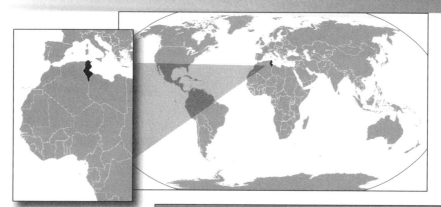

The Tunisian Republic is located on the Mediterranean coast of North Africa, between Algeria and Libya. Tunisia has promoted medical tourism for over a decade, well before other countries started, appealing largely to Europeans looking for warm, sunny beaches and inexpensive cosmetic surgery.

Tunisia Politics:

Unlike its less stable neighbors, which suffer from fundamentalist Islamic groups and dictatorial regimes, Tunisia is quite closely integrated with Europe and has a thriving tourist industry.

Tunisia Travel Requirements:

Passport and onward or return ticket required. Visa not required for stay of up to four months.

Now, the government of Tunisia has plans to make this a major national industry, going so far as to declare 2005 as the "Year of Health Tourism."

This small desert country has more than 80 private clinics that offer high-quality cosmetic surgery at prices about half of those in Europe or the U.S.

Typical costs:

Rhinoplasty (nose reshaping)	$2,140
Breast augmentation	$2,980
Upper and lower eyelid shaping	$2,020
Facelift	$4,080

Hammamet

Known as the most popular tourist resort town in Tunisia, Hammamet is often referred to as the "Tunisian Saint Tropez." The Arabic name of this coastal city on the Cape Bon peninsula means "baths" — an indication of its 2,000-year history as a health retreat. The houses of Hammamet are mostly white with touches of blue, framed by decorations of beautiful iron works. This town definitely has a bit of a "tourist scene," especially during July and August, when it plays host to the International Festival of Culture.

Bio Azur Thalasso Center

This spa is part of the five-star Royal Azur Hotel, which is in turn part of Les Orangers complex. This facility consists of six hotel units, all with a particular health focus and clientele (businesspersons, families, young adults, children), specializing in nutrition, skin, internal medicine, and physiotherapy. Perhaps the biggest draws are treatments for arthritis and obesity, including:

- Thalassotherapy
- Special herbal products
- Mud treatments
- Temperature-controlled baths
- Massages
- Wrappings with algae
- Clay or mud baths with essential oils
- Steam baths
- The Hammam bath (a Roman bath with heated sea water)

The spa also offers "underwater showers," which is rather hard to imagine until you realize they are referring to an underwater jet massage — in other words, a whirlpool bath.

Other features of the neighborhood include casinos, golf courses, tennis courts, indoor and outdoor swimming pools, camel and horseback riding, mini golf, and beautiful white-sand beaches. The hotel itself serves up many international and local dishes from its six main onsite restaurants, including a Moorish Cafe, a Grill-Pizzeria, and a Health Restaurant.

☎ 216-2-278-500
✆ 216-71-965-999
🌐 www.southtravels.com/africa/tunisia/royalazur/index.html

Tunis

Cosmetica Travel

This referral agency is directed by Houssem Ben Azouz, a former manager of the

Tunisian National Tourism Office in Amsterdam and London. Cosmetica Travel is a medical tourism service managed jointly by the Polyclinic Alyssa and Siroko Travel.

Package deals include:
- Surgery and related fees
- Prosthesis (if any)
- Compression garments
- 2 nights' stay at the clinic
- 5 nights at a five-star hotel on a half-board basis
- A "relaxing treatment" prior to the operation

📠 Cosmetica Travel
✉ Immeuble MINIAR
   Rue des Lacs de Mazurie apt1, B1
   Les Berges du Lac
   1053 Tunis
   Tunisia
☎ 216-71-965-196
☏ 216-71-965-197
🌐 www.cosmeticatravel.com/english
@ english.contact@cosmeticatravel.com

Polyclinique El Menzah

El Menzah has been in business for more than 25 years. This modern cosmetic surgery clinic is located in a fashionable residential part of Tunis, just a 10-minute drive from Tunis-Carthage International Airport. The clinic itself has hospitality suites where you can stay in an individual room or "Grand Luxe" accommodations. All rooms are air-conditioned and equipped with satellite TV. Alternatively, the clinic can make arrangements for a discounted stay at a number of partner hotels, such as the Yadis Ibn Khaldoun, near the relaxing nature of Belvédère Park, or the Phébus, on the coast.

📠 El Menzah Clinic
✉ 1, rue Apolo XI cité Mahrajene
   Tunis 1082
   Tunisia
☎ 216-98-306-896
☎ 216-71-841-522
☏ 216-71-785-110
   Skype Polyclinique.elmenzah

🌍 www.esthetiquecontact.com/home.php

@ polyclinique.elmenzah@gnet.tn

La Marsa Clinic

This combination of clinic and hotel is located in the La Marsa residential district
Tunis, about 15 minutes from Tunis Carthage airport, five minutes from the mythical
city of Carthage, and just over 500 yards from the Mediterranean Sea. *Marsa* means port
in Arabic — this was the summer vacation resort of the *beys* or kings during the Ottoman empire.

The clinic has four operating rooms run by a panel of 43 doctors.

The hotel has 45 rooms, in order of luxury from hospital room, double room, individual room, comfort room, and the suite.

🏥 La Marsa Clinic

✉ rue du Lac Malaren
Imm. Rihab App A201
Les Berges du Lac
1053 Tunis
Tunisia

☎ 216-71-89-40 06

☎ 216-71-28-77 52

📠 216-71-84-82 72

🌍 www.estetikatour.com/en/cosmetic_surgery_private_hospital_tunisia.shtml

@ info@estetikatour.com

Turkey

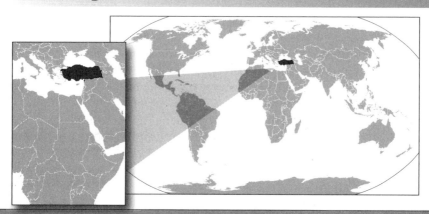

Turkey Politics:

Once the crown of the Ottoman Empire, Turkey is a bridge between Europe and Asia — where west meets east. Culturally, it is the most authoritarian of European nations and the most liberal of Islamic states.

Turkey Travel Requirements:

Passport and visa are required. Visas can be obtained at Turkish border crossing points for visits of up to three months or through a Turkish consular office in the U.S. Visa requires a completed application form and a passport with a minimum validity of three months. Visa fee is $20 for single entry and $65 for multiple entry (cash or money order only). Visa requires your valid passport, one completed application form, and SASE. For further information, contact the Consular Office of the Embassy of the Republic of Turkey, 2525 Massachusetts Ave., NW, Washington, DC 20008 (202/612-6740/41) or nearest Consulate: CA (323-937-0118), IL (312-263-0644), NY (212-949-0160), or TX (713-622-5849). Internet: www.turkishembassy.org

The Republic of Turkey straddles the Bosporus strait that separates Southeast Europe from Southwest Asia. Because of its geographical position Turkey has been a historical crossroads, the homeland of and battleground between several great civilizations, and a center of commerce.

Some typical costs for procedures:
Rhinoplasty (nose reshaping)..$2,700
Breast augmentation...$2,900

Upper and lower eyelid shaping $2,300
Facelift $2,700

Cosmetic Tourism Turkey

Originally formed as Dental Tourism Turkey, this service expanded in 2006 to include cosmetic surgery. It is owned by the IMCA Travel Agency. They promise to have selected the best clinics throughout Turkey and have screened them to assure quality standards. Services include airport pickup and transfer to hotel, introductions to the clinic, and daily contact to ensure you have everything you need, including arrangements for any excursions you're planning. The company is located in Izmir, on the Aegean coast, Turkey's third largest city; however, they service the entire country.

🏥 Cosmetic Tourism Turkey
✉ Akdeniz Cad. No:5 D:201 Pasaport
   Izmir
   Turkey
☎ 90-232-446-3034
📞 90-232-483-5946
🌐 www.cosmetictourismturkey.com
@ info@ctghealthcare.co.uk

Istanbul

This is one of the most pleasant, beautiful and culturally rich cities in the world.

Anadolu Health Center

This grand new medical complex has an even grander ambition: "To be the creator, applicator, and the forerunner of a new healthcare understanding in Turkey and in the neighbouring countries." The Anadolu Health Center is a fully equipped hospital with expertise in oncology, neurology, cardiac care, and women's health issues. Its association with Johns Hopkins University gives it considerable credibility in the medical tourism industry.

🏥 Anadolu Health Center
✉ Anadolu Caddesi No:1
   Bayramoglu Cikisi Cayirova Mevki
   Gebze 41400 Kocaeli
☎ 90-262-678-5000
📞 90-262-654-0055
🌐 www.anadolusaglik.org
@ internationalpatients@anadolusaglik.org

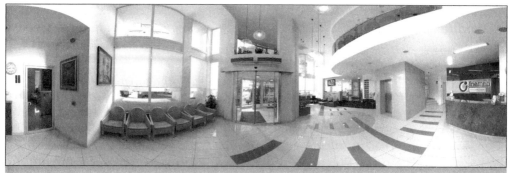

This panoramic view of the interior of Jinemed reveals a spacious, high-tech medical center.

Jinemed

Jinemed is a hospital with three strong specializations in medical tourism: gynecology, cosmetic surgery, and dentistry. English-speaking doctors attend to international patients. Jinemed works with a travel agency to prepare package prices that include hotel, airport transfers, all medical and surgical services, and local tours. Medical tourists are typically booked at the Seminal Hotel, a luxurious four-star hotel on Taksim Square in the heart of Istanbul.

Women's health

Jinemed excels in a large variety of women's healthcare, including:

- Gynecology
- Gynecologic oncology
- Laparoscopy
- High-risk pregnancy
- Infertility
- Dentistry
- Advanced plastic surgery

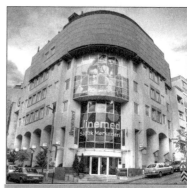

Jinemed Medical Center in Istanbul has become a global center for assisted fertility and cosmetic surgery.

Assisted reproductive technologies include some that are available in only a few clinics in the world:

- IUI (Intra-uterine insemination)
- IVF (In-vitro fertilization)
- IVM (In-vitro maturation)
- ICSI (Intracytoplasmic sperm injection)
- Assisted hatching
- Blastocyst transfer
- PGD (pre-implantation genetic diagnosis)

- Embryo biopsy
- Embryo freezing
- Frozen embryo transfer
- TESE (testicular biopsy from azospermic men)
- Ovarian cortex freezing

In Turkey, hospitals are allowed to transfer up to three embryos at each procedure, increasing chances of a successful pregnancy. The cost for a single IVF cycle is $3,000 (about one-third of the cost in the U.S.). A complete package price is available for $7,300 that includes:
- One IVF/ICSI cycle, including medication
- Two round-trip flight tickets from New York or Chicago to Istanbul
- Hotel accommodation for 17 nights
- Assisted hatching, blastocyst transfer, and embryo glue, if necessary
- Prepaid cell phone to reach the doctor at all times
- Airport and hotel transfers

Cosmetic surgery
Jinemed has three board-certified plastic surgeons who trained in the United States and United Kingdom They perform plastic surgery in both men and women, doing everything from hair implants to liposuctions, breast implants, and face lifting.

Sample procedures, required days in hospital and package prices

Procedure	Days	Cost
Eyelid surgery		
(2 eyelids, upper or lower)	4	$3,000
(4 eyelids, upper and lower)	4	$4,500
Mini abdominoplasty	3	$4,000
Full abdominoplasty	7	$5,500
Nose reshaping	7	$4,000–5,000
Breast lift	3	$5,000
Breast implant with prosthesis	3	$5,500
Breast reduction	5	$6,000
Hair transplantation	2	$3,000
Facelift	7	$5,000–9,000
Ear correction	3	$4,300

✆ Jinemed Hospital
✉ Nuzhetiye Caddesi Deryadil Sokak No 1
  Besiktas

Istanbul
Turkey
☎ 90-212-511-22-96
🌐 www.jinemed.com.tr
@ jinemedistanbul@gmail.com

International Health Tourism
A referral service for people desiring dental care, cosmetic surgery, eye treatment, and assisted fertility.
🖧 International Health Tourism
✉ Cumhuriyet Cad Beler Palas No 42/2
Kat: 4 D: 16
Taksim
Turkey
☎ 90-212-237-8464
📞 90-212-327-8452
🌐 www.internationalhealthtourism.com
@ nihan@internationalhealthtourism.com

Fethiye

This coastal resort on the western Mediterranean is a great place to get dental treatment.

Dental Tourism Turkey
Although it sounds like a referral service, this is a small dental clinic focused on medical tourism. All staff speak English, will arrange hotel and local transportation, and will even pick you up at the airport. They promise to "work out a complete programme for you, which will include day trips out (optional), relaxation time and, of course, a treatment schedule. All you need to do is drop us an email telling us what you want done, send us a panoramic x-ray of your teeth by post and we'll give you a quote on accommodation and treatment."
🖧 Dental Tourism Turkey
✉ No 178/7 Fetip Merkezi Gunlukbasi
Fethiye
Turkey
☎ 90-252-613-6636
📞 90-542-644-8157
🌐 www.dentalinturkey.com
@ info@dentalinturkey.com

Venezuela

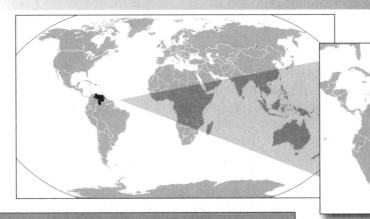

Venezuela Politics:

The two most interesting features of the political situation in Venezuela are 1) the leftist government, which has been sharply critical of the United States, and perhaps because of this has drawn support and closer relations with other Latin American countries, especially Cuba, and 2) the boom in oil revenue, which allows Venezuela to take this stance without suffering economically. Venezuela is generous with its oil reserves, offering it at discount prices to neighboring countries, and in Venezuela itself gas costs as little as 20 cents a gallon!

Venezuela Travel Requirements:

Passport, onward or return ticket, and proof of sufficient funds required. A visa not required for a stay of up to 90 days.

The Bolivarian Republic of Venezuela (*República Bolivariana de Venezuela*) is located on the northern tropical Caribbean coast of South America. Neighboring countries are Brazil to the south, Guyana to the east, and Colombia to the west.

Tourism has long been a big draw — one might say from the very beginning of European contact. When he arrived in 1498, Christopher Columbus was apparently so enthralled by Venezuela's landscape that he called it *Tierra de Gracia* ("Land of Grace"), which has become the country's nickname. Anyone who sees Angel Falls, the world's highest waterfall, would surely agree.

Venezuela now offers an additional draw — medical tourism, with a focus on cosmetic surgery.

Margarita Island

Isla Margarita, just 11 miles off the coast, is consistently described as laid back, and it is becoming very popular with those who want to escape the more heavily developed Caribbean tourist spots.

International Surgery Center

This is a referral service for a group of cosmetic and plastic surgery specialists. All are accredited by the Venezuelan Plastic, Reconstructive, Aesthetic and Maxillofacial Surgery Board, and therefore by the International Confederation of Plastic Reconstructive and Aesthetic Surgery. They report that they have patients from numerous countries, with about 60 percent requesting buttock implants.

The island's name does not come from the Spanish, as one might suppose, but from the Greek name for pearl — which Columbus found in abundance and immediately exploited. Margarita became a haven of pirates attracted by the pearl trade.

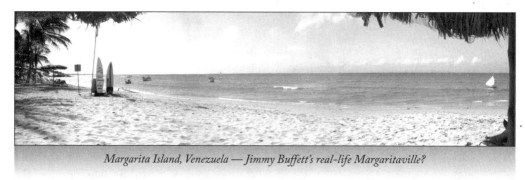

Margarita Island, Venezuela — Jimmy Buffett's real-life Margaritaville?

Medical tourism support includes:
- A bilingual escort provides daily visits
- Pre-travel medical evaluation
- Pre-travel advice on flights and transportation
- Arriving and departing assistance and transfers (airport, hotel, clinic)
- Accommodation advice
- Pre-surgery consultation, lab tests, cardiovascular evaluation, and x-rays
- Post-surgery check-ups
- Unlimited post-surgery email and phone support after patient returns back home

International Surgery Center
Calle El Torito
Playa El Angel, Pampatar
Isla Margarita
Venezuela
☎ 58-295-267-2955
🌐 www.internationalsurgery.com
@ margaritamedical@gmail.com

Vietnam

A top destination choice for:
alternative medicine, massage,
traditional Chinese medicine

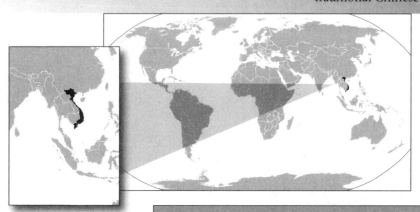

The Socialist Republic of Vietnam consists of the former communist North Vietnam and capitalist South Vietnam. Now the entire country is officially communist but becoming increasingly capitalist in orientation, and open to international trade and tourism. Along with the transition to communism came a name change for Saigon, which is now called Ho Chi Minh City after the revered revolutionary leader. However, the name hasn't stuck, and everyone seems to prefer the old name. Somehow, the popular musical *Miss Saigon* wouldn't sound quite as well named Miss Ho Chi Minh City.

Vietnam Politics:

What a difference a few decades can make. In 1975, Americans suffered a humiliating retreat, tarnished by memories that still linger. But Vietnam has changed profoundly in the past 30 years, and the old animosities have been replaced by a friendly openness.

Vietnam Travel Requirements:

Passport and visa are required. The visa requires an application form, passport-sized photo, and SASE. The visa fee should be paid by money order or cashier check, payable to the Embassy of Vietnam, 1233 20th St., NW, Suite 400, Washington, DC 20036 202-861-2293 or 861-0694). Internet: www.vietnamembassy-usa.org

In the last few years, Vietnam has become a popular medical tourism destination, noted for its traditional medicine, such as acupuncture, with a large number of skillful doctors. Unfortunately, relatively few of these physicians are fluent in English.

Saigon (Ho Chi Minh City, HCMC)

Columbia Asia Saigon International Clinic

D r. Nguyen Tai Thu, a world-renowned acupuncturist, suffers from a typical problem when it comes to tourists: they don't know how to pronounce his name. Many also don't know that the name order is reversed, so that the family name comes before the given names. If you are unsure about how to pronounce Nguyen, one of the most common Vietnamese names, just say "wen" and everyone will understand you.

… an overheard German medical tourist: "When will we wisit Dr. Nguyen?"

The Columbia Asia Saigon International Clinic is a multi-specialty clinic located in downtown Saigon. The facility was opened in 2000 to provide care to both the local population and resident foreigners, but it has expanded into medical tourism. It is affiliated with Columbia Asia Gia Dinh International Hospital, located nearby, and uses the services of this facility when necessary.

- Columbia Asia Saigon International Clinic
- 08 Alexandre de Rhodes, Dist 1
  HCM City
  Vietnam
- 84-08-823-8888
- 84-08-829-2295
- @ dzungvn@columbiaasia.com

PART I

Quotes are from: "Medical Tourism," *New York Times*, Sept. 13, 2002, and Mundia, M. Letter to editor, *New York Times*, Sept. 9, 2002

Chapter 1

Dr. David Brailer quote is from: Katie Hafner, "Treated for Illness, Then Lost in a Labyrinth of Bills." *New York Times*, Oct. 13, 2005

Bradley Thayer quote from: http://archive.wn.com/2005/09/26/1400/thailandhealth/

Meghan Stone quote from: www.healthadvocate.com/downloads/stories/2005/05_11-20(20Negotiating(20Doctor(20Bills_WSJ.pdf

Tom Raudaschl quote from: http://www.interactivecode.com/computer-consultants-5/indias-low-price-high-tech-care-14973/

Dr. Pont quote is from: Carreyrou, J. As medical costs sour, even insured face huge tab. *Wall Street Journal*, Nov 29, 2007.

Chapter 3

Peters WP, Rogers MC. Variation in Approval by Insurance Companies of Coverage for Autologous Bone Marrow Transplantation for Breast Cancer. *New Engl J Med* 1994; 330:473-477

Dr. Moelleken quote is from: "Medical Tourism" *New York Times*, September 13, 2002

A Real "Boob Job": http://www.thesun.co.uk/sol/homepage/news/article193239.ece

Chapter 4

Much of the discussion in this chapter is adapted from the following excellent articles: Relman AS. The new medical-industrial complex. N Engl J Med 1980; 303: 963–70.

"For-profit hospitals take over" — this information is taken from: Woolhandler S, Himmelstein DU. Costs of care and administration at for-profit and other hospitals in the United States. *New Engl J Med* 1997; 336: 769–74.

"national death rates for Medicare patients" — data taken from: Chen J, Radford MJ, Wang Y, Marciniak TA, Krumholz HM. Do "America's Best Hospitals" perform better for acute myocardial infarction? *New Engl J Med* 1999; 340: 286–92.

"...for-profit hospitals compared with their not-for-profit" data are taken from: Yuan Z, Cooper GS, Einstadter D, Cebul RD, Rimm AA. The association between hospital type and mortality and length of stay: a study of 16.9 million hospitalized Medicare beneficiaries. Med Care 2000; 38: 231–45

Tenet Healthcare Corporation — data taken from: Abelson R. Nurses' Association says in study that big hospital chain overcharges patients for drugs. The *New York Times* Nov. 24, 2002; Sect. 1:26.

"*characteristics of our major for-profit HMOs:*" *Much of this discussion is derived from: Geyman JP. The Corporate Transformation of Medicine and Its Impact on Costs and Access to Care. Journal of the American Board of Family Practice 2003; 16:443-454http://www.jabfm.org/cgi/content/full/16/5/443*

"Catholics can have a mass...": "For every problem, a cut-rate solution." *Wired*, Oct. 2006, p. 40

Nuevo Progreso: http://www.shop-progreso.com

Household healthcare budget data are from: Institute for the Future. *Health and healthcare 2010: The Forecast, The Challenge, 2nd Edition.* Jossey-Bass, 2001

Labyrinth of Bills quote from: Katie Hafner, "Treated for Illness, Then Lost in a Labyrinth of Bills." *New York Times*, Oct. 13, 2005 http://www.nytimes.com/2005/10/13/health/13paper.html

Commonwealth report data are from: Carreyrou, J. As medical costs sour, even insured face huge tab. *Wall Street Journal*, Nov. 29, 2007.

"medispas": "How med tourism will benefit — more considerate care." Medscape Medical News 2005, original from *SUNDAY TIMES* (UK), Feb. 15, 2004

Chapter 5

"Bra fat" and other surgery stories are derived from: Natasha Singer. "Do my knees look fat to you?" *New York Times*, June 15, 2006

http://www.nytimes.com/2006/06/15/fashion/thursdaystyles/15skin.html
U.S. Surgeon's fees are for 2006, from: http://www.implantinfo.com/faqs/1.21.html
Singer, N. "Is the 'Mom Job' Really Necessary? *New York Times*, Oct. 4, 2007

Chapter 6
Mexican dental care: http://www.shop-progreso.com *New York Times*, May 7, 2006

Chapter 7
Pear R. "Obesity Surgery Often Leads to Complications, Study Says." *New York Times*, July 24, 2006
http://www.nytimes.com/2006/07/24/health/24health.html

Chapter 8
Sunday Times, UK, December 28, 2003

Chapter 9
"Organs for sale." *Wired*, April 2007, p 48
Stem cells for joint replacement: "Advanced Knee Repair." *Wired*, Oct. 2006, p 44

Chapter 10
Rundle, R. "Beverly Hills and Surgeons Face Off Over Higher Taxes." Wall Street Journal, Oct. 5, 2007; Page B1

Chapter 11
Medical spas: "Reconstructing Beauty; Medical Spas Offer Holiday Experience." *Health Worlds Magazine*, Jan. 5, 2005

PART II

Argentina
The medical tourism blog: http://expat-argentina.blogspot.com/2005/07/medical-tourism-in-argentina.html

Barbados
Single Mothers By Choice can be found at: http://mattes.home.pipeline.com/

Costa Rica
"As soon as I stepped off the plane ..." posted by El Expatriado at *7/26/2005*; http://expat-argentina.blogspot.com/2005/07/medical-tourism-in-argentina.html

Croatia
testimonials are from: http://antiaging-europe.com/docs/testimonials.html

Czech Republic
Hotel in Tabor quote: http://www.bodiesbeautiful.co.uk/tummy_tuck_with_liposuction_2.html

Hungary
William O'Brien quoted in *International Herald Tribune*:
http://www.iht.com/articles/2005/05/23/news/meditour.php
Perfect Profiles: http://www.revahealth.com/consumer/browseproviders.aspx

India
The quote is from *Time* magazine, June 26, 2006

Also Available from Sunrise River Press:

The Anti-Cancer Cookbook:
How to Cut Your Risk with the Most Powerful, Cancer-Fighting Foods
by Julia B. Greer, MD, MPH

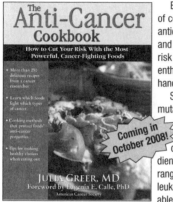

Eat broccoli sprouts to prevent bladder cancer…Eat more blueberries to reduce your risk of colon cancer…It seems that every day we hear new discoveries about various foods' anticancer properties. But the information comes in little bits, from all different directions, and it's hard to know how to put all this information to use in your own diet to reduce your risk of getting cancer. Now, Dr. Julia Greer – a physician, cancer researcher, and food enthusiast – pulls together everything you need to know about anti-cancer foods into one handy book: The Anti-Cancer Cookbook.

She explains what cancer is and how antioxidants work to prevent pre-cancerous mutations in your body's cells, and then describes in detail which foods have been scientifically shown to help prevent which types of cancer. She then shares her collection of more than 250 scrumptious recipes for soups, sauces, main courses, vegetarian dishes, sandwiches, breads, desserts, and beverages, all loaded with nutritious ingredients chock-full of powerful antioxidants that may significantly slash your risk of a broad range of cancer types, including lung, colon, breast, prostate, pancreatic, bladder, stomach, leukemia, and others. Dr. Greer even includes tips on how to cook foods to protect their valuable antioxidants and nutrients and how to make healthy anticancer choices when eating out. If you love good food and are looking for delicious ways to keep yourself and your family healthy and cancer-free, you'll find yourself reaching for The Anti-Cancer Cookbook time and time again. Softbound, 7.5 x 9 inches, 224 pages. **Item # SRP149**

Conquer Back & Neck Pain: Walk It Off!
A Spine Doctor's Proven Solutions for Finding Relief Without Pills or Surgery
by Mark Brown, MD, PhD

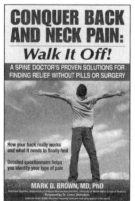

Every human being suffers from back pain at some point in life. In an effort to find relief, people turn to a wide variety of treatments, and to doctors who will prescribe narcotic painkillers. What they don't realize is that many of these treatments — especially narcotic drugs — actually interfere with their body's own ability to heal and overcome pain. When these treatments fail to help, they desperately conclude that surgery is their only option for relief. In his new book Conquer Back and Neck Pain: Walk It Off!, renowned spine surgeon Dr. Mark Brown, MD, PhD, explains exactly what causes back pain and why humans are so predisposed to spinal problems. He provides a detailed questionnaire that allows you to identify which of seven types of back pain you are experiencing, and then he explains each of those types in clear and easy-to-understand language.

Contrary to what you might expect from a spinal surgeon, Dr. Brown actually advocates against turning to surgery in most cases of spinal pain. In his 35 years of experience, he has found that the vast majority of back pain cases will resolve with minimal treatment. In fact, the very best thing you can do is to simply allow your body to heal itself by avoiding the many treatment pitfalls that people with back pain commonly fall into when looking for relief. Avoiding these mistakes, along with incorporating gentle aerobic exercise, will almost always allow you to "walk off" your back or neck pain naturally.

With an interesting collection of anecdotes and a frank discussion of the pitfalls that come with many of the back-pain treatments out there, Conquer Back and Neck Pain: Walk It Off! will give you fresh, new insight into how your back really works and how to finally find healthy relief from your back pain. Softbound, 6 x 9 inches, 168 pages. **Item # SRP601**